Advances and Diverse Applications of Biomaterials

Advances and Diverse Applications of Biomaterials

Edited by **Ralph Seguin**

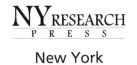

New York

Published by NY Research Press,
23 West, 55th Street, Suite 816,
New York, NY 10019, USA
www.nyresearchpress.com

Advances and Diverse Applications of Biomaterials
Edited by Ralph Seguin

International Standard Book Number: 978-1-63238-028-9 (Hardback)

Printed in the United States of America.

Contents

Preface

This book compiles reviews and original researches conducted by experts and scientists working in the field of biomaterials, covering a broad range of topics, from design to new applications. It offers readers the potentials of distinct synthetic and engineered biomaterials. This book elucidates different features of biomaterials and studies techniques used to produce biomaterials with the specific properties required for certain clinical and medical functions. It covers various topics like latest methods for characterization and evaluation of new materials, traditional applications in nanotechnology and tissue engineering, and new applications of these products. This book will be helpful for readers interested in this field.

This book has been the outcome of endless efforts put in by authors and researchers on various issues and topics within the field. The book is a comprehensive collection of significant researches that are addressed in a variety of chapters. It will surely enhance the knowledge of the field among readers across the globe.

It is indeed an immense pleasure to thank our researchers and authors for their efforts to submit their piece of writing before the deadlines. Finally in the end, I would like to thank my family and colleagues who have been a great source of inspiration and support.

Editor

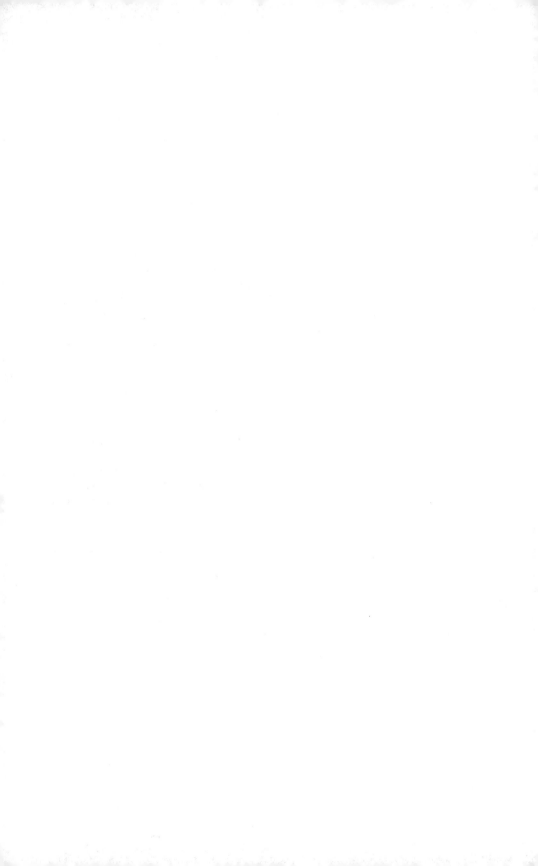

Characterization of Novel Biomaterials

Biomedical Applications of Materials Processed in Glow Discharge Plasma

V. Tereshko, A. Gorchakov, I. Tereshko,
V. Abidzina and V. Red'ko

Additional information is available at the end of the chapter

1. Introduction

There is exhaustive literature about interactions of charged particles with solid surfaces [l, 2]. For a long period only high energies were assumed to cause any significant modifications. However, low-energy ion bombardments (up to 5 keV) of metal and alloy samples were shown to be very efficient too: the increase of dislocation density (up to 10 mm in depth from the irradiated surface) was detected [3–7]. In fact, a bulk long-range modification of materials in the glow discharge plasma (GDP) took place. The above results were obtained by the use of transmission electron microscopy for well annealed samples with initially small dislocation density (armco-Fe, Ni3Fe, *etc.*) [4, 6]. For materials with initially increased dislocation density (unannealed copper, M2 high-speed steel, titanium alloys) reorganization of dislocation structure is the most considerable: either intensive formation of the dislocation fragments or grinding of the fragments with corresponding increase in their disorientation is observed. These reorganizations also take place well below the irradiated surface. When the ion energy decreases by 1 keV, the modified layer became even deeper [7].

The above results can only be explained by taking the nonlinear nature of atom interactions into account. The ion bombardment is assumed to induce nonlinear oscillations in crystal lattices leading to self-organization of the latter. Modelling shows the formation of new collective atom states. The observed phenomena include the redistribution of energy, clusterization, structure formation when the atoms stabilizes in new non-equilibrium positions, localized structures, auto-oscillations, and travelling waves and pulses [3–7].

The next step was to look at the influence of low-energy GDP on liquids. Water that occupies up 70 percent of the Earth's surface and is the main component of all living things was taken for investigation. Water molecules are able to create molecular associates using Van der Waals forces as well as labile hydrogen interactions [8–11]. Owing to hydrogen bonds molecules of water are capable to form not only random associates (one having no ordered structure) but clusters, i.e. associates having some ordered structure [9–11]. The network of hydrogen bonds and the high order of intermolecular cooperativity facilitate long-range propagation of molecular excitations [12, 13]. This allows, in principle, to consider water and water-based solutions as systems sensitive to weak external forces. Indeed, the study of luminescence at long time scale shows that the structural equilibrium in water is not stable: it changes after dissolution of small portions of added substances and after exposition of aqueous samples to UV and mild X-ray irradiation [14].

The results obtained by Lobyshev, *et al* opened up the new avenues to water and aqueous solutions as non-equilibrium systems capable of self-organization [14]. The key property of self-organization is, however, nonlinearity to which, in models of water, hasn't paid the required attention yet. The present paper is aimed to cover this flaw. Basic models of nonlinear chains that can be related to water structure were investigated. We observed self-organization processes resulting in the displacement of atoms and their stabilization in new positions, which can be viewed as the formation of water clusters.

In experiments, we exposed crop seeds, baking yeast and water to GDP. The results were very promising: the seed sprouts showed greater growth and the yeast showed greater metabolic activity compared to the control samples. The results on volunteers with different diseases, who either drunk the processed water or was injected intravenously with the processed physiological solution, were encouraging too. The diagnostics of volunteers' blood immune cells (lymphocytes and leukocytes) showed significant normalization of their state toward homeostasis.

Next part of this paper is devoted to the study of properties of implants processed in GDP. The modern medicine is characterized by active introduction of high technologies to clinical practice. It requires sufficient biocompatibility of implanted mechanical, electromechanical and electronic devices with natural tissues. The properties of materials are crucial, since insufficient biocompatibility can lead to the negative reactions to the implant from the side of surrounding tissues causing inflammatory processes, dysfunction of the endothelium, disturbance of homeostasis, destruction and the necrosis of bone tissue and so forth [15, 16]. The formation of hydrophilic coatings and the modification of chemical composition and topography of the implant surface make it possible to reduce the frequency of the development of negative processes. The bone, fibrous and endothelial tissues are uniquely structured, and the attempts to design the next generations of implants are focused on the development of unique nanotopography of the surface of implants based on the imitation of nature. Our and other studies showed the effectiveness of vacuum-plasma technology for improving biocompatibility and durability (mechanical and chemical) of implanted materials [17–19]. New avenues in the application of above technology to the titanium implants and their influence to surrounding tissues are explored in this paper.

2. Modelling atomic and molecular chains

Molecular dynamics were used to develop the model. To describe the atomic and molecular interactions, Morse (1) and Born-Mayer (2) potentials were chosen [2].

Morse potential takes the form

$$U(r) = J\left\langle \exp\left[-2\alpha\left(r - r_0\right)\right] - 2\exp\left[-\alpha\left(r - r_0\right)\right]\right\rangle \tag{1}$$

where J and α are the parameters of dissociation energy and anharmonicity respectively; $\Delta r = (r - r_0)$ is the displacement from an equilibrium.

Born-Mayer potential takes the form

$$U(r) = T \cdot e^{\frac{-r}{a}} \tag{2}$$

where T, a, and r are the energy constant, the shielding and atomic lengths respectively.

We assume the existence of multiple equilibria corresponding to thermodynamic as well non-thermodynamic branches. Expanding the potentials in a Taylor series (up to the fifth order term), find the interaction force

$$F = -\frac{dU(r)}{dr} = -K\Delta r + A\Delta r^2 - B\Delta r^3 + C\Delta r^4 - D\Delta r^5 \tag{3}$$

For the Morse potential

$$K = 2\alpha^2 J, \ A = 3\alpha^3 J, \ B = 2.3\alpha^4 J,$$
$$C = 1.25\alpha^5 J, \ D = 1.1\alpha^6 J \tag{4}$$

where K, A, B, C, D are the coefficients of elasticity, quadratic cubic, fourth and fifth orders nonlinearities respectively.

For the Born-Mayer potential

$$K = \frac{T}{a^2}, \ A = \frac{T}{2a^2}, \ B = \frac{T}{6a^4}, \ C = \frac{T}{24a^5}, \ D = \frac{T}{120a^6}. \tag{5}$$

The coefficient values are presented in Table 1.

Coefficient	Born-Mayer potential	Morse potential
K, N/m	$9{,}341 \bullet 10^4$	$1{,}140 \bullet 10^4$
A, N/m²	$1{,}951 \bullet 10^{15}$	$8{,}244 \bullet 10^{14}$
B, N/m³	$2{,}716 \bullet 10^{25}$	$3{,}046 \bullet 10^{25}$
C, N/m⁴	$2{,}836 \bullet 10^{35}$	$7{,}980 \bullet 10^{35}$
D, N/m⁵	$2{,}370 \bullet 10^{445}$	$3{,}385 \bullet 10^{446}$

Table 1. Coefficients for Morse and Born-Mayer potentials.

There are many models that describe water molecules [13]. The molecular structure of water is presented in Figure 1. The covalent and hydrogen bonds are marked by the grey springs and the bold lines respectively. For simplicity, in our simulations we consider a chain, i.e. 1D lattice, of water molecules (see the marked area of Figure 1).

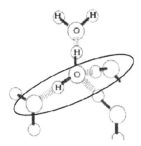

Figure 1. Molecular structure of water in a solid phase. The ellipse marks a piece of 1D chain used in simulations.

Considering only single component of $r = (x, y, z)$, say x, and viewing the atom as interacting nonlinear oscillators, the system equations take the form:

$$m\frac{d^2x_1}{dt^2} = -K'x_1 + Ax_1^2 - Bx_1^3 + Cx_1^4 - Dx_1^5 + K(x_2 - x_1) -$$

$$-A(x_2 - x_1)^2 + B(x_2 - x_1)^3 - C(x_2 - x_1)^4 + D(x_2 - x_1)^5 - \beta'\frac{dx_1}{dt},$$

$$m\frac{d^2x_i}{dt^2} = -K(x_i - x_{i-1}) + A(x_i - x_{i-1})^2 - B(x_i - x_{i-1})^3 + C(x_i - x_{i-1})^4 -$$

$$-D(x_i - x_{i-1})^5 + K(x_{i+1} - x_i) - A(x_{i+1} - x_i)^2 + B(x_{i+1} - x_i)^3 - C(x_{i+1} - x_i)^4 + \qquad (6)$$

$$+D(x_{i+1} - x_i)^5 - \beta'\frac{dx_i}{dt},$$

$$m\frac{d^2x_n}{dt^2} = -K(x_n - x_{n-1}) + A(x_n - x_{n-1})^2 - B(x_n - x_{n-1})^3 + C(x_n - x_{n-1})^4 -$$

$$-D(x_n - x_{n-1})^5 - K'x_n + Ax_n^2 - Bx_n^3 + Cx_n^4 - Dx_n^5 - \beta'\frac{dx_n}{dt},$$

where x_i, $i = 1,\ldots, n$ is displacement of i-th oscillator from the its equilibrium position, K′ is the coefficient of elasticity on the chain borders, and ß and ß′ are the damping factors inside the chain and on its borders respectively. The system (6) was solved by the Runge–Kutta method.

Relaxation processes of atoms after stopping the external influence were under investigation. Sources that gave impulses to atoms of the chains were both direct ion impact on the first atom of the chain (single impact) and random impacts on randomly chosen atoms of the chain (plasma treatment). In practice the atom bonds are important to keep unbroken, so all types of influences were low-energy ones.

2.1. Hydrogen atom chain

We carried out the simulations for chain consisting of 50 hydrogen atoms (Figure 2). Morse potential was chosen; N_i defines the number of i-th atoms. For single impact the first atom of the chain was displaced with velocity $V = 500$ m/s, which corresponds to 10^{-3} eV of the exposed energy. In case of plasma treatment the following atoms were exposed to low-energy impacts: atom N_1 ($V = 538$ m/s), atom N_{10} ($V = 1682$ m/s) and atom N_{30} ($V = 1237$ m/s).

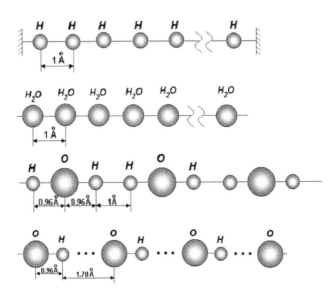

Figure 2. Chain of hydrogen atoms.

Figure 3 illustrates the atom displacements after the plasma treatment. The atoms are stabilized in the new positions that can be described as (nano)clusters (atoms N_{1-29} and N_{30-50}). After atom relaxation the simulations were continued fourth times longer, and the persistent stabilization was always observed.

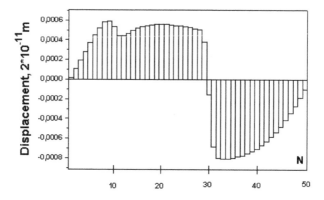

Figure 3. Displacement of 50 atoms of the excited nonlinear chain at the time of stabilization. N defines the atom number in the chain.

2.2. H–O–H molecule chain

We investigated the chain of H–O–H molecules shown in Figure 4. From two to eight molecules (6–24 atoms) were used. The equilibrium distances between H and O atoms inside the molecule are 0.96 Å, and the equilibrium distance between the molecules is 1 Å, which corresponds to … Single impact were assumed, and the velocity of the first atom was varied from 100 to 1600 m/s, which corresponds to 10^{-5}–10^{-2} eV of the exposed energy. Again, Morse potential was used.

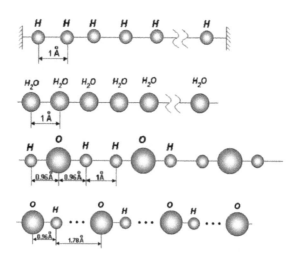

Figure 4. Atom chain of water consisting of hydrogen and oxygen atoms.

Figure 5 illustrates the atom displacements versus the velocity that the first atom received from external impact. In all cases significant shrinkage, or collapse, of the chains is observed. One can see that the length of the collapsed chain depends on the above velocity, the minimal length being detected at some low impact energies. For example, for the chain consisting of eight H–O–H molecules the minimal length of the chain was observed at $V = 1200$ m/s (see Fig. 5b).

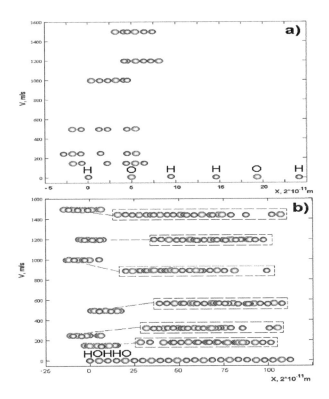

Figure 5. Atom displacements in the chain of H–O–H molecules versus the velocity received by the first atom: a) chain consisting of two molecules, b) chain consisting of eight molecules. In dashed areas the collapsed chains are shown enlarged.

2.3. 1D water molecule chain

Finally, we investigated the chain shown in Figure 6. It corresponds to the 1D cut of water molecule (see the area marked by the ellipse in Figure 1). The solid and dotted lines correspond to the covalent and hydrogen bonds respectively. As one can see the covalent bonds yields the equilibrium between O and H atoms at 0.96 Å whereas the hydrogen bonds yields the equilibrium at about twice longer distance (1.78 Å).

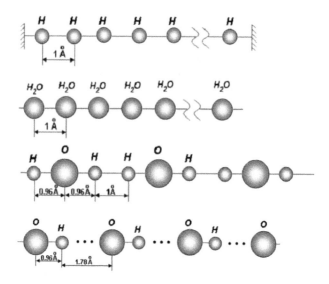

Figure 6. chain of water consisting of hydrogen and oxygen atoms. The solid and dotted lines mark the covalent and hydrogen bonds respectively.

In simulations we considered simple chain consisting of two 1D water molecules. The initial velocity of the first atom was taken at $V = 500$ m/s. The Morse and Born-Mayer potentials were used for this investigation.

Figure 7 represents the initial and final stabilized conditions of atom chains (after direct low-energy ion impact to the first atom of the chain) calculated with Born-Mayer (Figure 7a) and Morse (Figure 7b) potentials

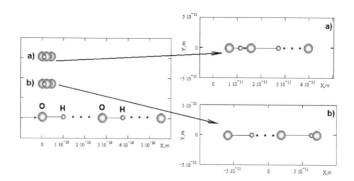

Figure 7. Initial and final positions of atoms of 1D water molecule after direct low-energy impact to the first atom (oxygen): a) Born-Mayer potential, b) Morse potential. The right figures show the enlarged final chains.

3. Biomedical applications

Biological objects are known for their high sensitivity to weak external fields. The evidence that electromagnetic fields can have "non-thermal" biological effects is now overwhelming. When the production of heat shock proteins is triggered electromagnetically it needs 100 million times less energy than when triggered by heat [20]. Low-frequency weak magnetic fields may lead to the resonant change of the rate of biochemical reactions although the impact energy is by ten orders of magnitude less than $k_B T$ where k_B is the Boltzmann constant and T is the temperature of the medium [21].

The therapeutic ability of the low intensity electromagnetic radiations is actively discussed [22]. The low-power millimeter wave irradiation and magnetic-resonance therapy are used in practical medicine already, which differ significantly from the drug treatment by the fact that they do not clog organism with the undesirable chemical compounds, i.e. xenobiotics. In this chapter we discuss the biomedical application of vacuum-plasma technologies.

3.1. Activating and therapeutic properties of water processed in GDP

To understand the above extreme sensitivity of living objects, investigations in influences of weak fields on water appear to be essential. Indeed, water plays a major role in biological processes. A man consumes about 2 l of drinking water a day. Water is the main component of human, animal, plant and generally every living being body. A new-born child body contains 97% of water, decreasing to 70–75% with aging. In particular, human brain consists of about 85% of water.

So, we performed experiments with water, crop seeds and baking yeast S. cerevisiae. The crop seeds and yeast were processed directly in GDP. Also, the untreated crop seeds and yeast were poured with the water processed in GDP. In all cases practically the same biotrophic effects were observed. Namely, the seed sprouts showed the growth in 3–4 times higher than the control samples. Both the processed yeast and the unprocessed one that immersed in the processed (by GDP) water showed greater metabolic activity compared to the control samples.

The obtained results allow suggesting that the discovered phenomena can be used for direct correction of pathological states. Therefore we processed water and physiological solution. The samples were exposed to low-energy ion irradiation in GDP of residual gases. The ion energy depends on the voltage in the plasma generator. The latter was kept at 1.2 keV while the current in the plasma generator was maintained at 70 mA. The temperature in the chamber was controlled during the irradiation process and did not exceed 298 K (25° C). The irradiation time was 60 minutes.

In test experiments, volunteers with different diseases either drunk the processed water or they were injected intravenously with the similarly processed physiological solution. The course of treatment included 3–5 sessions of 0.5 l physiological solution transfusion. The preliminary results appeared to be very promising. We were most interested in the therapeutic treatment of the global inflammatory processes such as cardio-vascular diseases and pancreatic (insular) diabetes complicated by the acute and chronic forms of atherosclerosis. Also, different types of oncology, say, leukemia, etc., were under investigation.

The blood immune cells were taken for diagnostics. The immune system is known as one of the leading homeostatic systems in the organisms. It may serve as a mirror that reflects practically all adaptations and pathological rearrangements. The immunocompetent cells, lymphocytes and leukocytes, have a set of properties that may be used as an indicator of the organism state. In addition, the structural organization of blood lymphocytes and leukocytes makes possible a most efficient use of microspectral analysis and different fluorescent probes for their studies [23].

We used the dual-wavelength microfluorimetry analysis. The selected cell populations (mono- and polynuclears of blood immunocytes) were mapped as clusters of points on the phase plane in coordinates of the red and green luminescence intensities, i.e. on the wavelengths I_{530} (abscissa) and I_{640} (ordinate). Figure 8 presents the above phase plane for an oncologic outpatient before and after the monthly course treatment. The black and grey pluses represent lymphocyte and leukocyte cells respectively. The white ellipses mark the distribution of fluorescent signals of lymphocytes (lower ellipse) and leukocytes (upper ellipse) in norm. As seen, the treatment results into significant normalization toward the homeostasis.

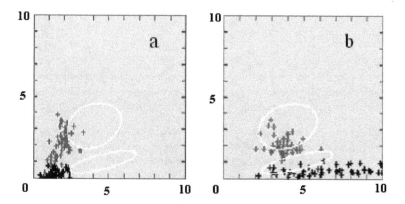

Figure 8. Dual-wavelength microfluorimetry analysis (abscissa and ordinate represent the luminescent intensity I_{530} and I_{640} respectively) of blood immunocytes of oncologic patient (second stage breast cancer). The state before (a) and after (b) the water treatment course (see the text). The black and grey pluses represent lymphocytes and leukocytes respectively. The white ellipses mark the distribution of fluorescent signals of lymphocytes (lower ellipse) and leukocytes (upper ellipse) in norm.

3.2. Biocompatibility of titanium alloys and stainless steel processed in GDP

Stainless steel, titanium and its alloys are among the most utilized biomaterials and are still the materials of choice for many structural implantable device applications [24, 25]. We processed both the titanium and stainless steel samples and investigated changing in their properties caused by GDP.

Current titanium implants face long-term failure problems due to poor bonding to juxtaposed bone, severe stress shielding and generation of debris that may lead to bone cell death and perhaps eventual necrotic bone [26–28]. Improving the bioactivity of titanium implants, especially with respect to cells, is a major concern in the near and intermediate future. Surface properties such as wettability, chemical composition and topography govern the biocompatibility of titanium. Conventionally processed titanium currently used in the orthopedic and dental applications exhibits a micro-rough surface and is smooth at the nanoscale. Surface smoothness on the nanoscale has been shown to favor fibrous tissue encapsulation [27–29]. An approach to design the next-generation of implants has recently focused on creating unique nanotopography (or roughness) on the implant surface, considering that natural bone consists of nanostructured materials like collagen and hydroxyapatite. Some researchers have achieved nano-roughness in titanium substrates by compacting small (nanometer) constituent particles and/or fibers [30]. However, nanometer metal particles can be expensive and unsafe to fabricate. For this reason, alternative methods of titanium surface treatment are desirable.

For the investigation of biocompatibility of implanted materials the tests *in vitro* with the cultures of different cells (fibroblasts, lymphocytes, macrophages, epithelial cells, *etc.*) are used. The influence of material is typically evaluated according to such indicators as adhesion, change in the morphological properties, inhibition of an increase in the cellular population, oppression of metabolic activity and others.

The adhesion of cells, as is known, plays exceptionally important role in the biological processes, such as formation of tissues and organs during embryogenesis, reparative processes, immune and inflammatory reactions, *etc.* Capability for movement is the characteristic property of fibroblasts, cells of immune system and cells, which participate in the inflammation. Moreover, in immunocytes and leukocytes it consists not only in the free recirculation in the blood stream or lymph but also in the penetration into vascular walls and active migration into the surrounding tissues. Adhesion and flattening of cells to the base layer always precede their locomotion. The degree of flattening is important preparatory step to the cell amoeboid mobility. We concentrate our attention on the above components in experiments with titanium alloys.

Titanium samples were cut into pieces (1 cm × 0.5 cm) and placed in a specially constructed plasma generator. They were exposed to glow discharge plasma by ions of the residual gases of the vacuum. The ion energy depended on the voltage in the plasmatron and did not exceed 1–10 keV. Irradiated fluence was 10^{17} ion•cm^{-2}. The temperature of the specimens was controlled during the irradiation process and did not exceed 343 K while the irradiation time varied from 5 to 60 minutes. Rutherford Backscattering Spectrometry (RBS) was used to study the changes after the irradiation. Cell adhesion to titanium samples was tested with L929 mouse connective tissue (fibroblasts-like cells). L929 cells were cultured in Dulbecco's modified Eagle's medium with 10% fetal bovine serum. Initial cell density was $5 \cdot 10^5$ cells/ml. The samples were placed into the sterile disposable 9 cm diameter tissue culture Petri dishes. 2 ml growth medium with cells were distributed into each Petri then incubated in the 5% CO_2 at 37° C for 2 hours. After that period, cultures were prepared for scanning electron microscopy (SEM).

RBS data for the irradiated sample show the presence of iron on the surface that occurred from high-carbon steel cathode as a result of secondary emission process (Figure. 9). Percentage of iron and thickness of the layer were calculated using RUMP, the program for simulation and analysis based on RBS and Elastic Recoil Detection techniques.

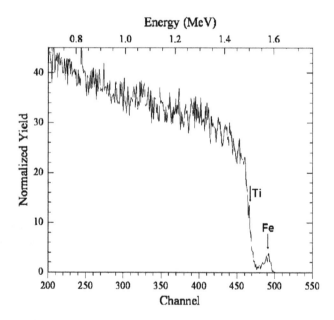

Figure 9. RBS spectrum of the titanium sample irradiated for 5 min at 10 kV.

The obtained data for different voltage and time of the irradiation are presented in Table 2.

Voltage, kV	Time of irradiation, min	Fe:Ti atomic ratio	Density of flattened cells per μm^2	Percentage of flattened cells	Increase factor in amount of all cells in comparison with control sample
0.4	60	0.0277:1	534±20	50.2±2.0	1.78
1.2	30	0.0560:1	413±9	43.7±0.9	1.63
10	5	0.0549:1	381±15	42.5±1.7	1.53
Control	0	0:1	26±8	4.4±1.5	1

Table 2. Data obtained from the experiments with titanium samples exposed to GDP.

Calculated data indicate an increase in the density of flattened cells as well as in the cell amount in comparison with the control sample. According to Table 2 one conclude that best adhesion (column 4) and most prolific cell attachment (column 5) correspond to the samples that were exposed to GDP for maximum time at minimum voltage. For this sample we observed less percentage of iron and thickness of the iron layer in comparison with others that were exposed to higher voltage plasma irradiation.

Figure 10 demonstrates SEM images of control and irradiated samples. In comparison with the control sample, analysis of cell attachment for the irradiated samples shows high confluence (attachment ratio) and better spreading.

We also performed experiments on the adhesion of immune-competent cells of human blood to the stainless steel samples. Figure 11 represents the microphotography of the healthy person lymphocytes and leukocytes adhered to the irradiated and non-irradiated plates. As can be seen from photographs, cells, which are located on the different samples, are essentially different. The morphology of leukocytes and lymphocytes, which were adhered to the irradiated material, indicates the expressed amoeboid mobility.

In the majority of the cases endoprosthetics is conducted not in the healthiest people. This fact is very important and it must be considered. Figure 12 displays the results of similar study of the blood nucleus of person who suffers from second stage hypertonia, coronary artery disease and atherosclerosis. From the above data one can conclude that the nature of adhesion of cells to the base layer depends on both the physico-chemical state of this base layer and the state of organism, the owner of cells.

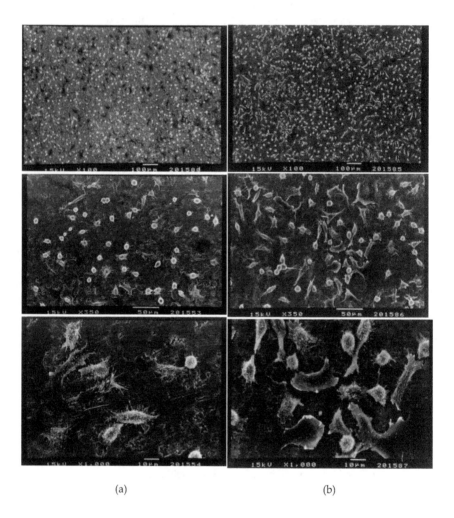

(a)   (b)

Figure 10. SEM images of cell attachment on (a) the control sample and (b) the titanium sample that was irradiated for 5 min at 10 kV.

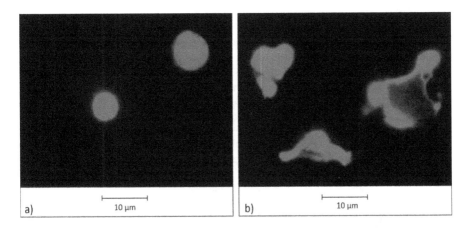

Figure 11. Luminescent microscopy (1000×) of lymphocytes and granulocytes of the blood of healthy donor adhered to (a) non-irradiated and (b) irradiated in GDP surface of the stainless steel samples. The cell nucleus fluorochromization is performed by propidium iodide (λ_{fl} = 615 nm).

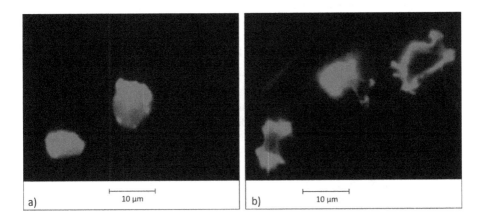

Figure 12. Luminescent microscopy (1000×) of lymphocytes and granulocytes of the blood of donor suffering from second stage hypertonia, coronary artery disease and atherosclerosis. The cell nuclei are adhered to (a) non-irradiated and (b) irradiated in GDP surface of the stainless steel samples. The fluorochromization is performed by propidium iodide (λ_{fl} = 615 nm).

4. Discussion and conclusions

Studying the homogeneous chains, like the hydrogen atom chain, exposed to low energies we observed clusterization. It is important to stress that this is truly self-organization phenomenon induced by an external excitation. The chains utilize the excitation energy to initialize nonlinear oscillations and redistribute the energy throughout the chain, which leads to the pattern formation. In the case of multiple impacts on randomly chosen atoms (so-called plasma processing) the atom displacements are by an order higher than in the case of single impact. Thus, the plasma treatment leads to more active self-organization processes and atom rearrangements.

In the cases of inhomogeneous chains containing H and O atoms another type of structures is developed. The shrinkage of chains is so significant that we can say about the collapsed structures. This collapse is observed irrespective of the choice of the atom interaction potentials, whereas the collapsed chain patterns are found to depend on the latter.

To conclude, the performed simulations demonstrated that the system nonlinearity is, in fact, the main reason for the development of self-organization processes leading to significant modifications even in case of low-energy impacts.

In experiments with water and biological objects processed in GDP significant biotrophic effects were detected. The crop seeds and yeast processed directly or indirectly (being immersed in the water processed in GDP) showed markedly greater metabolic activity compared to the control samples. Using the water and the physiological solutions processed in GDP we observed significant therapeutic effects in the test treatments of cardiovascular, oncologic and other diseases. The obtained results suggest the use of discovered phenomena for direct corrections of pathological states by shifting a body state towards its homeostasis. Understanding the mechanisms of the latter will be our next priority.

Next part of this study is devoted to experiments with the titanium alloys and stainless steel exposed to GDP. The experiments with titanium samples reveal an increase in the density of flattened (to the sample surface) cells as well as in the cell amount in comparison with the control sample. These are nothing but preparatory step to the cell amoeboid mobility. Indeed, adhesion and flattening of cells to the base layer always precede their locomotion. According to the results, best adhesion and most prolific cell attachment correspond to the samples that were exposed to GDP for maximum time at minimum voltage. Similar results were obtained in the experiments with stainless steel samples: the morphology of leukocytes and lymphocytes, which were adhered to the irradiated material, indicated the expressed amoeboid mobility. The results with the blood nucleus of person who suffers from several diseases revealed some deviations in the morphology of adhered cells compared to the healthy blood. Thus, the nature of adhesion of cells to the base layer depends on both the physico-chemical state of this base layer and the state of organism, the owner of cells. This circumstance determines even more stringent requirements for the material of the implants.

Author details

V. Tereshko[1*], A. Gorchakov[2], I. Tereshko[3], V. Abidzina[3] and V. Red'ko[4]

*Address all correspondence to: valery.tereshko@uws.ac.uk

1 School of Computing, University of the West of Scotland, Paisley, UK

2 MISTEM, Mogilev, Belarus

3 Department of Physics, Belarusian-Russian University, Mogilev, Belarus

4 Department of Physical Methods of Control, Belarusian-Russian University, Mogilev, Belarus

References

[1] Ziegler, J. F, Biersack, J. P, & Littmark, U. The Stopping and Range of Ions in Solids. New York: Pergamon; (1985).

[2] Eckstein, W. Computer Simulation of Ion-Solids Interaction. Berlin: Springer; (1991).

[3] Tereshko, I. V, Khodyrev, V. I, Tereshko, V. M, Lipsky, E. A, Goncharenya, A. V, & Ofori-sey, S. Self-organizing processes in metals by low-energy ion beams. Nucl. Instr. and Meth. B (1993). , 80, 115-119.

[4] Tereshko, I. V, Khodyrev, V. I, Lipsky, E. A, Goncharenya, A. V, & Tereshko, A. M. Materials modification by low-energy ion irradiation. Nucl. Instr. and Meth. B (1997). , 128, 861-864.

[5] Tereshko, I. V, Glushchenko, V. V, & Tereshko, A. M. Computer simulation of the defect structure formation in crystal lattices by low-energy ion irradiation. Comput. Mater. Sci. (2002). , 24, 139-143.

[6] Tereshko, I, Abidzina, V, Tereshko, A, & Elkin, I. Nanostructural evolution of steel and titanium alloys exposed to glow discharge plasma. Nucl. Instr. and Meth. B (2007). , 261, 678-681.

[7] Tereshko, I. V, Abidzina, V. V, Elkin, I. E, Tereshko, A. M, Glushchenko, V. V, & Stoye, S. Formation of nanostructures in metals by low-energy ion irradiation. Surf. & Coat. Tech. (2007). , 201, 8552-8556.

[8] Stillinger, F. N. Water revisited. Science (1980). , 209(4455), 451-457.

[9] Liu, K, Cruzan, J. D, & Saykally, R. J. Water clusters. Science (1996). , 271(5251), 929-933.

[10] Keutsch, F. N, & Saykally, R. J. Water clusters: untangling the mysteries of the liquid, one molecule at a time. PNAS (2001). , 98(19), 10533-10540.

[11] Galamba, N. Cabral BJC. The changing hydrogen-bond network of water from the bulk to the surface of a cluster: a Born-Oppenheimer molecular dynamics study. J. Am. Chem. Soc. (2008). , 130, 17955-17960.

[12] Luck, W. A. The importance of cooperativity for the properties of liquid water. J. Mol. Struct. (1998).

[13] Shelton, D. P. Collective molecular rotation in water and other simple liquids. Chem. Phys. Lett. (2000).

[14] Lobyshev, V. I, Shikhlinskaya, R. E, & Ryzhikov, B. D. Experimental evidence for intrinsic luminescence of water. J. Mol. Liquids (1999).

[15] Park, J. B, & Lakes, R. S. Biomaterials: An Introduction. New York: Plenum; (1992).

[16] Ratner, B. D, Hoffman, A. S, Schoen, F. J, & Lemons, J. E. editors. Biomaterials Science: Introduction to Materials in Medicine. New York: Academic; (1996).

[17] Abidzina, V, Deliloglu-gurhan, I, Ozdal-kurt, F, Sen, B. H, Tereshko, I, Elkin, I, Budak, S, Muntele, C, & Ila, D. Cell adhesion study of the titanium alloys exposed to glow discharge. Nucl. Instr. and Meth. B. (2007). , 261, 624-626.

[18] Mandl, S, & Rauschenbach, B. Improving the biocompatibility of medical implants with plasma immersion ion implantation. Surf. Coat. Technol. (2002).

[19] Lopez-heredia, M. A, Legeay, G, Gaillard, C, & Layrolle, P. Radio frequency plasma treatments on titanium for enhancement of bioactivity. Acta biomater. (2008). , 4, 1953-1962.

[20] Blank, M, & Goodman, R. Stimulation of stress response by low frequency electromagnetic fields: possibility of direct interaction with DNA. IEEE Trans. Plasma Sci. (2000). , 28, 168-172.

[21] Binhi, V. N, & Savin, A. V. Effects of weak magnetic fields on biological systems: physical aspects. Physics- Uspekhi (2003). , 46(3), 259-291.

[22] Betskii, O. V, Devyatkov, N. D, & Kislov, V. V. Low intensity millimeter waves in medicine and biology. Crit. Rev. Biomed. Eng. (2000).

[23] Gorchakov, A. M, & Karnaukhov, V. N. Melenets YuV, and Gorchakova FT. Identification of pathological conditions by luminescence analysis of immunocompetent blood cells. Biophysics (1999). , 44(3), 550-555.

[24] Hermawan, H, & Ramdan, D. Djuansjah JRP. Metals for biomedical applications. In: Fazel R, editor. Biomedical Engineering- From Theory to Applications. Rijeka: In-Tech; (2011). , 411-430.

[25] Williams, D. F. Titanium for medical applications. In: Brunette DM, Tengvall P, Textor M, Thomsen P, editors. Titanium in Medicine. Berlin: Springer; (2001). , 13-24.

[26] Buser, D, Nydegger, T, Oxland, T, Cochran, D. L, Schenk, R. K, Hirt, H. P, Snétivy, D, & Nolte, L. P. Interface shear strength of titanium implants with a sandblasted and acid-etched surface: a biomechanical study in the maxilla of miniature pigs. J. Biomed. Mater. Res. (1999). , 45(2), 75-83.

[27] Kaplan, F. S, Hayes, W. C, Keaveny, T. M, Boskey, A, & Einhorn, T. A. Biomaterials. In: Simon SP, editor. Orthopedic Basic Science. Columbus: American Academy of Orthopedic Surgeons; (1994). , 460-478.

[28] Kaplan, F. S, Hayes, W. C, Keaveny, T. M, Boskey, A, Einhorn, T. A, & Iannotti, J. P. Form and function of bone. In: Simon SP, editor. Orthopedic Basic Science. Columbus: American Academy of Orthopedic Surgeons; (1994). , 127-185.

[29] Boyan, B. D, Dean, D. D, Lohmann, C. H, Cochran, D. L, Sylvia, V. L, & Schwartz, Z. The titanium-bone cell interface in vitro: the role of the surface in promoting osteointegration. In: Brunette DM, Tengvall P, Textor M, Thomsen P, editors. Titanium in Medicine. Berlin: Springer; (2001). , 561-586.

[30] Webster, T. J, & Ejiofor, J. U. Increased osteoblast adhesion on nanophase metals: Ti, Ti6Al4V, and CoCrMo. Biomaterials (2004). , 25, 4731-4739.

Chapter 2

Degradation of Polyurethanes for Cardiovascular Applications

Juan V. Cauich-Rodríguez, Lerma H. Chan-Chan,
Fernando Hernandez-Sánchez and
José M. Cervantes-Uc

Additional information is available at the end of the chapter

1. Introduction

Polyurethanes are a family of polymers used in a variety of biomedical applications but mainly in the cardiovascular field due to their good physicochemical and mechanical properties in addition to a good biocompatibility. Traditionally, segmented polyurethanes (SPUs), have been used in cardiovascular applications (Kuan et al., 2011) as permanent devices such as pacemaker leads and ventricular assisting devices; however, due to their great chemistry versatility, SPUs can also be tailored to render biodegradable systems for the tissue engineering of vascular grafts and heart valves. Therefore many research work have been focused on varying the chemical composition to enhance biostability or more recently to control the biodegradability of polyurethanes depending on specific applications in the cardiovascular field (Bernacca et al., 2002; Stachelek et al., 2006; Thomas et al., 2009; Wang et al., 2009; Hong et al., 2010; Arjun et al., 2012; Styan et al., 2012). In this way, polyurethanes for biomedical applications can be classified in two main types, according their relative stability in the human body as either biostables or biodegradables. In this chapter, general aspects of polyurethanes chemistry are presented first and then, the various types of degradations that can affect these polymers both *in vivo* and simulated *in vitro* conditions. Emphasis is also made on the mechanism of degradation under various conditions and the techniques used for following the changes in their properties.

2. Chemistry of polyurethanes

2.1. Synthesis of polyurethanes

Polyurethanes (PU's) properties depend both on the method of preparation and the mono‐mers used. In general, PU's can be prepared in one shot process or more commonly by a two step method, especially for the case of segmented polyurethanes (SPU's). These materials are thermoplastic block copolymers of the (AB)n type consisting of alternating sections of hard segments, composed of a diisocyanate and a low molecular weight diol chain extender, and soft segments, generally composed of various types of polyols, also called macrodiols. In the two steps method for SPU synthesis, a prepolymer is first obtained and then chain extended as illustrated in Figure 1. In the first step, an excess of the diisocyanate reacts with the soft segment polyol to form the prepolymer. Here, the characteristic urethane linkages are formed through the reaction between the isocyanate groups and the hydroxyl-terminat‐ed end groups of the polyol. In the second step, the low molecular weight chain extender is used to link the prepolymer segments yielding a high molecular weight polymer. During this stage, additional urethane functional groups are formed when using a diol chain ex‐tender whereas ureas are produced when a diamine is used.

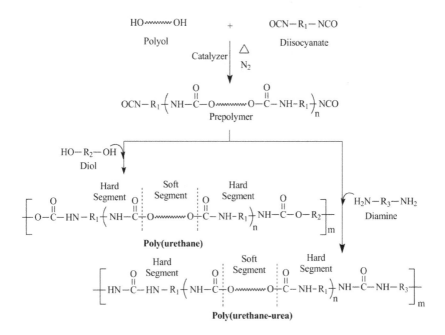

Figure 1. Standard two-step reaction to prepare segmented poly (urethane)s and poly(urethane-urea)s

The properties of polyurethanes as those shown in Figure 1 depend on the various types of monomers that are used during their manufacturing (see Table 1). Historically, biostable polyurethanes were first developed by using polyether type of polyol and different aromatic diisocyanates. Further developments in this area were focused on the substitution of the polyether macrodiol by novel hydrocarbon, polycarbonate or siloxane macrodiols (Gunatillake et al., 2003) or a combination of these which in general are responsible for the flexibility of the SPUs (Król, 2007). In addition to the polyol chemical composition, their molecular weight and concentration have an important effect in the polyurethane behavior. They can be incorporated in various concentrations but up to 50-75% of the polyol is common.

Commercial and experimental polyurethanes have been synthesized by the combination of the aforementioned monomers. Poly(tetramethylene oxide) (PTMO) is the most common polyether in conventional medical formulations (Silvestri et al., 2011). Thus, for example, the Pellethane® 2363 80A and Elasthane™ 80A are poly(ether-urethane)s obtained by the reaction of PTMO, MDI and BD monomers; Tecoflex® by Thermedics is also a poly(ether-urethane) synthesised by the reaction of PTMO, HMDI and BD monomers while Biomer® is a poly(ether-urea-urethane) synthesized from PTMO, MDI and ethylenediamine. Bionate®, Myo Lynk™ and Chronoflex are polyurethanes prepared with polycarbonate diol. These commercial polyurethanes are typical examples of biostables polymers.

The use of vegetable raw materials containing hydroxyl groups such as starch, castor oil, vegetable oil, natural rubber, cellulose, etc, makes possible to obtain biodegradable polyurethanes (Krol, 2007; Aranguren et al. 2012). However, ester polyol commonly used to synthesize biodegradable polyurethanes are polycaprolactone, polylactic acid and adipate polyols. Polyethyleneglycol is a polyether which has been copolymerized with poly lactic acid and/or polycaprolactone because its higher hydrofilicity can accelerate the biodegradation when this is required (Guan et al., 2005b; Wang et al., 2011b).

The most frequently used diisocyanates in the synthesis of biodegradable polyurethanes for biomedical applications are aliphatic or cycloaliphatic as MDI and TDI which can release carcinogenic and mutagenic aromatic diamines (Heijkants et. al., 2005). Aliphatic diisocyanates are less reactive than the aromatic counterparts but have a greater resistance to hydrolysis compared to aromatic diisocyanates, although this resistance frequently results in lower mechanical properties (Gogolewski, 1989).

In general, there are two types of compounds that are generally used as chain extenders, diols or diamines, which can either be aliphatic or aromatic, depending on the required properties in the synthesized polyurethanes. New chain extenders, including amino acids have been also used during polyurethane synthesis as isocyanates can react vigorously with amine, alcohol, and carboxylic acids (Thomson, 2005). These novel chain extenders have been used to synthesize biodegradable polyurethanes (Skarja et al., 1998; Marcos-Fernández et al., 2006; Sarkar et al., 2007).

Monomeric component	Type	Chemical compound	Type of polyurethanes
Polyol (macrodiols)	Polyethers	Poly(ethylene oxide) (PEO)	Biostables, Biodegradables (Sarkar et al., 2009; Lu et al., 2012)
		Poly(propylen oxide) (PPO)	Biostables, Biodegradables (Francolini et al., 2011)
		Poly(tetramethylene oxide) (PTMO)	Biostables (Silvestri et al., 2011; Jiang et al., 2012)
		Poly(caprolactone) (PCL)	Biodegradables (Sarkar et al., 2009; Lu et al., 2012)
		Poly(lactic acid) (PLA)	Biodegradable (Wang et al., 2011a)
		Poly hydroxyalkanoates (PHA)	Biodegradables (Li et al., 2009; Liu et al., 2009)
		Poly(ethylene adipate) (PEA)	Biodegradables (Macocinschi et al., 2009)
	Others	Poly(carbonate) (PCU)	Biostables (Spirkova et al., 2011)
		Polybutadiene (PBD)	Biostables (Thomas et al., 2009)
		Poly(dimethylsiloxane) (PDMS)	Biostables (Park et al., 1999; Madhavan et al., 2006)
Diisocyanate	Aromatic	Methylene diphenyl diisocyanate (MDI)	Biostables (Gunatillake et al., 1992; Styan et al., 2012)
		2,4-toluene diisocyanate (TDI)	Biostables (Labow et al., 1996; Basak et al., 2012)
	Aliphatic	4,4'-methylene bis(cyclohexyl isocyanate) (HMDI)	Biostables, Biodegradables (Thomas et al., 2009; Chan-Chan et al., 2010)
		1,6- hexamethylene diisocyanate (HDI)	Biostables, Biodegradables (Wang et al., 2011a; Baudis et al., 2012)
		1,4-butane diisocyanate (BDI)	Biostables, Biodegradables (Heijkants et al., 2005; Hong et al., 2010)
		Isophorone diisocyanate (IPDI)	Biostables, Biodegradables (Jiang et al., 2007; Ding et al., 2012; He et al., 2012)
		L-lysine ethyl ester diisocyanate (LDI)	Biodegradable (Abraham et al., 2006; Guelcher et al., 2008; Han et al., 2009; Wang et al., 2011b)
Chain Extender	Diols	Ethylene glycol (EG)	Biostables, Biodegradables (Król, 2007)
		Diethylenglycol	
		1,4-butanediol (BD)	
		1,6-hexanediol (HD)	
	Diamines	Aliphatic diamines	
		Aromatic diamines	
	Others	Amino acids	Biodegradables (Kartvelishvili et al., 1997; Skarja et al., 1998; Marcos-Fernández et al., 2006; Sarkar et al., 2007; Chan-Chan et al., 2012)

Table 1. Common monomers used in the synthesis of biostable and biodegradable polyurethanes

During polyurethane synthesis, several side reactions may occur leading to branching, crosslinking, or changes in the stoichiometry of reactants. For example, undesirable branching and crosslinking may occur at elevated temperatures between isocyanates and urethanes (Allophanate formation) and isocyanates and ureas (Biuret reactions). Furthermore, the presence of water causes isocyanate groups to form unstable carbamic acids, which subsequently decompose to amines with the liberation of CO_2 gas (see Figure 2). These newly formed amines react with isocyanates to form ureas, thus changing reactant stoichiometry and leading to lower molecular weight polymers. Additives are sometime used for improving specific properties of the polyurethane, for example Vitamin E and Santowhite®, two hindered phenolic antioxidants, prevents oxidative chain scission and crosslinking of poly(ether urethane) by capturing oxygen radicals (Schubert et al., 1997; Christenson et al., 2006). Di-tert-butylphenol and bisphosphonates have been incorporated to promote bromoalkylation of urethane nitrogens in prepolymerized polyurethanes to inhibit the oxidation or calcification (Alferiev et al., 2001; Stachelek et al., 2007). Other compounds as fluorocarbon or polydimethylsiloxane end groups have been attached to the surface of polyurethanes in order to enhance their biostability and hemocompatibility (Ward et al., 2007; Xie et al., 2009; Jiang et al., 2012).

In general, monomer type and stoichiometry, type and concentration of catalyzer, temperature and moisture, and the use of additives are important in parameters for controlling the properties of these polymers.

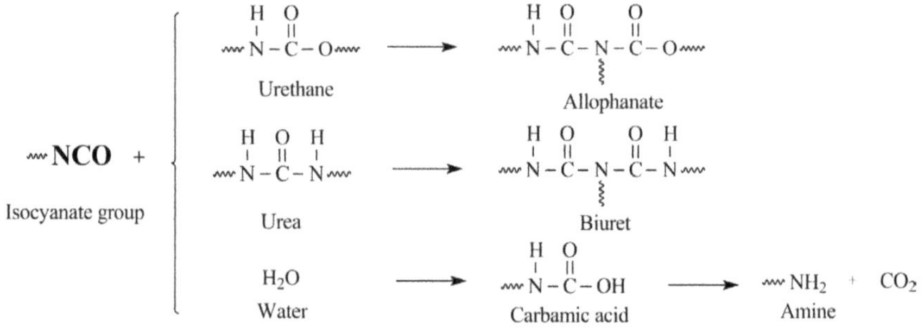

Figure 2. Secondary reactions involved during polyurethane synthesis

3. *In vivo* degradation

SPU's traditionally has been used in medical devices due to their excellent mechanical properties and an acceptable hemocompatibility. However, in the long term they suffer from poor biostability (Santerre et al., 2005). The main reason of this behavior is that living tissues are a very aggressive environment and even when the degradation of these polymers can be simulated by *in vitro* experiments, after *in vivo* usage they can be severally degraded. The *in vivo* failure of polymeric cardiovascular devices has been attributed to a combination of hydrolysis, oxidation, environmental stress cracking and calcification. However, depending on the composition of the polymer one of these predominate over the other.

Polymer degradation in the biological environment results from the synergistic effects of the enzymes present in biological fluids, oxidizing agents and mechanical loads. For example, α-2-macroglobulin, cholesteryl esterase, A2 fosfolipase, K protease and B Cathepsin are enzymes that are known to degrade polyurethanes (Zhao et al., 1993; Dumitriu, 2002). Even when some enzymes require very specific biological substrates, some of them seem to recognise and act over non biological substrates such as polymers (Santerre et al., 2005). White blood cells play also an important role in the *in vivo* degradation. Some experiments conducted using implanted metallic cages have shown that neutrophiles, monocytes, monocyte derived macrophages (MDM) attach to polymer surfaces, leading to the presence of multinucleated giant cells and foreign body reaction. It is generally accepted that one of the immediate immune responses by the body is the release of reactive oxygen species (ROS). In addition, neutrophils and monocytes release hypochlorous acid (HClO) and lysosomal hydrolases as part of their reaction to foreign surfaces. It has been also reported that activated MDM release ROS leading to the formation of hydrogen peroxide (Christenson et al., 2006; McBane et al., 2007). In addition, during the inflammatory reaction macrophages are able to lower the local pH up to 4. This condition can be simulated by following the ISO 10993 section 5.

Suntherland et al. (Sutherland et al., 1993) suggested that poly(ether urethanes) (PEU) cannot be significantly degraded by preformed products of phagocytic cells (such as cationic proteins and proteases) or by activated oxygen species such as superoxide and hydrogen peroxide. In view of the chemically stable nature of PEU, they hypothesized that the *in vivo* degradation of these materials might involve attack by chlorine-based and/or nitric oxide (NO)-derived oxidants, major oxidative products of activated phagocytes. Therefore, they exposed Pellethane to polymorphonuclear neutrophils (PMN) isolated from heparinized venous blood drawn from normal adult donors. The results reported support the idea that PMN-generated chlorine compounds are likely responsible for initial damage to PEU after brief implantation and in addition to macrophage-derived NO and/or peroxynitrite (ONOO-).

Van Minen et al. (van Minnen et al., 2008) studied the *in vivo* (26 weeks of subcutaneous implantation in rats and 2.5 years in rabbits) degradation of porous aliphatic SPU based on butanediisocyanate, DL-lactide-co-caprolactone soft segments and extended with BD-BDI-BD block urethane. After 1 week macrophages were observed along with giant cells and after 4 week phagocytosis was observed. The number of these cells was reduced with time but after 3 years fragments of the polymer remained. Furthermore, few macrophages were observed in the lymph nodes suggesting their local degradation.

Adhikari et al. (Adhikari et al., 2008) studied the *in vivo* degradation of two-part injectable biodegradable polyurethane prepolymer systems (prepolymer A and B) consisting of lactic acid and glycolic acid based polyester star polyols, pentaerythritol (PE) and ethyl lysine diisocyanate (ELDI) using sheep femoral cortical defect model. No adverse acute or chronic inflammatory tissue response was noted in the interface tissues of the pre-cured polymer implants. By 6 weeks, there was direct apposition of new bone to the polymers. New bone and fibrovascular tissue was also observed within the porous spaces of the precured polymers by 6 weeks, and fluorochrome analysis suggested that this bone had started to be laid down at between 4 and 5 weeks. The polymer without β-tricalcium phosphate (TCP) showed histological evidence of some degradation by 6 weeks with progressive increase in polymer loss by 12 and 24 weeks. The polymer with β-TCP showed no evidence of degradation at 6 weeks and only minimal loss at 12 weeks. By 12 weeks, there had been considerable degradation of the polymers and at week 24, polymer was completely degraded.

The *in vivo* degradation of segmented poly(urethane urea)s (SPUUs) with hard segments derived only from methyl 2,6-diisocyantohexanoate (LDI) and PCL, PTMC (polytrimethylene carbonate), P(TMC-co-CL), P(CL-co-DLLA), or P(TMC-co-DLLA) as soft segment was conducted by Asplund et al. (Asplund et al., 2008). The *in vivo* study of SPUU-PCL using male Sprague-Dawley rats displayed the typical foreign body response seen with most inert polymeric implant materials. The reaction at 1 week thus displayed an infiltration of ED1 positive macrophages closest to the implant surface, an outside layer of fibroblasts and some collagen formation. At 6 weeks, the foreign body capsule had matured, displaying lower numbers of interfacial macrophages and an increased amount of collagen in the fibrotic capsule. The thickness of the foreign body capsule was similar to the controls. These observations seemed also to be reflected in the number of ED1 positive macrophages, as well as in the total number of cells throughout the reactive capsule.

Hafeman et al. (Hafeman et al., 2008) synthesized polyurethane scaffolds by one-shot reactive liquid molding of hexamethylene diisocyanate trimer (HDIt) or lysine triisocyanate (LTI) and a polyol as hardener. Trifunctional polyester polyols of 900-Da and 1,800-Da molecular weight were prepared from a glycerol starter and 60% ε-caprolactone, 30% glycolide, and 10% D,L-lactide monomers, and stannous octoate catalyst. Tissue response was evaluated by subcutaneous implantation in male Sprague-Dawley rats for up to 21 days. During this time, initial infiltration of plasma progressed to the formation of dense granulation tissue. All of the implants showed progressive invasion of granulation tissue with little evidence of an overt inflammatory response or cytotoxicity. Fibroplasia and angiogenesis appeared to be equivalent among the different formulations. Extracellular matrix with dense collagen fibers progressively replaced the characteristic, early cellular response. The LTI scaffolds exhibited a greater extent of degradation at 21 days, although the incorporation of PEG into the HDIt scaffold accelerated its degradation significantly. Degradation rates were much higher *in vivo*. With time, each of the materials showed signs of fragmentation and engulfment by a transient, giant cell, foreign body response. After the remnant material was resorbed, giant cells were no longer evident.

Khouw et al. (Khouw et al., *2000*) reported that the foreign body response to degradable materials differs between rats and mice. van Minnen et al., (van Minnen et al., 2008) also suggested that it is possible that the response between rats and rabbits differs as well, due to the faster degradation in the rabbit. This may be related to differences at the enzymatic or cellular level, but also to the highly mobile and well vascularized skin of the rabbit, as compared to the rat.

3.1. Calcification

Mineralization or calcification (formation of various types of calcium phosphates such as apatite) is a well documented event in various medical devices, especially in those used in the cardiovascular field. Calcification is in fact, the most common macroscopic cause of failure in heart valves including those made of polyurethanes (Santerre et al., 2005). Even when calcification has been identified in heart valves, *in vitro* experiments on SPU showed little mineralization and associated exclusively to failure regions, indicating that the SPU's have a lower intrinsic capacity for calcification compared to bovine bioprosthesis (Bernacca et al., 1997).

3.2. Thrombosis

Plasma protein adsorption is well accepted as one of the first events to occur when blood is in contacts with a biomaterial. These adsorbed proteins mediate the subsequent interactions of cells and platelets with the surface and may induce thrombus formation, which remains one of the major problems associated with the long-term use of blood-contacting medical devices. The surface properties of the implanted materials are determinant in protein adsorption and biological interactions with the material. The effects of various physicochemical properties such as surface hydrophilicity/hydrophobicity balance, surface charge density, ability to form hydrogen bonds, and chemical composition of biomaterials on protein adsorption as well as subsequent blood platelet adhesion have been investigated (Xu et al., 2010).

Antithrombogenicity is one of the essential requirements for a vascular graft, but it is very difficult to achieve. There are two common approaches employed to attain this goal. One is to develop biomaterials with inherent antithrombogenicity or to use surface modified biomaterials with an anticoagulant. The other approach is to quickly and completely endothelialize the inner surface of the tubular scaffolds, thereby, reducing thrombogenicity (Yan et al., 2007).

Thrombosis is a leading cause of vascular graft failure in small-diameter prostheses, where it leads to decreased flow or occlusion. In addition to inducing acute or subacute failure of grafts, it may be a cause of late failure owing to thrombosis superimposed on stenosis due to other causes of vessel narrowing, such as intimal hyperplasia. Methods to improve vascular grafts (e.g., antithrombotic therapy) have been shown to be beneficial in decreasing graft occlusion after surgery. Agents known to inhibit thrombogenesis or promote anticoagulation (e.g., heparin, prostaglandin E1, hirudin, dipyridamole, tissue factor pathway inhibitor and aspirin) have also been bound to the lumen of the synthetic vessels (Wang et al., 2007; Lu et al., 2012).

3.3. Environmental stress cracking and metal ion oxidation

Traditionally, SPUs have been used as permanent devices such as pacemaker leads insulation and ventricular assisting devices. When used as pacemaker lead insulators, they substitute silicone rubbers and have been used as biostable polymer for outer or inner insulated coating of coaxial bipolar pacemakers. Unfortunately, decades of experience showed that they were degraded by environmental stress cracking (ESC) or metal ion oxidation (MIO) or even autooxidation (AO) within a period of 28 and 34 months.

Environmental stress cracking includes crack formation and propagation on the surface of the polyurethane (Santerre et al., 2005). However, this type of degradation is a combination of the *in vivo* chemical degradation with the presence of mechanical stresses. In other words, polymer chain scission caused by the chemical degradation, create microscopic defects that are augmented by the presence of mechanical loads, leading to the formation of cracks on the surface (Wiggins et al., 2003). ESC it is also enhanced by the presence of residual stresses in the polymeric surface introduced during manufacturing and not eliminated during polymer annealing (Santerre et al., 2005).

The generally accepted *in vivo* degradation MIO mechanism involves the presence of hydrogen peroxide (H_2O_2) produced by a variety of inflammatory cells (McBane et al., 2007; Chandy et al., 2009) and divalent metal ion such as Co^{2+} released from the lead. This reaction is known as the Haber-Weiss reaction and yields hydroxyl radicals that can attack α-methylene groups in the polyether (PTMO based polyurethanes) to render hydroperoxydes with decompose in the presence of divalent cations rendering carbonyl groups that can accelerate (catalyse) further this decomposition (Kehrer, 2000; Wiggins et al., 2001). Polyether diol based polyurethanes are prone to oxidation and environmental stress cracking (ESC) (Król, 2007). However, polycarbonate based-polyurethanes (PCNUs) have been proven superior to polyether and polyester PUs, especially in terms of reduced ESC and metal ion oxidation (MIO), although they are still susceptible to hydrolysis (McBane et al., 2007).

Environmental stress cracking, calcification and thrombosis only became evident after a sufficiently long-term implantation of several years. For biodegradable PUs, which are designed to degrade in a relative short period (several months), the effective degradation mechanisms are hydrolysis with or without the assistance of enzymatic catalysis (Chen et al., 2012).

4. *In vitro* degradation to simulate *in vivo* degradation

In vivo experimentation using an animal model is not always available for elucidating the degradation mechanism of polyurethanes. Instead, various *in vitro* experiments have been designed to simulate their *in vivo* degradation. Among these tests, hydrolytic degradation has been conducted using distilled water (at elevated temperature), strong acids and alkalies, and sometimes physiological conditions using Phosphate Buffer Saline (PBS) as degradating media.

4.1. Hydrolytic degradation

Degradation of segmented polyurethanes through hydrolysis depends strongly not only on the chemical composition of the soft segment, when is the major component, but also on the rigid segment chemistry. It is generally accepted that water absorption is a necessary condition for hydrolytic degradation of materials. Therefore, in a typical hydrolytic degradation test the rate of water absorption (or sample weight gain) can be correlated with sample weight loss (Mondal et al., 2012).

The presence of labile ester linkages in PCL containing polyurethanes makes them susceptible to degradation in the presence of water (Gunatillake et al., 1992; Nakajima-Kambe et al., 1999; Kannan et al., 2006). This type of reactions is catalysed by the presence of acids or alkaline compounds. In some cases, the acid is produced by the degradation of the soft segment; caproic acid in the case of PCL or lactic acid in the case of PLA. Polyester urethanes are more prone to hydrolytic degradation although they are more resistant to oxidative environments as can be observed in Table 2, where PCL based polyurethanes (BSPU1 and BSPU2) and a commercial polyether polyurethane (Tecoflex) are compared (Chan-Chan et al., 2010).

	H_2O	NaOH 5M	HCl 2N	H_2O_2 30 wt.%
BSPU1*	1.46 ± 0.08	63.42 ± 7.63	82.70 ± 2.60	13.08 ± 3.35
BSPU2*	6.15 ± 1.35	87.23 ± 4.76	52.65 ± 13.26	19.07 ± 7.01
Tecoflex	0.63 ± 0.3	1.66 ± 0.66	1.48 ± 1.62	2.16 ± 1.47

* BSPU's were prepared with PCL, HMDI and either butanediol (BSPU1) or dithioerythritol (BSPU2) as chain extenders.

Table 2. Polyurethane mass loss (%) after degradation under hydrolytic and oxidative accelerated conditions

Because of the susceptibility of the ester groups to hydrolysis, biodegradable poly(ester urethanes) degrade *in vitro* through bulk erosion via chain scission. During hydrolysis, new carboxylic acid groups are formed that auto-catalyze the degradation, leading to faster degradation in the bulk than at the surface. Thus, a decrease in molecular weight preceding the loss of mechanical properties and weight loss is typical for such degradation. In addition, an increase in crystallinity is observed, if the soft segment contains a crystalline fraction. Polyesters in the soft segment will, therefore, increase the effect of hydrolysis compared with polyether or polycarbonates (Ma et al., 2012).

Tanzi et al. (Tanzi et al., 1991) degraded various commercial polyurethanes used in the cardiovascular field among them Cardiothane 51, Pellethane 2363 80A, Estane 5714 Fl, Estane 58810 and Biomer. The degradation was conducted in water or alkaline borate buffer (pH 10) at 37°C, 60°C and 85°C from 96 h to 168 h. They found that after hydrolytic degradation in distilled water at 85°C for 96 h, borate buffer during 96 h at 60°C and borate buffer during 168 h at 37°C there were no changes in tensile properties although a reduction in molecular weight was reported.

Polyester urethanes based on methylene-bis(4-phenylisocyanate) (MDI), BD and polyadipate diol were prepared by Pretsch (Pretsch et al., 2009) and accelerated degradation studied in distilled water at 80°C where the degradation process was followed by DSC. It was found that the intensities of the melting peaks and therefore the crystallinity of the soft segments increase after one day. Then, two main degradation scenarios were proposed: first, a hydrolytic scission of polymer chains in the molten soft segments take place, which is accelerated by the "high" immersion temperature; second, and on top of it, there is an annealing effect. For example, the domains of segmented polyurethane elastomers may become unstable at high temperatures and mixing of hard and soft segments is enforced.

Wang et al. (Wang et al., 2011a) prepared segmented polyurethanes based on poly(D,L-lactic acid)diol, hexamethylene diisocyanate (HDI) and with either peperazine (SPU-P), 1,4-butanediol (SPU-O) or 1,4-butanediamine (SPU-A) as chain extenders. The degradation process was conducted in double distilled water at 37°C and 50 rpm. For these SPUs, acidic groups from the degradation of PDLLA and BD could reduce the pH value of medium, while the dissolution of the hard segment (amide group and carbamide) could alkalize the medium; after 12 weeks, the pH values of SPU-O, SPU-A and SPU-P were 2.57, 3.87 and 3.71, respectively. These results suggest that the chain extender can play a main role in the degradation mechanism as using an alkaline chain extender can neutralize the acidity, the hydrophilicity and hydrolysis sensitivity of these bonds.

4.2. Oxidative degradation

Polyether urethanes (PEU) are readily degraded by oxidative conditions (Stachelek et al., 2006). Furthermore, the presence of metallic ions such as cobalt accelerates this process (Gunatillake et al., 1992; Dumitriu, 2002; Santerre et al., 2005). The MIO mechanism was reproduced in vitro by immersing a lead into a hydrogen peroxide solution. In a different in vitro test, a sealed PEU tube containing cobalt metal in the center was immersed into a 3% hydrogen peroxide solution and MIO was observed on the inner surface of the tube. The cobalt ion and hydrogen peroxide react to form hydroxyl radicals, simulating the oxidative radicals present at the material-macrophage interface.

Takahara et al. (Takahara et al., 1991) degraded SPU's based on MDI, BD (50% rigid segment content) and various polyols using 0.1 M $AgNO_3$ oxidative solution. They found a reduction in mechanical strength of those SPU's based on PTMO due to surface cracking related to ether scission upon oxidation.

Suntherland et al. (Sutherland et al., 1993) degraded Pellethane 2363 80A using 10 mM HClO in phosphate buffer (PB) at 25°C. In addition, peroxynitrite (ONOO-) degradation was achieved via the oxidation of hydroxylamine in an oxygen atmosphere at elevated pH. They observed a significant reduction in molecular weight, increase in polydispersity index and an increasing content of oxygenated species on the polymer surface.

Tanzi et al. (Tanzi et al., 2000) studied the oxidative degradation of polyether (Pellethane 2363 80A) and polycarbonate (Corethane 80A, Bionate 80A and Chronoflex AL 80A) urethanes in 0.5 N nitric acid (acidic) and sodium hypochlorite (4% Cl_2, alkaline) up to 14 days at 50°C and under constant strain (100%). It was found that PEU were more degraded under alkaline oxidation (HClO) mainly in the absence of applied strain while PCU was more affected by HNO_3.

Our own work using Tecoflex as model PEU degraded in H_2O_2 did not show significant changes in FTIR absorptions and only small differences in the bands located at
3330 cm^{-1} and 1660 cm^{-1} were observed (see Figure 3), although this was clear when the
polyol was tested alone. However, TGA revealed that their degradation temperature
were lowered and the amorphous content determined by XRD only exhibited a little
changes (Chan-Chan et al., 2010).

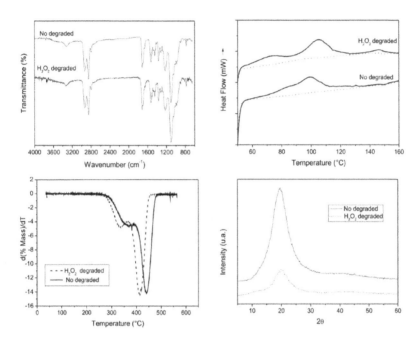

Figure 3. Chemical and structural changes in Tecoflex after degradation under oxidative conditions

4.3. Degradation in physiological media

Poly(ester urethane)urea (PEUU) and poly(ether ester urethane)urea (PEEUU) from polycaprolactone, polycaprolactone-b-polyethylene glycol-b-polycaprolactone, BDI and putrescine were prepared by Guan et al. (Guan et al., 2005a) and degraded in phosphate buffered
saline (PBS, pH=7.4) at 37°C; scaffold degradation was related to the porosity and polymer
hydrophilicity. The scaffolds exhibited progressive mass loss over the 8-week period ranging from 13.3% to 20.7% for PEUU scaffolds and from 25.4% to 47.3% for PEEUU scaffolds.
In this study, the polymer films and scaffolds did not show evidence of an autocatalytic effect during the monitored degradation process. Furthermore, the presence of BDI and 1,4-
butanediamine in the hard segment of PU yielded putrescine as degradation product, which

is already present in the body and has been implicated as an important mediator of cellular growth and differentiation in response to growth factors.

Two gelatin based poly(ester urethane) were prepared by Sarkar et al. (Sarkar et al., 2006) using polyethylene lactate ester diol as a soft segment, and degraded in phosphate buffer saline solution (pH 7.4) at 37°C in a Biochemical Oxygen Demand (BOD) incubator shaker. It was found that the weight loss (up to 45.7% in 30 days) occurred due to the hydrolytic degradation of the gelatin based polyester urethane scaffold by PBS solution and it was proportional to the gelatin content.

Sarkar et al. (Sarkar et al., 2008) prepared segmented polyurethanes using polyethylene glycol (PEG) or poly caprolactone diol (PCL) as the soft segment while hexamethylene diisocyanate (HDI) or dicyclohexylmethane 4,4-diisocyanate (HMDI) were used with desaminotyrosyl tyrosine hexyl ester (DTH) as the chain extender in the rigid component. For degradation in PBS (0.1M, pH 7.4 containing 200 mg of sodium azide) samples were incubated at 37°C. It was found that PEG-based polyurethanes degrade at a faster rate compared with PCL-based polyurethanes due to their hidrophillicity and that this effect was marked when using high molecular weight PEG. It was also found that more amorphous SPU (i.e. exhibiting more phase mixing and therefore more urethane linkages H-bonded with the soft segment), such as those prepared with HMDI, degrade faster as they absorb more water.

Knight et al. (Knight et al., 2008) studied new hybrid thermoplastic polyurethane (TPU) system that incorporates an organic, biodegradable poly(D,L-lactide) soft block with a hard block bearing the inorganic polyhedral oligosilsesquioxane (POSS) moiety and degraded them in PBS buffer at 37 °C over a 2 months period. They found that less than 4% of the original mass elutes from the sample after a month in the buffer, most likely from chain ends on the surface of the sample undergoing hydrolysis. Although only a small mass loss was observed, the molecular weight of the samples dropped dramatically after only one week to 40% of the initial molecular weight.

Biodegradable ionic polyurethanes (PUs) were synthesized from methylene di-p-phenyl-diisocyanate (MDI), polycaprolactone diol (PCL-diol) and N,N-bis (2-hydroxyethyl)-2-aminoethane-sulfonic acid (BES) by Zhang et al. (Zhang et al., 2008). *In vitro* degradation of the PUs was evaluated by recording the samples' weight loss, molecular weight changes, and mechanical properties changes over time in PBS buffer solution at 67°C to accelerate degradation. Although there was a 20% molecular weight reduction, degradation rate was lower in those PUs containing sulfonic acid compared to PU's without this chain extender. This was explained in terms of their higher phase separation.

Segmented polyurethane based on poly(ε-caprolactone), ethyl lysine diisocyanate or hexamethylene diisocyanate in combination with ethylene glycol or ester from ethylene glycol and lactic acid (2-hydroxyethyl 2-hydroxypropanoate) were degraded *in vitro* (0.1 M phosphate buffered saline at 37°C in a shaken incubator set at 50 rpm (ASTM F 1635)) over a 1 year period (Zhang et al., 2008). It was found that all polyurethanes exhibited considerable molecular weight decrease over the test period and ester chain extender polyurethanes showed the highest mass loss and that it was directly proportional to hard segment not to the PCL used as soft segment.

Guelcher et al. (Guelcher et al., 2008) prepared injectable polyurethanes by two-component reactive liquid molding of low-viscosity quasi-prepolymers derived from lysine polyisocyanates and poly(3-caprolactone-co-DL-lactide-co-glycolide) triols and degraded porous discs by incubation in PBS at 37°C and 5% CO_2 for 2, 4, 6, and 8 months. They found that these polymers degrade by hydrolysis of ester linkages to yield α-hydroxy acids and soluble urethane fragments. Furthermore, the materials prepared from PCL triol exhibit minimal (e.g., <5%) degradation after 8 months. However, materials prepared from P6C3G1L (triol synthesized from a glycerol starter and a mixture of monomers comprising 60% caprolactone, 30% glycolide, and 10% DL-lactide) exhibit 15-27% mass loss after 8 months.

Multi-block poly(ether ester urethane)s consisting of poly[(R)-3-hydroxybutyrate] (PHB), poly(propylene glycol) (PPG), and poly(ethylene glycol) (PEG) were prepared by Loh et al. (Loh et al., 2007). The poly(PEG/PPG/PHB urethane) copolymer hydrogels were hydrolytically degraded in phosphate buffer at pH 7.4 and 37°C for a period of up to 6 months. The degradation products in the buffer were characterized by GPC, ^{1}H NMR, MALDI-TOF, and TGA. The results showed that the ester backbone bonds of the PHB segments were broken by random chain scission, resulting in a decrease in the molecular weight. In addition, the constituents of degradation products were found to be 3-hydroxybutyric acid monomer and oligomers of various lengths (n= 1–5).

Multiblock poly(ether ester urethane)s comprising of poly(lactic acid) (PLA), poly(ethylene glycol) (PEG), and poly(propylene glycol) (PPG) segments and hexamethylene diisocyanate were synthesized by Loh et al. (Loh et al., 2008). Their degradation process in pH 7.4 buffer solution (8.0 g of NaCl, 0.2 g of KCl, 1.44 g of Na_2HPO_4, and 0.24 g of $K_2H_2PO_4$ in 1 L of solution) was studied over a period of 3 months. Multi-modal GPC profiles of these polymers suggested that the polymer degrades in fragments with molecular weight of about 2000, 4000, 6000 and 8000 g/mol. These gels degraded at a much faster rate than the previously reported PEG-PPG-PHB poly(ester urethane) thermogels, which were reported to degrade over a period of 6 months.

Degradation of segmented poly(urethane urea)s (SPUUs) with hard segments derived only from methyl 2,6-diisocyanatehexanoate (LDI) and PCL, PTMC, P(TMC-co-CL), P(CL-co-DLLA) or P(TMC-co-DLLA) as soft segment was conducted by Asplund et al. (Asplund et al., 2008). For the hydrolysis study, sterile and nonsterile samples were placed in 40 mL PBS buffer solution (pH 7.4) and put in an oven at 37°C. Degradation was studied after 5, 10, 15, and 20 weeks and analyses performed in triplicate for each sample. The effect of sterilization was studied after 10 weeks of hydrolysis. Physical ageing was studied after 5 and 15 weeks at 50°C. They found that the degradation rate was dependant on the soft segment structure, with a higher rate of degradation for the polyester-dominating PUUs exhibiting a substantial reduction in intrinsic viscosity. A tendency of reduction of tensile strength and strain hardening was seen for all samples. Also, loss in elongation at break was detected, for PUU-P(CL-DLLA) it went from 1600% to 830% in 10 weeks. Gamma radiation caused an initial loss in inherent viscosity and induced more rapid hydrolysis compared with nonsterilized samples, except for PUU-PTMC.

Yeganeh et al. (Yeganeh et al., 2007) prepared epoxy terminated polyurethanes from glycidol and isocyanate-terminated polyurethanes made from poly(ε-caprolactone) (PCL) or poly(ethylene glycol) (PEG) and 1,6-hexamethylene diisocyanate. Degradation studies were performed using tris buffered saline solutions (TBS; 0.05, 0.1molL^{-1} NaCl, pH 7.4) and incubated at 37°C up to 6 months. They observed that degradation rates correspond to their water-absorbing ability, with faster degradation in the more absorbent polymers while the weight loss, due to hydrolytic degradation, increased as the amount of PEG content increased. A possible explanation is that following dissolution of some PEG segments, there will be an increase in the porosity of the blends, leading to a greater surface area for water to access the ester bonds of hydrophobic PCL, which dominates the degradation rate. Other possible explanations include an increase in the hydrophilicity of the surface, which accelerates degradation, or an increase in the mobility of the PCL molecules, which could also facilitate hydrolytic degradation. Also the rate of hydrolysis was raised with increasing time, which might result from the augmentation content of hydrophilic hydroxyl, amine, and carboxylic groups generated at the surface during degradation.

Wang et al. (Wang et al., 2008) prepared novel biodegradable and biocompatible poly(ester-urethane)s by *in situ* homogeneous solution polymerization of poly(3-caprolactone) diol, dimethylolpropionic acid (DMPA), and methylene diphenyl diisocyanate in acetone followed by solvent exchange with water. The hydrolytic degradation test was conducted on buffer solution (pH=7.4) at 37°C up to 12 weeks and showed that the degradation rate was little affected by the DMPA content in the range investigated, but was observed to be influenced by the hard segment content.

Hong et al. (Hong et al., 2010) synthesized poly(ester carbonate)urethane ureas (PECUUs) using a blended soft segment of poly(caprolactone) (PCL) and poly(1,6-hexamethylene carbonate) (PHC), 1,4- butane diisocyanate and putrescine as chain extender. They found that degradation of PECUUs in aqueous buffer (PBS at 37°C) and subcutaneous implantation in rats (Adult female Lewis rats) was slower than poly(ester urethane)urea but faster than poly(carbonate urethane)urea (PCUU). Over a period of 56 days, poly(ether urethane)ureas (PEUU) exhibited a 9% mass loss in addition to a reduction in inherent viscosity, while all of the PECUUs and PCUU did not show detectable loss of mass. *In vivo* it was observed that the majority of the PEUU scaffold was degraded, and loose connective tissue occupied the implant area with few observed putative macrophages. For the PECUU 50/50 scaffolds, more remnant material was seen with darker violet staining of the putative infiltrating macrophages and fibroblasts.

Chan-Chan et al. (Chan-Chan, et al. 2012) synthesized new polyester poly(urethane-urea)s and their molecular weight changes during PBS degradation were monitored by gel permeation cromatography (GPC) (see Figure 4). Significant weight loss was not observed at six months but bulk degradation was corroborated by this analytical technique.

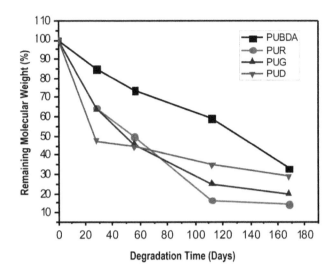

Figure 4. Molecular weight reduction in polyurethanes based on butanediamine (PUBDA), arginine (PUR), glycine (PUG) and aspartic acid (PUD).

4.4. Enzymatic degradation

Huang et al. (Huang et al., 1979) reported that a low molecular weight poly(ester-urea), poly(L-phenyl alanine/ethylene glycol/1,6-hexane diisocyanate), and a model diesterdiurea, dimethyl diphenyl alanine hexamethylene urea, were hydrolyzed by chymotrypsin at pH 8. They also observed degradation with papain latex (pH 6.5, PBS) of the model diesterdiurea.

Takahara et al. (Takahara et al., 1992) degraded SPU's based on MDI, BD and various poly-ols using papain (80 U/mL) and papain activating solution (0.05 M cysteine, 0.02 EDTA, pH=6.5) in sodium acetate buffer solution. In this study it was found that PEO based poly-urethanes exhibited the larger mass loss from all the SPU's studied in addition to a reduc-tion in Young's modulus and tensile strength due to a reduction in molecular weight.

Labow et al. (Labow et al., 1996) degraded in elastase (from human neutrophils or pancreat-ic porcine) a poly(ester-urea-urethane) containing [14C]toluene diisocyanate (TDI), poly(cap-rolactone) and ethylenediamine as well as a poly(ether-urea-urethane) containing [14C]TDI, poly(tetramethylene oxide) and ethylenediamine (ED). They used neutrophils, which con-tain elastolytic activity, as they are present during the inflammatory response. Ten-fold more radioactive carbon was released when porcine pancreatic elastase was incubated with [14C]TDI/PCL/ED than when human neutrophil elastase was used. Ten-fold less radioactive carbon was released when [14C]TDI/PTMO/ED was incubated with porcine pancreatic elas-tase (PPE) as compared to [14C]TDI/PCL/ED. Radioactive carbon release data for [14C]TDI/PCL/ED polymer incubated with trypsin, a possible contaminant in pancreatic porcine elastase showed no significant release of radioactive carbon by the same number of units of trypsin which would be present in the commercial PPE preparation used in the biodegradation experiments.

Skarja and Woodhouse (Skarja et al., 2001) studied degradable segmented polyurethanes containing a phenylalanine diester chain extender and degraded them in buffer chymotrypsin and trypsin solutions for up to 28 days. In this study it was found that the presence of phenylalanine resulted in an increased susceptibility to enzyme-mediated while the magnitude of degradation and erosion was highly variable and was dependent on soft segment type (PCL or PEO) and molecular weight (500-2000 g/mol).

It is well-known that the segmented poly(urethane ureas) prepared from 4,4-diphenylmethane diisocyanate, oligotetramethylene glycol, and diamines are not easily hydrolyzed by enzymes. This was further extended by Thomas and Jayabalan (Thomas et al., 2001) who reported that completely aliphatic poly(urethane urea) based on 4,4-methylene bis-cyclohexyl isocyanate/hydroxy terminated polybutadiene/1,6-hexamethylene diamine did not degrade in papain after 30 days at 37°C.

Labow et al. reported that cholesterol esterase cleaved polyetherurethanes at the most probable site susceptible to hydrolytic cleavage, which is the urethane bonds, resulting in the release of free amine (Labow et al., 2002). Santerre's group has also reported the degradation of polycarbonate polyurethanes with cholesterol esterase (Tang et al., 2002). Both the carbonate and urethane bonds were cleaved, resulting in many products ranging in molecular weight from 150 to 850 g/mol, as identified by GC–MS.

Yamamoto et al. (Yamamoto et al., 2007) degraded with different thiol proteases (papain, bromelain, and ficin) and Protease K and chymotrypsin, lysine diisocyanate (LDI) based poly(urethanes) and segmented poly(urethane ureas). For this, 1 mg of enzyme was added into the test tube coated with the polymer at 37°C and the total organic carbon (TOC) measured. From ^{1}H NMR results, it was evident that the pendant methyl ester group in LDI was rapidly hydrolyzed, followed by slow hydrolysis of urethane bonds in the backbone chain while the susceptibility of urea bonds to papain was very low. Before 50 h almost 30% of the PU has been degraded, with ethylene glycol exhibiting the highest rate of degradation; thiol proteases were most effective for all SPUUs. LDI/PTMO (Mw=2000 g/mol)/1,3-propylendiamine (PDA) (2/1/1), which does not contain degradable soft segments (caprolactone block), showed degradation by various proteases. This fact strongly suggests that the cleavage of the hard segment (urethane and/or urea) by these proteases occurred. For the SPUU the expected water-soluble degradation products are diamine, α-hydroxy caproic acid, and its low molecular oligomers, in addition to lysine derivatives.

Hafeman et al. (Hafeman et al., 2011) investigate the effects of esterolytic and oxidative conditions on scaffold degradation by incubating in 1 U/mL cholesterol esterase (CE), 1 U/mL carboxyl esterase (CXE), and 10 U/mL lipase (L) hydrogen peroxide (20 wt% hydrogen peroxide (H_2O_2) in 0.1 M cobalt chloride ($CoCl_2$), and buffer alone (0.5 M monobasic sodium phosphate buffer with 0.2% w/w sodium azide) and measured the mass loss for 10 weeks at 37°C. Polyurethane scaffolds were prepared by one-shot reactive liquid molding of hexamethylene diisocyanate trimer (HDIt) or lysine triisocyanate (LTI) and a polyol as hardener. Trifunctional polyester polyols of 900-Da molecular weight were prepared from a glycerol starter and 60% ε-caprolactone, 30% glycolide, and 10% D,L-lactide monomers (6C), ($t_{1/2}$ = 20 days) and 70% caprolactone, 20% glycolide, and 10% lactide (7C) ($t_{1/2}$ = 225 days) and stannous octoate catalyst. Incubation with esterases slightly accelerated degradation relative to PBS. Differences in degradation between the three candidate enzymes at any given time point were not significant. In contrast, incubation with medium that created an oxidative microenvironment had a more significant effect on the polyurethane degradation rate, especially for the LTI-based materials, except the 6C/HDIt (hexamethylene diisocyanate trimer) + PEG, which interestingly degraded faster in the presence of cholesterol and carboxyl esterase than in oxidative medium.

A new family of water borne polyurethanes (WBPU) were synthesized by Jiang et al. (Jiang et al., 2007) using isophorone diisocyanate (IPDI), polycaprolactone (PCL), polyethylene glycol (PEG) and BD:Lysine (1:1) as the chain extender. The polyurethane was then enzymatically degraded in PBS (pH = 7.4) with a solution mixture including PBS 60.0 ml, 0.1% $MgCl_2$ 15.0 ml and Lipase AK (10 mg/ml) 15.0 ml and then incubated with shaking for certain time at 55°C, which was the optimum temperature for enzyme activities of Lipase AK. An increased degradation was observed as decreasing of the amount of PEG in soft segments of WBPU, as judged from the change of tensile properties with time, owing to Lipase AK only interacting with PCL soft segments in these polymers structures. This result reveals that the degradation rate is proportional to the PCL content, and inverse proportion to the PEG content in the WBPUs. Depending on the PCL content, degradation started even at 6 h in the presence of Lipase AK.

A polyurethane was synthesized with LDI, PCL, and BD in the presence of dilaurate as catalyst by Han et al. (Han et al., 2009) and then degraded in PBS with a solution mixture including 4.0 mL PBS, 1.0 mL 0.1 wt.% $MgCl_2$ and 1.0 mL Lipase AK (10 mg/mL) in water at 50°C. It was found that loss mass decreased with increasing the PCL soft segment content in hydrolytic degradation in PBS. Because PCL is hydrophobic in comparison with the polar hard segment, increasing its content would decrease water uptake of PU films, and then decrease mass loss. In contrast, in the presence of Lipase AK the mass loss was observed to be increased with increasing the PCL soft segment content.

Biodegradable polyurethanes were prepared by Wang et al., using PLA-PEG-PLA as soft segment, and L-lysine ethyl ester diisocyanate (LDI) and 1,4-butanediol (BD) as rigid segment (Wang et al., 2011b). These polymers were degraded in PBS (0.1 M PBS with 0.9% NaCl and 0.02% NaN_3, pH 7.4, 6 and 5) and enzymatic (0.1mg/ml lipase from porcine pancreas in 0.1 M PBS with 0.9% NaCl and 0.02% NaN_3, pH 7.4) solutions at 37 °C to simulate *in vivo* dynamic tissue environment. PU samples demonstrated rapid degradation in 96 h (more than 90%) which might be attributed to hydrophilicity of PEG segments, low number-average molecular weight and microphase separation degree of these polyurethanes and enzyme functions. The enzymatic degradation rate was higher than hydrolytic degradation rate, verifying that Lipase from porcine pancreas can accelerate hydrolysis on these polyurethanes.

A series of pH-sensitive biodegradable polyurethanes (pHPUs) were designed and synthe-sized using pH-sensitive macrodiol (poly(ϵ-caprolactone)-hydrazone-poly-(ethylene glycol)-hydrazone-poly(ϵ-caprolactone) diol (PCL-Hyd-PEG-Hyd-PCL)), L-lysine ethyl ester diisocyanate (LDI) and L-lysine derivative tripeptide as chain extender by Zhou et al. (Zhou et al., 2011). The polyurethanes could be cleaved in acidic media (pH ~ 4-6) as well as de-graded in PBS (100 mM, and pH 7.4) overnight at room temperature and enzymatic solution (Lipase AK (10 mg/mL, 2 mL) in PBS buffer solution with 0.1 wt % $MgCl_2$ (2 mL) and then incubated with cyclic shaking at 52.5°C). It was found that the hydrolysis rates of the two samples observed in Lipase AK PBS are higher than that in PBS i.e. 31.1% and 35.9% of weight loss are detected after hydrolytic and enzymatic degradation for 144 h of pHPU4 (pHPU prepared with LDI/macrodiol/tripeptide 3.15/2/1), respectively. The results indicate that the pHPUs are also facile to degrade in enzymatic solution, which is in agreement with reported literatures that Lipase AK is able to accelerate the PCL-based polymers biodegra-dation. Polymers with more pH sensitive macrodiol and lower crystallinity degraded even faster. The importance of studying these materials (pH-sensitive biodegradable polyur-ethanes) lies in the fact that they been used for intracellular multifunctional antitumor drug delivery (Zhou et al. 2012).

Elliott et al. (Elliott et al., 2002) determined mechanism of enzymatic degradation by HPLC/MS. Prior to product separation and identification, residual enzyme (chymotrypsin) was removed from the incubation solution samples. This process was necessary since the chymotrypsin could interfere with the accurate detection of the degradation products in the high performance liquid chromatography (HPLC) columns, and because proteins have a tendency to aggregate and then later precipitate during the gradient run, thereby causing additional difficulties in data acquisition. The results of the tandem mass spectrometry (MS/MS) analysis indicated that chymotrypsin may act to cleave urea bonds adjacent to L-phenylalanine residues. This is a significant finding since it confirms that the polyurethanes are susceptible to selective enzymatic degradation in the hard segment. Traditionally, this domain of the polyurethane has been considered a relatively stable group. The materials used in this study, however, were especially developed to encourage degradation of the hard segment rather than relying solely on degradation of the soft segment. Hence, the re-sults of this study confirm that this goal was achieved. The cleavage of urea bonds by chy-motrypsin is an important finding as it contradicts results of a previous study with similar chemistry that found that urea bonds adjacent to L-phenylalanine residues were not cleaved. However, since the level of chymotrypsin activity was not stated in the other study, it may be possible that the right conditions were not presented in order to degrade the urea bond (Elliott et al., 2002).

4.5. Lipid degradation

Lipid absorption has been reported to occur in many medical devices such as heart valves made of silicon, leading to their calcification. In addition, fatigue properties of SPU have been reduced by lipid absorption.

Takahara et al. (Takahara et al., 1992) degraded SPU´s based on MDI, BD and various polyols using 0.25 % phophatidyl choline and 0.1% M cholesterol liposome solution during 28
days at 37°C. They found that SPU based on PDMS disintegrated under these conditions
while PTMO based SPUs exhibited a severe reduction in tensile strength and elongation.
These results were not related to the presence of a specific chemical group in the soft segment as PEO based SPU´s were not affected.

4.6. Compost biodegradation

Synthetic poly(ester urethanes) are known to be degraded by microbes mainly due to the
presence of ester linkages, being more susceptible those containing long chains rather than
short polyester chains. Lactic acid based polyester urethanes have been degraded with compost inoculum (thermophilic-stage household waste compost was added to 100 ml of ASTM
solution and the CO_2 evolved was followed by Hiltunen et al. (Hiltunen et al., 1997). The
data showed that poly(ester-urethanes) did not biodegrade at 25°C but when the temperature was raised, biodegradation was accelerated. At 37°C the stereo structure of polymer
chains had a strong effect on biodegradation. This temperature was below the glass transition temperature of poly(ester-urethanes) but about the same as the glass transition temperature of prepolymer chains. The lower the glass transition temperature of prepolymer, the
faster the biodegradation. Urethane bonds probably break first, and after that the properties
of lactic acid prepolymer chains determine the biodegradation behavior. All poly(ester-urethane) samples biodegraded well at 55°C, and the percentage of biodegradation varied between 45 and 77% in 55 days. At 60°C the poly(ester-urethanes) biodegraded well and they
reached even higher levels of biodegradation than Biopac™ and lactic acid. The biodegradation varied from 45 to 77% in 55 days.

Polyurethanes based on MDI and PCL with different molecular weights were prepared by
Watanabe et al. (Watanabe et al., 2009) and degraded by soil burial test at 28°C. It was found
that biodegradation rate of the polyurethanes increased as the number of average molecular
weight (Mn) of poly(caprolactone) diol used increased from 500 to 1000 (urethane content
11.9 to 7.6 wt % respectively), whereas it decreased as the Mn of poly(caprolactone) diol increased from 1200 to 2000 (4.2 wt % of urethane content). Furthermore, when 2000 PCL triol
was used led to a high degradation ratio.

4.7. Thermal degradation of polyurethanes

Although the thermal degradation of both polyurethanes (PU) and segmented polyurethanes (SPU) has been extensively investigated due to their wide range of applications, studies on thermal decomposition of polyurethanes used specifically in
biomedical field such as catheters, heart valves, vascular prostheses, etc., are less common as generally these materials are not subjected to high temperatures during their *in
vivo* performance [Cervantes-Uc et al. 2009]. In some cases, these studies are used to investigate the composition and stability of the remaining material after the chemical hydrolysis and oxidation of SPU [Chan-Chan et al. 2010] as well as to determine the soft
and hard segment ratio of polyurethanes.

The thermal degradation of polyurethanes allows determination of the proper conditions for manipulating and processing them and for obtaining high-performance products that are stable and free of undesirable by-products; if not processed properly, commonly by extrusion or by injection moulding, the PU's would generate toxic products to the human body, which is very critical in biomedical applications [Gomes Lage et al. 2001].

It is well known that polyurethanes are not thermal stable polymers and that the onset degradation temperature of the urethane bond depends on the type of isocyanate and alcohol used. It is a general rule that the more easily formed polyurethanes are less stable, i.e. more easily dissociated when compared with more difficulty formed ones [Petrovic et al. 1994]. Petrovic reported that the degradation temperature for these materials ranged from 120°C to 250°C depending on their structure [Petrovic et al. 1994]; however, literature reports processing temperatures closer to 180°C [Guignot 2002].

Polyurethanes are thermally degraded through three basic mechanisms. First, by urethane bond dissociation into its starting components (isocyanate and alcohol); secondly, by breaking the urethane bond with formation of primary amines, carbon dioxide and olefins; and finally, splitting the urethane bond into secondary amine and carbon dioxide [Petrovic et al. 1994; Cervantes-Uc et al. 2009].

5. Degradation mechanism

The nature of PU chemistry is central to understand why some PUs undergo faster degradation than others (Santerre et al., 2005). However, the degradation mechanism of polyurethanes depends on not only the PU chemistry structure but also the degradation environment, i.e. in the presence of water, acidic, alkaline or oxidative conditions, or in the presence of enzymes. Generally, the characterization of the by-products during the degradation of the polyurethane is the key to understand the mechanisms of degradation. Identification of degradation products is an important issue but of equal interest is the eventual toxicity of the degradation products. If the biomaterial degrades, either spontaneously or due to biological activity, components can leach into surrounding tissues and cause an inflammatory response if not easily metabolized by natural pathways. Therefore, it is compulsory to identify the major species produced at different stages of degradation and the kinetics of their formation (Azevedo et al., 2005).

Accelerated degradation has been used to determinate stability of non degradable polyurethanes (Gunatillake, 1992) but it can be used to provide valuable information about degradation mechanism of resorbable polyurethanes. In this context, both soluble products and solid residues can be studied with different analytical techniques and tests to determine their composition.

The main techniques used to evaluate the degradation of biomaterials can be divided into surface analysis (infrared spectroscopy, X-ray photoelectron spectroscopy, contact angle measurements), which are more appropriated to monitor the changes occurring in the first stages of degradation, and bulk analysis (determination of changes in molecular weight, weight loss, temperature transitions, mechanical properties) for characterizing the later stage of degradation (Azevedo et al., 2005).

In general, polyesterurethanes are susceptible to hydrolytic degradation because of ester groups in the soft segments while polyetherurethanes are susceptible to oxidative degradation. Furthermore, it has been observed that ester linkages hydrolyze about a magnitude faster than urethane linkages, and it has been shown that urea linkages hydrolyze faster than urethane, although at slightly acidic conditions. Figure 5 shows the possible mechanism of hydrolytic degradation of various functional groups present in polyurethanes.

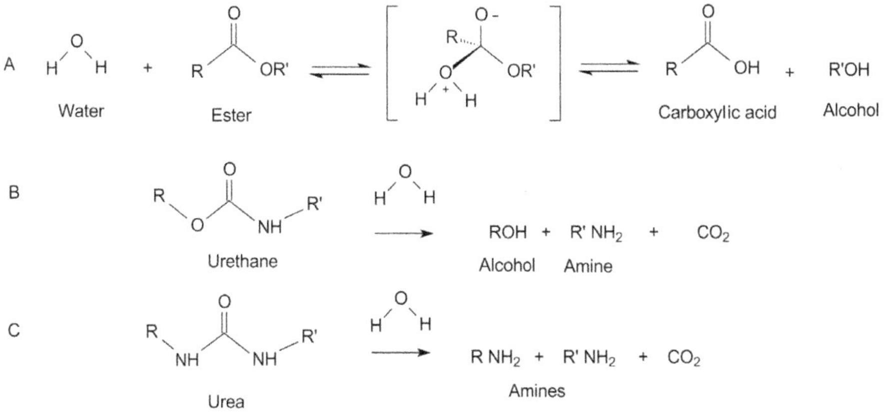

Figure 5. Hydrolytic degradation mechanism of polyesters (A), poly(urethane) (B) and poly(ureas) (C).

In spite of this, the degradation rate of the poly(ester urethane) based on PCL was found to be slow (i.e., 15% weight loss in 11 weeks (Wang et al., 2008). Furthermore, IR spectra for the degradation products of the LDI/PCL and LDI (lysine methyl ester diisocyanate)/P6C3G1L (triol synthesized from a glycerol starter and a mixture of monomers comprising 60% caprolactone, 30% glycolide, and 10% DL-lactide) materials after 2 and 8 months in PBS (Guelcher et al., 2008) shows an absorption band at approximately 1070-1050 cm^{-1}, which is assigned to C-O stretching vibrations in alcohols and carboxylic acids. This observation implies that the polyurethanes degrade by hydrolysis of ester linkages to yield α-hydroxy acids and is further supported by the appearance of the strong peaks at 1675-1650 cm^{-1}, which correspond to the COO asymmetric stretching vibration associated with carboxylic acid salts. Therefore, it is possible under these conditions that phosphate salts of carboxylic acids will form in the PBS solution due to the reaction of carboxylic acids with the basic phosphate salts present in PBS. Hydrolysis of LDI/PCL containing poyurethanes networks in sodium hydroxide solutions has been reported to yield L-lysine as a degradation product; however, the presence of L-lysine in the degradation products under physiological conditions was not confirmed.

Other studies reported the presence of lysine in the degradation products from lysine-derived polyurethanes networks.

Segmented polyurethane based on poly(ε-caprolactone), ethyl lysine diisocyanate or hexamethylene diisocyanate in combination with ethylene glycol or ester from ethylene glycol and lactic acid (2-hydroxyethyl 2-hydroxypropanoate) with greater hard segment content (HS) liberate higher amine concentrations during their degradation (Tatai et al., 2007). Amine concentration was determined using a spectrophotometer by acquiring the A_{570} (absorbance at 570 nm) of the test sample and by quantifying the detected concentration with use of the standard curve. This being expected, on the assumptions that PUs with higher HS contained more urethane bonds. To detect amine groups using this technique, a degradation product must undergo hydrolysis at its respective urethane linkage. Since this process is somewhat slower than that of ester bond hydrolysis, it seems that part of the degradation product may still contain urethane segments.

Hafeman et al. (Hafeman et al., 2011) investigate the effects of esterolytic and oxidative conditions on scaffold degradation by incubating in 1 U/mL cholesterol esterase (CE), 1 U/mL carboxyl esterase (CXE), and 10 U/mL lipase (L) hydrogen peroxide (20 wt% hydrogen peroxide (H_2O_2) in 0.1 M cobalt chloride ($CoCl_2$), and buffer alone (0.5 M monobasic sodium phosphate buffer with 0.2% w/w sodium azide) and analysed the degradation products by HPCL. Hydrolysis of ester bonds was anticipated to yield α-hydroxy acids (e.g., hydroxycaproic, lactic, and glycolic acids), which was confirmed by HPLC. The lysine triisocyanate (LTI) scaffolds produced more α-hydroxy acids than trimer of hexamethylene diisocyanate (HDIt) scaffolds. The 7C/LTI (triol synthesized from a glycerol starter and a mixture of monomers comprising 70% caprolactone, 30% glycolide and 10% lactide) formulation, which degraded more slowly due to the longer polyester half-life, yielded lower concentrations of α-hydroxy acids than the 6C/LTI (60% caprolactone, 30% glycolide and 10% lactide) formulation. Inclusion of polyethylene glycol (PEG) in the 6C/HDIt scaffold reduced the amount of α-hydroxy acids in the degradation medium due to the replacement of 50% of the polyester with PEG. Several unidentified peaks appeared in the HPLC spectra, which are conjectured to be adducts of α-hydroxy acids and either lysine or ethanolamine connected by urethane or urea bonds. Oxidation of urethane and urea bonds was predicted to yield lysine and ethanolamine from LTI scaffolds, and cyanuric acid from HDIt scaffolds. Both lysine and ethanolamine were detected in the degradation products from LTI scaffolds when incubated in PBS; however, cyanuric acid was not detected in the degradation products from HDIt scaffolds. The amount of lysine recovered from 6C/LTI scaffolds was significantly greater than that from 7C/LTI scaffolds after 14 weeks, which is consistent with the faster *in vitro* degradation of the 6C/LTI materials. At 36 weeks, 18% of the lysine incorporated in the 6C/LTI scaffolds was recovered, while 100% of the original mass had degraded to soluble degradation products. This suggests that the majority of the lysine was incorporated in soluble urethane and urea adducts with α-hydroxy adducts. The recovery of ethanolamine arises from the hydrolysis of the ester group in LTI and a urethane bond. Ethanolamine was not detected (<0.001 µg/mg polyurethane) until 14 weeks, and at later time points the ethanolamine concentration increased with time. The recovery of ethanolamine upon complete dissolution of the 6C/LTI scaffold at 36 weeks was 9%.

Suntherland et al. (Sutherland et al., 1993) degraded Pellethane 2363 80A with either HClO or ONOO. An oxidative reaction involving the ether or ester moieties of PEU would be reflected by a decrement in the urethane-aliphatic ester and/or aliphatic ether stretching peaks on ATR/FTIR analysis. Indeed, a substantial decrement in the aliphatic ether stretching at 1105-1110 cm^{-1} relative to the urethane-aliphatic ester peak at 1075 cm^{-1} has been observed in implanted material. In fact, the intensity of both aliphatic ether and urethane-aliphatic ester peaks decreases after long-term implantation, suggesting that both groups are oxidized *in vivo*. PEU previously exposed to HClO exhibited a decrement in the signal from the urethane-aliphatic ester.

FTIR has been used to determine the composition of residues after degradation. In this sense, hydrolytic degradation of polyester urethanes affects carbonyl bands at 1730 cm^{-1}. Soluble products of the ester scission are carboxyl acids and alcohols that can be observed between 2500 and 3500 cm^{-1}. Pérez et al. (Pérez et al., 2006) studies showed that urea bonds derived from amino acids can be hydrolyzed in basic conditions but after more prolonged period than ester groups, this degradation was monitored by capillary electrophoresis-ion trap-mass.

Oxidative degradation has been generally associated with poly(ether-urethane)s, since many studies have determined that these polymers degrade by mean alpha-hydrogen abstraction adjacent to oxygen in polyethers and polycarbonates (Christenson et al., 2004; Xie et al., 2009). In contrast, few works related to oxidative degradations on polyester polyurethanes has been done, and even less has studied the mechanism of degradation of polyurethane ureas. However recent studies about oxidative degradations of PCL and polyester poly(urethane urea)s PCL based have showed ester, urethane and urea groups are susceptible to oxidative degradation (Sabino, 2007; Sarkar et al., 2007; Hafeman et al., 2011). This mechanism is illustrated in Figure 6.

A $-CH_2-O-CH_2-$ +   •OH $\longrightarrow$ $-CH_2-O-\overset{\bullet}{C}H-$ + H_2O

B $-CH_2-OCOO-CH_2-$ +   •OH $\longrightarrow$ $-CH_2-OCOO-\overset{\bullet}{C}H-$ + H_2O

C $-Ph-NHCOO-CH_2-$ +   •OH $\longrightarrow$ $-Ph-NHCOO-\overset{\bullet}{C}H-$ + H_2O

Figure 6. Mechanism of oxidative degradation by H_2O_2 in poly(ether urethanes) (A), poly(carbonate urethanes) (B) and aromatic polyurethanes (C).

Oxidative degradation using HClO is less commonly pursued but it may be clinically more relevant as hipochlorous anions can be produced by neutrophils. These conditions can be simulated *in vitro* and the suggested mechanisms of the polyurethane degradation can be depicted in Figure 7.

$$R-\overset{\overset{\displaystyle O}{\|}}{C}-O-\overset{\overset{\displaystyle H}{|}}{\underset{\underset{\displaystyle H}{|}}{C}}-R \xrightarrow{ClO^-} R-\overset{\overset{\displaystyle O}{\|}}{C}-O^- \quad + \quad O=\overset{\overset{\displaystyle H}{|}}{C}-R \quad + \quad H^+ \quad + \quad Cl^-$$

Figure 7. Mechanism of oxidative degradation in polyurethanes by means of HClO

Degradation of polyurethanes with H_2O_2 (30% v/v) does not seem to affect ester bonds but affect urea bonds as observed by FTIR. The wide band of 3650-3400 cm^{-1} and a small peak in 930 cm^{-1} corresponding to carboxylic acid confirm scission of urea groups as shown in Figure 8. Other bands such as those at 1298 cm^{-1} show some crosslinking by C-N bonds and an increase in PCL crystallinity, as the 1143 y 1189 cm^{-1} bands, corresponding to amorphous and crystalline PCL, changed (Chan-Chan, 2012).

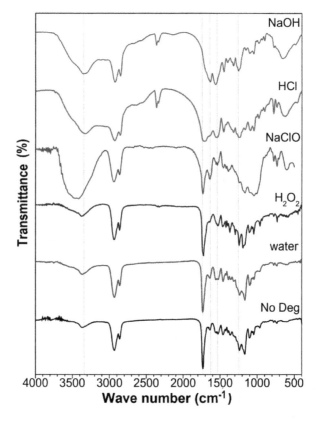

Figure 8. FTIR spectra of poly(urethane ureas) degraded in various media.

6. Conclusions

Polyurethanes are very versatile polymers that found application in the biomedical field, especially in cardiovascular applications. In spite of their good physicochemical and mechanical properties and acceptable biocompatibility they are prone to degradation under different conditions. These conditions range from hydrolysis, oxidation, metal induced oxidation, environmental stress cracking, enzyme-assisted degradation, etc. which can be found *in vivo* during the useful life of the device. In order to simulate these, *in vitro* approaches has been followed. Thanks to this information today it is well accepted that polyurethanes are no longer inert materials placed within the body. However, this disadvantage can be used to modulate their degradation to a rate that can be controlled mainly by their composition, and be used in the design of tissue engineering scaffolds.

Acknowledgements

This work was supported by CONACYT (México) Grant 79371, and Fondo Mixto CONACYT-Gobierno del Estado de Yucatán, Grants 108160 and 170132.

Author details

Juan V. Cauich-Rodríguez, Lerma H. Chan-Chan, Fernando Hernandez-Sánchez and José M. Cervantes-Uc

Centro de Investigación Científica de Yucatán A.C., Grupo de Biomateriales e Ingeniería de Tejidos, Mexico

References

[1] Abraham, G. A., A. Marcos-Fernández and J. San Román (2006). Journal of Biomedical Materials Research Part A 76(4): 729-736.

[2] Adhikari, R., P. A. Gunatillake, I. Griffiths, L. Tatai, M. Wickramaratna, S. Houshyar, T. Moore, R. T. M. Mayadunne, J. Field, M. McGee and T. Carbone (2008). Biomaterials 29(28): 3762-3770.

[3] Alferiev, I., N. Vyavahare, C. Song, J. Connolly, J. Travis Hinson, Z. Lu, S. Tallapragada, R. Bianco and R. Levy (2001). Biomaterials 22(19): 2683-2693.

[4] Aranguren M.I., J.F. González, M.A. Mosiewicki. (2012) Polymer Testing 31 (1): 7-15.

[5] Arjun, G. N. and P. Ramesh (2012). Journal of Biomed Materials Research Part A: Polymer Chemistry. DOI: 10.1002/jbm.a.34255

[6] Asplund, B., C. Aulin, T. Bowden, N. Eriksson, T. Mathisen, L. M. Bjursten and J. Hilborn (2008). Journal of Biomedical Materials Research Part B: Applied Biomaterials 86(1): 45-55.

[7] Azevedo, H. S. and R. L. Reis, Eds. (2005). Boca Raton, FL, CRC Press. pp.177-201.

[8] Basak, P. and B. Adhikari (2012). Materials Science and Engineering: C 32(8): 2316-2322.

[9] Baudis, S., S. C. Ligon, K. Seidler, G. Weigel, C. Grasl, H. Bergmeister, H. Schima and R. Liska (2012). Journal of Polymer Science Part A: Polymer Chemistry 50(7): 1272-1280.

[10] Bernacca, G. M., I. Straub and D. J. Wheatley (2002). Journal of Biomedical Materials Research 61(1): 138-145.

[11] Bernacca, G. M., T. G. Mackay, R. Wilkinson and D. J. Wheatley (1997). Journal of Biomedical Materials Research 34(3): 371-379.

[12] Cervantes-Uc J.M., J.I. Moo-Espinosa, J.V. Cauich-Rodríguez, A. Ávila-Ortega, H. Vázquez-Torres, A. Marcos-Fernández, J. San Román. (2009). Polymer Degradation and Stability 94 (10) 1666-1677.

[13] Chan-Chan, L. H., R. Solis-Correa, R. F. Vargas-Coronado, J. M. Cervantes-Uc, J. V. Cauich-Rodríguez, P. Quintana and P. Bartolo-Pérez (2010). Acta Biomaterialia 6(6): 2035-2044.

[14] Chan-Chan, L. H. (2012). PhD Thesis, Centro de Investigación Científica de Yucatán. Mérida, México.

[15] Chen, Q., S. Liang and G. A. Thouas (2012). Progress in Polymer Science. DOI: 10.1016/j.progpolymsci.2012.05.003.

[16] Christenson, E. M., J. M. Anderson and A. Hiltner (2006). Journal of Biomedical Materials Research Part A 76A(3): 480-490.

[17] Christenson, E. M., M. Dadsetan, M. Wiggins, J. M. Anderson and A. Hiltner (2004). Journal of Biomedical Materials Research Part A 69(3): 407-416.

[18] Da Silva, G. R. (2010). Polymer Degradation and Stability 95(4): 491-499.

[19] Ding, M., J. Li, H. Tan and Q. Fu (2012). Soft Matter 8(20): 5414-5428.

[20] Dumitriu, S. S. (2002). USA, Marcel Dekker.

[21] Elliott, S., J. Fromstein, J. PSanterre and K. Woodhouse (2002). Journal of Biomaterials Science, Polymer Edition 13(6): 691-711.

[22] Francolini, I., F. Crisante, A. Martinelli, L. D'Ilario and A. Piozzi (2012). Acta Biomaterialia 8(2): 549-558.

[23] Gogolewski, S. (1989). Colloid & Polymer Science 267(9): 757-785.

[24] Gomes Lage L and Y. Kawano (2001). Journal of Applied Polymer Science 79(5): 910-919.

[25] Guan, J., K. L. Fujimoto, M. S. Sacks and W. R. Wagner (2005a). Biomaterials 26(18): 3961-3971.

[26] Guan, J., M. S. Sacks, E. J. Beckman and W. R. Wagner (2002). Journal of biomedical materials research 61(3): 493-503.

[27] Guan, J., M. S. Sacks, E. J. Beckman and W. R. Wagner (2004). Biomaterials 25(1): 85-96.

[28] Guan, J. and W. R. Wagner (2005b). Biomacromolecules 6(5): 2833-2842.

[29] Guelcher, S. A., A. Srinivasan, J. E. Dumas, J. E. Didier, S. McBride and J. O. Hollinger (2008). Biomaterials 29(12): 1762-1775.

[30] Guignot C., N. Betz, B. Legendre, A. Le Moel and N. Yagoubi (2002). Journal of Applied Polymer Science 85(9): 1970-1979.

[31] Gunatillake, P. A., D. J. Martin, G. F. Meijs, S. J. McCarthy and R. Adhikari (2003). Australian journal of chemistry 56(6): 545-557.

[32] Gunatillake, P. A., G. F. Meijs, E. Rizzardo, R. C. Chatelier, S. J. McCarthy, A. Brandwood and K. Schindhelm (1992). Journal of Applied Polymer Science 46(2): 319-328.

[33] Hafeman, A. E., B. Li, T. Yoshii, K. Zienkiewicz, J. M. Davidson and S. A. Guelcher (2008). Pharmaceutical research 25(10): 2387-2399.

[34] Hafeman, A. E., K. J. Zienkiewicz, A. L. Zachman, H. J. Sung, L. B. Nanney, J. M. Davidson and S. A. Guelcher (2011). Biomaterials 32(2): 419-429.

[35] Han, J., B. Chen, L. Ye, A. Zhang, J. Zhang and Z. Feng (2009). Frontiers of Materials Science in China 3(1): 25-32.

[36] He, X., Z. Zhai, Y. Wang, G. Wu, Z. Zheng, Q. Wang and Y. Liu (2012). Journal of Applied Polymer Science 126(S1): E354-E361.

[37] Heijkants, R. G. J. C., R. V. Calck, T. G. Van Tienen, J. H. De Groot, P. Buma, A. J. Pennings, R. P. H. Veth and A. J. Schouten (2005). Biomaterials 26(20): 4219-4228.

[38] Hiltunen, K., J. V. Seppälä, M. Itävaara and M. Härkönen (1997). Journal of Polymers and the Environment 5(3): 167-173.

[39] Hong, Y., J. Guan, K. L. Fujimoto, R. Hashizume, A. L. Pelinescu and W. R. Wagner (2010). Biomaterials 31(15): 4249-4258.

[40] Huang, S. J., D. A. Bansleben and J. R. Knox (1979). Journal of Applied Polymer Science 23(2): 429-437.

[41] Jiang, G., X. Tuo, D. Wang and Q. Li (2012). Journal of Materials Science: Materials in Medicine DOI: 10.1007/s10856-012-4670-y.

[42] Jiang, X., J. Li, M. Ding, H. Tan, Q. Ling, Y. Zhong and Q. Fu (2007). European Polymer Journal 43(5): 1838-1846.

[43] Kannan, R. Y., H. J. Salacinski, M. Odlyha, P. E. Butler and A. M. Seifalian (2006). Biomaterials 27(9): 1971-1979.

[44] Kartvelishvili, T., G. Tsitlanadze, L. Edilashvili, N. Japaridze and R. Katsarava (1997). Macromolecular Chemistry and Physics 198(6): 1921-1932.

[45] Kehrer, J. P. (2000). Toxicology 149(1): 43-50.

[46] Khouw I. M. S. L., P. B. van Wachem, G. Molema, J. A. Plantinga, L. F. M. H. de Leij, M. J. A. van Luyn. (2000). Journal of Biomedical Materials Research 52: 439–446.

[47] Knight, P. T., K. M. Lee, H. Qin and P. T. Mather (2008). Biomacromolecules 9(9): 2458-2467.

[48] Król, P. (2007). Progress in materials science 52(6): 915-1015.

[49] Kuan, Y. H., L. P. Dasi, A. Yoganathan and H. L. Leo (2011). International Journal of Biomaterials Research and Engineering 1(1):1-17.

[50] Labow, R. S., D. J. Erfle and J. P. Santerre (1996). Biomaterials 17(24): 2381-2388.

[51] Labow, R. S., Y. Tang, C. B. Mccloskey and J. P. Santerre (2002). Journal of Biomaterials Science, Polymer Edition 13(6): 651-665.

[52] Li, Z., X. Yang, L. Wu, Z. Chen, Y. Lin, K. Xu and G. Q. Chen (2009). Journal of Biomaterials Science, Polymer Edition 20(9): 1179-1202.

[53] Liu, Q., S. Cheng, Z. Li, K. Xu and G. Q. Chen (2009). Journal of Biomedical Materials Research Part A 90(4): 1162-1176.

[54] Loh, X. J., S. H. Goh and J. Li (2007). Biomaterials 28(28): 4113-4123.

[55] Loh, X. J., Y. X. Tan, Z. Li, L. S. Teo, S. H. Goh and J. Li (2008). Biomaterials 29(14): 2164-2172.

[56] Lu, H., P. Sun, Z. Zheng, X. Yao, X. Wang and F.-C. Chang (2012). Polymer Degradation and Stability 97(4): 661-669.

[57] Lu, Y., L. Shen, F. Gong, J. Cui, J. Rao, J. Chen and W. Yang (2012). Polymer International 61(9): 1433-1438.

[58] Ma, Y., D. Yang, W. Shi, S. Li, Z. Fan, J. Tu and W. Wang (2012). Polymer Engineering & Science DOI:10.1002/pen.23269.

[59] Macocinschi, D., D. Filip, S. Vlad, M. Cristea and M. Butnaru (2009). Journal of Materials Science: Materials in Medicine 20(8): 1659-1668.

[60] Madhavan, K. and B. S. R. Reddy (2006). Journal of Polymer Science Part A: Polymer Chemistry 44(9): 2980-2989.

[61] Marcos-Fernández, A., G. A. Abraham, J. L. Valentín and J. S. Román (2006). Polymer 47(3): 785-798.

[62] May-Hernández, L., F. Hernández-Sánchez, J. L. Gomez-Ribelles and R. Sabateri - Serra (2011). Journal of Applied Polymer Science 119(4): 2093-2104.

[63] McBane, J. E., J. P. Santerre and R. S. Labow (2007). Journal of Biomedical Materials Research Part A 82A(4): 984-994.

[64] Mondal, S. and D. Martin (2012). Polymer Degradation and Stability 97(8): 1553-1561.

[65] Nakajima-Kambe, T., Y. Shigeno-Akutsu, N. Nomura, F. Onuma and T. Nakahara (1999). Applied microbiology and biotechnology 51(2): 134-140.

[66] Park, J. H., K. D. Park and Y. H. Bae (1999). Biomaterials 20(10): 943-954.

[67] Pérez, P., C. Simó, C. Neusüss, M. Pelzing, J. San Román, A. Cifuentes and A. Gallardo (2006). Biomacromolecules 7(3): 720-727.

[68] Petrovic Z., Z. Zavargo, J. H. Flynn, W. J. Macknight (1994). Journal of Applied Polymer Science 51(6):1087–1095.

[69] Pretsch, T., I. Jakob and W. Müller (2009). Polymer Degradation and Stability 94(1): 61-73.

[70] Sabino, M. A. (2007). Polymer Degradation and Stability 92(6): 986-996.

[71] Santerre, J. P., K. Woodhouse, G. Laroche and R. S. Labow (2005). Biomaterials 26(35): 7457-7470.

[72] Sarkar, D., J.-C. Yang, A. S. Gupta and S. T. Lopina (2009). Journal of Biomedical Materials Research Part A 90A(1): 263-271.

[73] Sarkar, D., J. C. Yang and S. T. Lopina (2008). Journal of Applied Polymer Science 108(4): 2345-2355.

[74] Sarkar, D. and S. T. Lopina (2007). Polymer Degradation and Stability 92(11): 1994-2004.

[75] Sarkar, S., A. Chourasia, S. Maji, S. Sadhukhan, S. Kumar and B. Adhikari (2006). Bulletin of Materials Science 29(5): 475-484.

[76] Schubert, M. A., M. J. Wiggins, J. M. Anderson and A. Hiltner (1997). Journal of Biomedical Materials Research 34(4): 493-505.

[77] Silvestri, A., P. Serafini, S. Sartori, P. Ferrando, F. Boccafoschi, S. Milione, L. Conzatti and G. Ciardelli (2011). Journal of Applied Polymer Science 122(6): 3661-3671.

[78] Skarja, G. and K. Woodhouse (2001). Journal of Biomaterials Science, Polymer Edition 12(8): 851-873.

[79] Skarja, G. and K. Woodhouse (1998). Journal of Biomaterials Science, Polymer Edition 9: 271-295.

[80] Spirkova, M., J. Pavlicevic, A. Strachota, R. Poreba, O. Bera, L. Kaprálková, J. Baldrian, M. Slouf, N. Lazic and J. Budinski-Simendic (2011). European Polymer Journal 47(5): 959-972.

[81] Stachelek, S. J., I. Alferiev, H. Choi, C. W. Chan, B. Zubiate, M. Sacks, R. Composto, I. W. Chen and R. J. Levy (2006). Journal of Biomedical Materials Research Part A 78(4): 653-661.

[82] Stachelek, S. J., I. Alferiev, J. Fulmer, H. Ischiropoulos and R. J. Levy (2007). Journal of Biomedical Materials Research Part A 82A(4): 1004-1011.

[83] Styan, K. E., D. J. Martin, A. Simmons and L. A. Poole-Warren (2012). Acta Biomaterialia 8(6): 2243-2253.

[84] Sutherland, K. and J. Mahoney (1993). Journal of Clinical Investigation 92(5): 2360.

[85] Takahara, A., A. J. Coury, R. W. Hergenrother and S. L. Cooper (1991). Journal of Biomedical Materials Research 25(3): 341-356.

[86] Takahara, A., R. W. Hergenrother, A. J. Coury and S. L. Cooper (1992). Journal of Biomedical Materials Research 26(6): 801-818.

[87] Tang, Y., R. Labow, I. Revenko and J. Santerre (2002). Journal of Biomaterials Science, Polymer Edition 13(4): 463-483.

[88] Tanzi, M., L. Ambrosio, L. Nicolais, S. Iannace, L. Ghislanzoni and B. Mambrito (1991). Clinical materials 8(1-2): 57-64.

[89] Tanzi, M. C., S. Farè and P. Petrini (2000). Journal of Biomaterials Applications 14(4): 325-348.

[90] Tatai, L., T. G. Moore, R. Adhikari, F. Malherbe, R. Jayasekara, I. Griffiths and P. A. Gunatillake (2007). Biomaterials 28(36): 5407-5417.

[91] Thomas, V. and M. Jayabalan (2001). Journal of Biomedical Materials Research 56(1): 144-157.

[92] Thomas, V. and M. Jayabalan (2009). Journal of Biomedical Materials Research Part A 89(1): 192-205.

[93] Thomson, T. (2005). Boca Raton, Fl, CRC. pp.35-53.

[94] van Minnen, B., M. B. M. V. Leeuwen, G. Kors, J. Zuidema, T. G. v. Kooten and R. R. M. Bos (2008). Journal of Biomedical Materials Research Part A 85A(4): 972-982.

[95] Wang, F., Z. Li, J. L. Lannutti, W. R. Wagner and J. Guan (2009). Acta Biomaterialia 5(8): 2901-2912.

[96] Wang, W., Y. Guo and J. U. Otaigbe (2008). Polymer 49(20): 4393-4398.

[97] Wang, X., P. Lin, Q. Yao and C. Chen (2007). World Journal of Surgery 31(4): 682-689.

[98] Wang, Y., C. Ruan, J. Sun, M. Zhang, Y. Wu and K. Peng (2011a). Polymer Degradation and Stability 96: 1687-1694.

[99] Wang, Z., L. Yu, M. Ding, H. Tan, J. Li and Q. Fu (2011b). Polymer Chemistry 2(3): 601-607.

[100] Ward, R., J. Anderson, R. McVenes and K. Stokes (2007). Journal of Biomedical Materials Research Part A 80(1): 34-44.

[101] Watanabe, A., Y. Takebayashi, T. Ohtsubo and M. Furukawa (2009). Journal of Applied Polymer Science 114(1): 246-253.

[102] Wiggins, M. J., J. M. Anderson and A. Hiltner (2003). Journal of Biomedical Materials Research Part A 66A(3): 463-475.

[103] Wiggins, M. J., B. Wilkoff, J. M. Anderson and A. Hiltner (2001). Journal of Biomedical Materials Research 58(3): 302-307.

[104] Xie, X., R. Wang, J. Li, L. Luo, D. Wen, Y. Zhong and C. Zhao (2009). Journal of Biomedical Materials Research Part B: Applied Biomaterials 89B(1): 223-241.

[105] Xu, L. C. and C. A. Siedlecki (2010). Journal of Biomedical Materials Research Part A 92(1): 126-136.

[106] Yamamoto, N., A. Nakayama, M. Oshima, N. Kawasaki and S.-i. Aiba (2007). Reactive and Functional Polymers 67(11): 1338-1345.

[107] Yan, Y., X. H. Wang, D. Yin and R. Zhang (2007). Journal of bioactive and compatible polymers 22(3): 323-341.

[108] Yeganeh, H., H. Jamshidi and S. Jamshidi (2007). Polymer International 56(1): 41-49.

[109] Zhang, C., X. Wen, N. R. Vyavahare and T. Boland (2008). Biomaterials 29(28): 3781-3791.

[110] Zhao, Q., A. McNally, K. Rubin, M. Renier, Y. Wu, V. Rose-Caprara, J. Anderson, A. Hiltner, P. Urbanski and K. Stokes (1993). Journal of Biomedical Materials Research 27(3): 379-388.

[111] Zhou, L., D. Liang, X. He, J. Li, H. Tan, J. Li, Q. Fu, Q. Gu. (2012) Biomaterias 33 (9): 2734-2745.

[112] Zhou, L., L. Yu, M. Ding, J. Li, H. Tan, Z. Wang and Q. Fu (2011). Macromolecules 44(4): 857-864.

Chapter 3

Mechanical Properties of Biomaterials Based on Calcium Phosphates and Bioinert Oxides for Applications in Biomedicine

Siwar Sakka, Jamel Bouaziz and Foued Ben Ayed

Additional information is available at the end of the chapter

1. Introduction

Calcium phosphates (CaP) have been sought as biomaterials for reconstruction of bone defect in maxillofacial, dental and orthopaedic applications [1-31]. Calcium phosphates have been used clinically to repair bone defects for many years. Calcium phosphates such as hydroxyapatite ($Ca_{10}(PO_4)_6(OH)_2$, HAp), fluorapatite ($Ca_{10}(PO_4)_6F_2$, FAp), tricalcium phosphate ($Ca_3(PO_4)_2$, TCP), TCP-HAp composites and TCP-FAp composites are used for medical and dental applications [3, 10-29]. In general, this concept is determined by advantageous balances of more stable (frequent by hydroxyapatite or fluorapatite) and more resorbable (typically tricalcium phosphate) phases of calcium phosphates, while the optimum ratios depend on the particular applications. The complete list of known calcium phosphates, including their major properties (such, the chemical formula, solubility data) is given in Table 1. The detailed information about calcium phosphates, their synthesis, structure, chemistry, other properties and biomedical applications have been comprehensively reviewed recently in reference [24].

Calcium phosphate-based biomaterials and bioceramics are now used in a number of different applications throughout the body, covering all areas of the skeleton. Applications include dental implants, percutaneous devices and use in periodontal treatment, treatment of bone defects, fracture treatment, total joint replacement (bone augmentation), orthopedics, cranio-maxillofacial reconstruction, otolaryngology and spinal surgery [32-35]. Depending upon whether a bioresorbable or a bioactive material is desired, different calcium orthophosphates might be used.

In the past, many implantations failed because of infection or a lack of knowledge about the toxicity of the selected materials. In this frame, the use of calcium phosphates is logical due to their similarity to the mineral phase of bone and teeth [36-40]. However, according to available literature, the first attempt to use calcium phosphates as an artificial material to repair surgically-created defects in rabbits was performed in 1920 [41]. More than fifty years later, the first dental application of a calcium phosphate (erroneously described as TCP) in surgically-created periodontal defects [42] and the use of dense HAp cylinders for immediate tooth root replacement were reported [43]. Since Levitt et al. described a method of preparing an apatite bioceramics from FAp and suggested its possible use in medical applications in 1969[44]. According to the available databases, the first paper with the term "bioceramics" in the abstract was published in 1971 [45], while those with that term in the title were published in 1972 [46-47]. However, application of ceramic materials as prostheses had been known before [48-49]. Further historical details might be found in literature [50]. Commercialization of the dental and surgical applications of Hap-based bioceramics occurred in the 1980's, largely through the pioneering efforts by Jarcho [51], de Groot [52] and Aoki [53]. Due to that, HAp has become a bioceramic of reference in the field of calcium phosphates for biomedical applications. Preparation and biomedical applications of apatites derived from sea corals (coralline HAp) [54–56] and bovine bone were reported at the same time [57]. Since 1990, several other calcium phosphate cements have been developed [58-62], injectable cements have been formulated [63], and growth factors have been delivered via these cements [64]. The tetracalcium phosphate [TTCP: $Ca_4(PO_4)_2O$] and dicalcium phosphate anhydrous [DCPA: $CaHPO_4$] system was approved in 1996 by the Food and Drug Administration (FDA) for repairing craniofacial defects in humans, thus becoming the first TTCP–DCPA system for clinical use [65]. However, due to its brittleness and weakness, the use of TTCP–DCPA system was limited to the reconstruction of non-stress-bearing bone [66-67]. To expand the use of TTCP–DCPA system to a wide range of load-bearing maxillofacial and orthopedic repairs, recent studies have developed natural biopolymers that are elastomeric, biocompatible and resorbable [68]. Calcium phosphates in a number of forms and compositions are currently either in use or under consideration in many areas of dentistry and orthopedics. For example, bulk materials, available in dense and porous forms, are used for alveolar ridge augmentation, immediate tooth replacement and maxillofacial reconstruction [35, 69]. Other examples include orbital implants (Bio-Eye) [70-71], increment of the hearing ossicles, spine fusion and repair of bone defects [72-73]. In order to permit growth of new bone onto bone defects, a suitable bioresorbable material should fill the defects. Otherwise, in-growth of fibrous tissue might prevent bone formation within the defects [69-73]. Today, a large number of different calcium phosphate bioceramics for the treatment of various defects are available on the market.

The performance of living tissues is the result of millions of years of evolution, while the performance of acceptable artificial substitutions those man has designed to repair damaged hard tissues are only a few decades old. Archaeological findings exhibited in museums showed that materials used to replace missing human bones and teeth have included animal or human (from corpses) bones and teeth, shells, corals, ivory (elephant tusk), wood, as well as some metals (gold or silver). For instance, the Etruscans learned to substitute missing teeth with bridges made from artificial teeth carved from the bones of oxen, while in ancient Phoenicia loose teeth were bound together with gold wires for tying artificial ones to neighboring teeth.

Compound	Acronym	Formula	Ca/P	pK_s [a]
Monocalcium phosphate monohydrate	MCPM	$Ca(H_2PO_4)_2.H_2O$	0.5	1.14
Monocalcium phosphate anhyrous	MCPA	$Ca(H_2PO_4)_2$	0.5	1.14
Dicalcium phosphate dihydrate	DCPD	$CaHPO_4.2H_2O$	1	6.59
Dicalcium phosphate anhydrous	DCPA	$CaHPO_4$	1	6.90
Aporphous calcium phosphates	ACP	$Ca_xH_y(PO_4)_z.nH_2O$ n = 3-4.5; 12-20%H_2O	1.2-2.2	b
Octacalcium phosphate	OCP	$Ca_8(HPO_4)_2(PO_4)_4.5H_2O$	1.33	96.6
α- Tricalcium phosphate	α-TCP	α- $Ca_3(PO_4)_2$	1.5	25.5
β- Tricalcium phosphate	β-TCP	β- $Ca_3(PO_4)_2$	1.5	28.9
Calcium-deficient Hydroxyapatite	CDHAp	$Ca_{10-x}(HPO_4)_x(PO_4)_{6-x}(OH)_{2-x}$ (0 < x < 1)	1.5-1.67	85
Hydroxyapatite	HAp	$Ca_{10}(PO_4)_6(OH)_2$	1.67	116.8
Fluorapatite	FAp	$Ca_{10}(PO_4)_6F_2$	1.67	120
Oxapatite	OAp	$Ca_{10}(PO_4)_6O$	1.67	69
Tetracalcium phosphate	TTCP	$Ca_4(PO_4)_2O$	2	38-44

[a]: Solubility at 25°C (pK_s = -$logK_s$);

[b] : Cannot be measured precisely.

Table 1. Calcium phosphates and their major properties [3, 24]

Calcium phosphates are established materials for the augmentation of bone defects. They are available as allogenic, sintered materials. Unfortunately, these calcium phosphates exhibit relatively poor tensile and shear properties [74]. In practice, the strength of the calcium phosphate cements is lower than that of bone, teeth, or sintered calcium phosphate bioceramics [75] and, together with their inherent brittleness, restricts their use to non-load bearing defects [76] or pure compression loading [74]. Typical applications are the treatment of maxillo-facial defects or deformities [77] and cranio facial repair [78] or augmentation of spine and tibial plateau [74]. A successful improvement of the mechanical properties would significantly extend the applicability of calcium phosphates [79] and can be achieved by forming composite materials [80]. Second phase additives to the calcium phosphate composites have been either fibrous reinforcements or bioinert oxides that interpenetrate the porous matrix.

Hydroxyapatite and other calcium phosphates bioceramics are important for hard tissue repair because of their similarity to the minerals in natural bone, and their excellent biocompatibility and bioactivity [81-86]. When implanted in an osseous site, bone bioactive materials such as HAp and other CaP implants and coatings provide an ideal environment for cellular reaction and colonization by osteoblasts. This leads to a tissue response termed osteoconduction in which bone grows on and bonds to the implant, promoting a functional interface [81, 84, 87]. Extensive efforts have significantly improved the properties and performance of HAp and other CaP based implants [88-92]. Calcium phosphate cements can be molded or injected to form a scaffold in situ, which can be resorbed and replaced by new bone [93, 65-67]. Chemically, the vast majority of calcium phosphate bioceramics is based on HAp, β-TCP, α-TCP and/or biphasic calcium phosphate (BCP), which is an intimate mixture of either β-TCP - HAp [94-100] or α-TCP - HAp [101-111]. The preparation technique of these calcium phosphates has been extensively reviewed in literature [1, 4, 37, 102-104]. When compared to both β- and α-TCP, HAp is a more stable phase under physiological conditions, as it has a lower solubility (Table 1) [37, 109-110]. Therefore, the BCP concept is determined by the optimum balance of a more stable phase of HAp and a more soluble TCP. Due to a higher biodegradability of the β - or α -TCP component, the reactivity of BCP increases with the TCP-HAp the increase in ratio. Thus, in vivo bioresorbability of BCP can be controlled through the phase composition [95]. As implants made of calcined HAp are found in bone defects for many years after implantation, bioceramics made of more soluble calcium phosphates is preferable for the biomedical purposes [94-110]. HAp has been clinically used to repair bone defects for many years [3]. However, Hap has poor mechanical properties [3]. Their use at high load bearing conditions has been restricted due to their brittleness, poor fatigue resistance and strength.

The main reason behind the use of β-TCP as bone substitute materials is their chemical similarity to the mineral component of mammalian bone and teeth [1-3]. The application of tricalcium phosphate as a bone substitute has received considerable attention, because it is remarkably biocompatible with living bodies when replacing hard tissues and because it has biodegradable properties [1-29]. Consequently, β-TCP has been used as bone graft substitutes in many surgical fields such as orthopedic and dental surgeries [3, 11-12, 16-17]. This use leads to an ultimate physicochemical bond between the implants and bone-termed osteointegration. Even so, the major limitation to the use of β-TCP as load-bearing biomaterial is their mechanical properties which make it brittle, with poor fatigue resistance [3, 10, 21-29]. Moreover, the mechanical properties of tricalcium phosphate are generally inadequate for many load-carrying applications (3 MPa – 5 MPa) [3, 10, 20-29]. Its poor mechanical behaviour is even more evident when used to make highly porous ceramics and scaffolds. Hence, metal oxides ceramics, such as alumina (Al_2O_3), titania (TiO_2) and some oxides (e.g. ZrO_2, SiO_2) have been widely studied due to their bioinertness, excellent tribological properties, high wear resistance, fracture toughness and strength as well as relatively low friction [19, 21-22, 29-31]. However, bioinert ceramic oxides having high strength are used to enhance the densification and the mechanical properties of β-TCP. In this chapter, we will try to improve the strength of β-TCP by introducing a bioinert oxide like alumina. This is because there are few articles reporting the toughening effects of an inert oxide (like alumina (Al_2O_3)) on the mechanical proper-ties of β-TCP [22, 27, 29]. Alumina has a high strength and is bio-inert with human tis-sues [19, 22, 27, 29]. In order to improve the biocompatibility of alumina and the strength of tricalcium phosphate effectively, and in order to search for an approach to produce high performances of alumina-tricalcium phosphate composites, β-TCP is intro-duced with different percentages in the alumina matrix. The aim of our study is to elabo-rate and characterize the TCP-Al_2O_3 composites for biomedical applications.

This chapter proposes to study the sintering of the alumina-tricalcium phosphate compo-sites at various temperatures (1400°C, 1450°C, 1500°C, 1550°C and 1600°C) and with differ-ent percentages of β-TCP (10 wt%, 20 wt%, 40 wt% and 50 wt%). The characterization of biomaterials will be realized by using dilatometry analysis, differential thermal analysis (DTA), X-ray diffraction (XRD), magic angle spinning nuclear magnetic resonance (MAS NMR), scanning electron microscopy analysis (SEM) and by using the mechanical proper-ties, such as rupture strength (σ_r) of these biomaterials.

2. Materials and methods

The synthesized tricalcium phosphate and alumina (Riedel-de Haën) were mixed in order to prepare biomaterial composites. The β-TCP powder was synthesized by solid-state reaction from calcium carbonate ($CaCO_3$) and calcium phosphate dibasic anhydrous ($CaHPO_4$) [27]. Stoichiometric amounts of high purity powders such as $CaHPO_4$ (Fluka, purity ≥ 99%) and $CaCO_3$ (Fluka, purity ≥ 98.5%), were sintered at 1000°C for one hour to obtain the β-TCP ac-cording to the following reaction:

$$2\,CaHPO_4(s) + CaCO_3(s) \quad \rightarrow \quad Ca_3(PO_4)_2(s) + H_2O(g) + CO_2(g) \tag{1}$$

The β-TCP and the alumina powders were mixed in an agate mortar. The powder mixtures were milled in ethanol for 24 hours. After milling, the mixtures were dried in a rotary vac-uum evaporator and passed through a 70-mesh screen. After drying the powder mixtures at 80°C for 24 hours, they were molded in a cylinder having a diameter of 20 mm and a thick-ness of 6 mm, and pressed under 150 MPa. The green compacts were sintered at various temperatures for different lengths of time in a vertical furnace (Pyrox 2408). The heating rate is 10°C min^{-1}. The size of the particles of the powder was measured by means of a Micromer-itics Sedigraph 5000. The specific surface area (SSA) was measured using the BET method and using N_2 as an adsorption gas (ASAP 2010) [112]. The primary particle size (D_{BET}) was calculated by assuming the primary particles to be spherical:

$$D_{BET} = 6 \,/\, S\rho \tag{2}$$

where ϱ is the theoretical density and S is the surface specific area.

The microstructure of the sintered compacts was investigated using the scanning electron microscope (Philips XL 30) on the fractured surfaces of the samples. The grains' mean size was measured directly using SEM micrographs. The powder was analyzed by using Xray diffraction (XRD). The Xray patterns were recorded using the Seifert XRD 3000 TT diffractometer. The Xray radiance was produced by using CuK_α radiation (λ = 1.54056 Å). The crystalline phases were identified with the powder diffraction files (PDF) of the International Center for Diffraction Data (ICDD). Linear shrinkage was determined using dilatometry (Setaram TMA 92 dilatometer). The heating and cooling rates were 10°C min^{-1} and 20°C min^{-1}, respectively. Differential thermal analysis (DTA) was carried out using about 30 mg of powder (DTATG, Setaram Model). The heating rate was 10°C min^{-1}. The ^{31}P and ^{27}Al magic angle spinning nuclear magnetic resonance (^{31}P MAS NMR) spectra were run on a Brucker 300WB spectrometer. The ^{31}P and ^{27}Al observational frequency were 121.49 MHz and 78.2 MHz, respectively. The ^{31}P MAS-NMR chemical shifts were referenced in parts per million (ppm) referenced to 85 wt% H_3PO_4. The ^{27}Al MAS-NMR chemical shifts were referenced to a static signal obtained from an aqueous aluminum chloride solution.

The Brazilian test was used to measure the rupture strength of biomaterials [113-114]. The rupture strength (σ_r) values were measured using the Brazilian test according to the equation:

$$\sigma_r = \frac{2 \cdot P}{\Pi \cdot D \cdot t} \tag{3}$$

where P is the maximum applied load, D the diameter, t the thickness of the disc and σ_r the rupture strength (or mechanical strength).

3. Results and discussion

3.1. Characterization of different powders

The X-ray diffraction analysis of β-TCP powder and α-alumina powder are presented in Figure 1. As it can be noticed from this figure, the X-ray diffraction pattern of tricalcium phosphate powder reveals only peaks of β-TCP (ICDD data file no. 70-2065) without any other phase (Figure 1a). Consequently, the XRD pattern obtained from the alumina powder illustrates α phase peaks relative to ICDD data file no. 43-1484 (Figure 1b).

The ^{31}P MAS-NMR solid spectrum of the tricalcium phosphate powder is presented in Figure 2a. We observe the presence of several peaks of tetrahedral P sites (at 0.36 ppm, 1.46 ppm and 4.83 ppm), while there are other peaks (at -7.43 ppm, -9.09 ppm and -10.35 ppm) which reveal a low quantity of calcium pyrophosphate which was formed during the preparation of the β-TCP.

The ^{27}Al MAS-NMR solid spectrum of the alumina powder is presented in Figure 2b. We notice the presence of two peaks which are characteristic of aluminum: one peak at 7.36 ppm corresponding to octahedral Al sites (Al^{VI}) and the other at 37.36 ppm which corresponds to pentahedral Al sites (Al^{V}). The results obtained for ^{31}P MAS-NMR and ^{27}Al MAS-NMR are similar to those previously reported by different authors [14, 22, 25-28, 31].

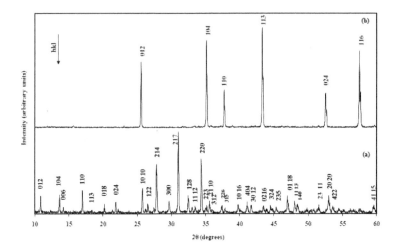

Figure 1. The XRD patterns of: (a) β-TCP powder and (b) α-Al$_2$O$_3$ powder

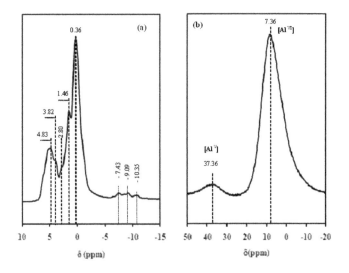

Figure 2. The ^{31}P MAS-NMR spectra of: (a) β-TCP and the ^{27}Al MAS-NMR spectra of: (b) α-Al$_2$O$_3$

The experimental characteristics of the different powders used in this study are illustrated in Table 2. Table 2 summarizes the SSA, the DTA measurements, the sintering temperature and the theoretical density of the different powders. The powder particles are assumed to be spherical; the size of the particles can be calculated using Eq. (2). The results from the average grain size obtained by the SSA (D_{BET}) and from the average grain size obtained by granulometric repartition (D_{50}) are presented in Table 2. Compared with those of the β-TCP powder, the grains of the alumina powder have a dense morphology. These (D_{BET}) values obtained by the SSA do not correspond to those obtained from the granulometric repartition (Table 2). The discrepancy may be due to the presence of agglomerates which are formed during the preparation of the β-TCP powder at 1000°C.

Compounds	SSA (m^2/g) ± 1.0	D_{BET} (µm) ± 0.2	D_{50} (µm)[a] ± 0.2	DTA measurements (endothermic peak)	T(°C)[b]	d[c]
TCP	0.70	2.79	6	1100°C-1260°C (β → α)	1000 - 1300	3.070 (β)
				1470°C (α → α')		2.860 (α)
Alumina	2.87	0.53	3	-	1400 - 1600	3.98 (α)

[a] mean diameter,

[b] : sintering temperature domain,

[c] : theoretical density

Table 2. Characteristics of the powders used in the study

Differential thermal analysis studies of the different powders used in this study detected a potential phase change during the sintering process. The DTA thermogram of β-TCP, α-Al_2O_3 and different Al_2O_3 - TCP composites are presented in Figure 3. The DTA curve of alumina reported no process relative to the sintering temperature (Figure 3a). Figure 3b shows the DTA curve of β-TCP. The DTA thermogram of β-TCP shows two endothermic peaks, relative to the allotropic transformations of tricalcium phosphate (Figure 3b). The peak between 1100°C – 1260°C is related to the first allotropic transformation of TCP (β to α), while the last peak at 1470°C is related to the second allotropic transformation of TCP (α to α'). As a matter of fact, this result is similar to the result previously reported by Destainville et al. and Ben Ayed et al. [9, 14]. Figure 3c shows the DTA curve of Al_2O_3-50 wt% TCP composites. This DTA curve is practically similar to the one shown in Figure 3b. Indeed, the DTA thermogram of the composites also shows two endothermic peaks. Figure 3 (d), (e) and (f) illustrate the DTA curves of Al_2O_3–40 wt% TCP composites, Al_2O_3–20 wt% TCP composites and Al_2O_3–10 wt% TCP composites, respectively. The DTA thermograms of each composites show only one endothermic peak between 1100°C and 1260°C, which are relative to the allotropic transformation of TCP (β to α). In these curves, we notice that the endothermic peak relative to a second allotropic transformation of TCP (α to α') has practically disappeared when the percentage of the alumina increases in the Al_2O_3 - TCP composites (Figure 3(d), (e) and (f)).

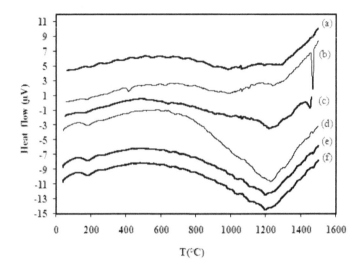

Figure 3. DTA curves of (a) α-Al$_2$O$_3$, (b) β-TCP, (c) Al$_2$O$_3$ – 50 wt% TCP composites, (d) Al$_2$O$_3$ – 40 wt% TCP composites, (e) Al$_2$O$_3$ – 20 wt% TCP composites and (f) Al$_2$O$_3$ – 10 wt% TCP composites

Figure 4 shows the dilatometric measurements of the different powders used in this study (β-TCP, α-Al$_2$O$_3$ and Al$_2$O$_3$ - TCP composites). A large sintering domain was observed for the three powders (β-TCP, alumina and composites). The sintering temperature of the initial powder began at about 900°C and at about 1400°C for the β-TCP and alumina (Figure 4a-b and Table 2). The sintering temperature of Al$_2$O$_3$-50 wt% TCP composites began at 1100°C (Figure 4c). It is to be noted that the presence of 50 wt% TCP in the alumina matrix decreases the sintering temperature of the alumina by around 300°C (Figure 4c). This variation of the sinterability is relative to the difference between the physicochemical compositions of these powders and the mixture of their different composites.

3.2. The mechanical properties of alumina–tricalcium phosphate composites

The influence of the sintering temperature on the rupture strength of Al$_2$O$_3$-TCP composites is shown in Figure 5. The mechanical resistance of Al$_2$O$_3$-TCP composites is studied at various temperatures (1400°C, 1450°C, 1500°C, 1550°C, 1600°C) for one hour with different percentages of β-TCP (50 wt%, 40 wt%, 20 wt% and 10 wt%). Thus, Figure 5 illustrates the rupture strength of the Al$_2$O$_3$-TCP composites relative to the percentages of the alumina and the sintering temperature. Consequently, the rupture strength of Al$_2$O$_3$ mixed with 10 wt% β-TCP reached its maximum value when sintered at 1600°C for one hour; it then decreased with the increase of this percentage. This is how the rupture strength of the Al$_2$O$_3$-10 wt% TCP composites reached 13.5 MPa.

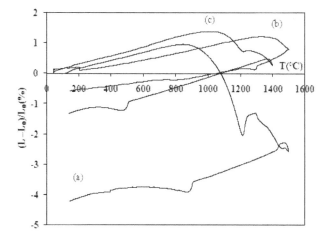

Figure 4. Linear shrinkage versus temperature of: (a) β-TCP, (b) α-Al$_2$O$_3$ and (c) Al$_2$O$_3$ – 50 wt% TCP composites

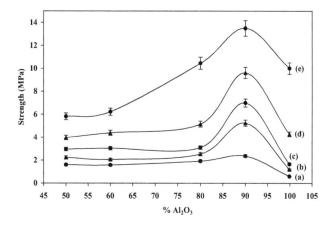

Figure 5. The rupture strength of the TCP-Al$_2$O$_3$ composites sintered for 1 hour at various temperatures: (a) 1400°C, (b) 1450°C, (c) 1500°C, (d) 1550°C and (e) 1600°C

Figure 6 shows the evolution of the rupture strength of the Al$_2$O$_3$ - 10 wt% TCP composites sintered at various temperatures (1500°C, 1550°C and 1600°C) for different sintering times (0 min, 30 min, 60 min and 90 min). The optimum value of the rupture strength was indeed obtained after an hour-long sintering process at 1600°C. Thus, the mechanical resistance of the samples reached 13.5 MPa.

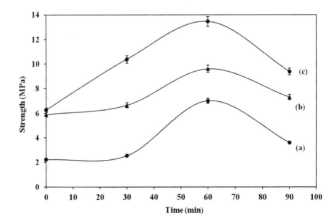

Figure 6. The rupture strength of the Al₂O₃–10 wt% TCP composites sintered for different lengths of time at various temperatures: (a) 1500°C, (b) 1550°C and (c) 1600°C

In this study, we showed that the presence of different amounts of alumina in the β-TCP improves the mechanical properties of Al₂O₃-TCP composites. In fact, the mechanical properties of Al₂O₃-10 wt% TCP composites reached the optimum value by being sintered at 1600°C for one hour. Thus, the rupture strength of these composites reached 13.5 MPa. Table 3 displays several examples of the mechanical properties of the calcium phosphates and the bone tissues. In comparison, we notice that the properties of Al₂O₃-10 wt% TCP composites are close to those of pure β-TCP, pure Fap and TCP-33.16 wt% Fap composites, which have a rupture strength of 5.3 MPa, 14 MPa and 13.7 MPa, respectively [15, 21, 25]. However, the mechanical properties of our composites are more closely comparable to those of the pure Fap and the TCP–33.16 wt% Fap composites (Table 3). Generally, the values found for the mechanical strength of our composites are not identical to those in Table 3, because the authors have used different mechanical modes other than the Brazilian test. In addition, many factors influence the mechanical properties of the samples such as: the use of particular initial powders as well as the conditions of the treatment process.

The sintering of materials is a complex process, involving the evolution of the microstructure through the action of several different transport mechanisms such as: surface diffusion, evaporation- condensation, grain boundary diffusion [3]. However, producing dense TCP–Al₂O₃ composites with a fine uniform microstructure through the sintering process does not seem to be a routine process because the β-TCP has a lower sinterability and a lower sintering temperature than those of pure alumina.

Materials	σ_r (a) (MPa)	σ_c (b) (MPa)	σ_f (c) (MPa)	References
β-TCP	4-6	-	92	[21,27]
Fap	10-14	-	-	[15]
Hap	-	5.35	-	[115]
TCP - 75 wt% Al$_2$O$_3$	8.60	-	-	[27]
TCP – 26.52 wt% Fap	9.60	-	-	[21]
TCP – 26.52 wt% Fap- 5 wt% Al$_2$O$_3$	13.60	-	-	[22]
TCP – 33.16 wt% Fap	13.70	-	-	[25]
Hap – TCP (40:60)	-	4.89	-	[115]
Al$_2$O$_3$ - 26.5 wt% Fap	21.7	-	-	[31]
Cortical bone	-	130-180	50-150	[1, 2]
Cancellous bone	-	2-12	-	[1, 2]

(a): Rupture strength (Brazilian test),

(b): compressive strength

(c): Flexural strength.

Table 3. Literature examples of the mechanical properties of calcium phosphates bioceramics and bone tissues

3.3. Characterization of alumina-tricalcium phosphate composites after the sintering process

Figure 7 shows the ^{31}P MAS-NMR spectra of the Al$_2$O$_3$-TCP composites obtained after the sintering process for 1 hour at 1550°C with different percentages of β-TCP (50 wt%, 40 wt%, 20 wt% and 10 wt%). The addition of 50 wt% Al$_2$O$_3$ to the TCP matrix shows the presence of several peaks which are assigned to the tetrahedral environment of P sites (1.03 ppm; 1.93 ppm; 3.50 ppm and 4.84 ppm) (Figure 7a). In fact, the increasing of the percentage of alumina in the TCP matrix decreases the number of the tetrahedral phosphorus site peaks which are reduced to a large single peak with 90 wt% alumina (Figure 7 b-d). Moreover, the tetrahedral environment of the phosphorus in tricalcium phosphate is not changed after the sintering process with different percentages of alumina. But the effect of the addition of alumina to the β-TCP matrix provokes the structural rearrangement of the coordination of phosphorus in β-TCP. Similar results were previously reported in literature [14, 26-27, 31].

The ^{27}Al MAS-NMR spectra of Al$_2$O$_3$-TCP composites sintered for 1 hour at 1550°C with different percentages of β-TCP (50 wt%, 40 wt%, 20 wt% and 10 wt%) are shown in Figure 8. The chemical shifts at 35 ppm and at 7.3 ppm indicate the presence of octahedral Al sites (Al^{VI}) and pentahedral Al sites (Al^V), respectively. The peak of pentahedral Al sites increases with the increase of the percentage of alumina in the Al$_2$O$_3$-TCP composites (Figure 8 b-8d). We notice especially the appearance of another octahedral Al peak at 18.6 ppm for alumina sintered with 40 wt% and 20 wt% of β-TCP (Figure 8 b-d). The aluminum in the alumina is primarily in one pentahedral Al site (35 ppm) and in one octahedral Al site (7.3 ppm) (Figure 8e). For the alumina sintered with different percentages of β-TCP (50 wt%, 40 wt%, 20 wt% and 10 wt%), the spectra show two octahedral aluminum environments: AlO_6 at about 7.3 ppm and at 18.6 ppm (Fig 8b-d). Indeed, the intensity of the octahedral signal at 18.6 ppm increases with the percentage of alumina. The estimated concentrations of AlO_5 and AlO_6 are reported in Table 4. During the sintering process, the aluminum in the Al_2O_3-TCP composites provokes the structural rearrangement of the coordination of aluminum. Similar results were provisionally reported by different authors [22, 27, 31]. Indeed, these authors show that the coordination of the aluminum in octahedral sites was forced to change into another coordination in pentahedral sites [31]. The same authors point out that the structural rearrangement of the coordination of aluminum was probably produced by the formation of calcium aluminates which was produced after the sintering process and the reaction between calcium phosphates and alumina [31]. In conclusion, the ^{31}P magic angle scanning nuclear magnetic resonance analysis of different composites reveals the presence of tetrahedral P sites, while the [27]Al magic angle scanning nuclear magnetic resonance analysis shows the presence of both octahedral and pentahedral Al sites.

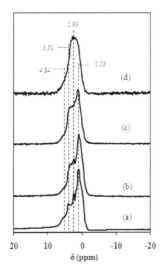

Figure 7. The ^{31}P MAS-NMR spectra of the Al_2O_3-TCP composites sintered for 1 hour at 1550°C with different percentages of β-TCP: (a) 50 wt%, (b) 40 wt%, (c) 20 wt% and (d) 10 wt%

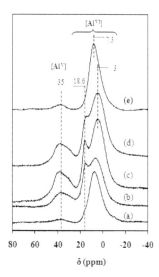

Figure 8. The ^{27}Al MAS-NMR spectra of the Al$_2$O$_3$-TCP composites sintered for 1 hour at 1550°C with different percentages of β-TCP: (a) 50 wt%, (b) 40 wt%, (c) 20 wt%, (d) 10 wt% and (e) 0 wt%

Compounds	AlO$_5$ (%)	AlO$_6$ (Type 1) (%)	AlO$_6$ (Type 2) (%)
δ (ppm)	30-40	7	18
TCP - 50 wt % Al$_2$O$_3$	0.50	99.50	
TCP - 60 wt % Al$_2$O$_3$	15.38	65.37	19.25
TCP - 80 wt % Al$_2$O$_3$	19.71	67.81	12.48
TCP- 90 wt % Al$_2$O$_3$	14.85	73.71	11.44
Al$_2$O$_3$	1.40	98.60	

Table 4. Properties of pentahedral and octahedral Al sites in the Al$_2$O$_3$-TCP composites sintered with different percentages of β-TCP at various temperatures for 1 hour

Figure 9 presents XRD patterns of Al$_2$O$_3$-TCP composites sintered at 1550°C for 1 hour with different percentages of β-TCP. Besides, the spectra show the characteristic peaks of β-TCP (ICDD data file no. 70-2065) and α- Al$_2$O$_3$ (ICDD data file no. 43-1484). This analysis shows that the peak of alumina is predominant in the elaboration of any composite.

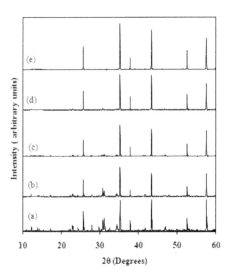

Figure 9. The XRD patterns of the Al$_2$O$_3$-TCP composites sintered at 1550°C for 1 hour with different percentages of β-TCP: (a) 50 wt%, (b) 40 wt%, (c) 20 wt%, (d) 10 wt% and (e) 0 wt%

The SEM technique helps to investigate the texture and porosity of any biomaterial. Figure 10 shows the fracture surface of the Al$_2$O$_3$-TCP composites sintered at 1550°C for 1 hour with different percentages of β-TCP. These micrographs show the coalescence between β-TCP grains produced with all the percentages of added alumina (Figure 10 a-d). The samples sintered with 50 wt%, 40 wt% and 20 wt% β-TCP present cracks and an important intragranular porosity (Figure 10 a-c). This result is a proof of the fragility of the composites elaborated with the different percentages of alumina as shown in Figure 10a-c. In fact, the microstructure of the composites shows different cracks relative to the allotropic transformation of TCP (β to α) (Figure 10 a-c). But the intensity of the cracks in the composites decreases with the increase in the percentage of β-TCP (Figure 10 a-d). Thus, the absence of micro-cracking and the reduction of the sizes of the pores in the Al$_2$O$_3$-10 wt% TCP composites explain the increase in the rupture strength of the samples (Figure 10 d$_1$-d$_2$). Indeed, the composites present excellent mechanical properties and a good aptitude for sinterability (Figure 10 d$_1$-d$_2$). The SEM micrographs of the alumina sintered without β-TCP shows an intergranular porosity (Figure 10e).

The effects of the sintering temperature on the microstructure of the Al$_2$O$_3$-10 wt% TCP composites are presented in Figure 11. The SEM micrographs show the coalescence between the grains with the increase of the sintering temperature. At 1500°C, the samples present an important intergranular porosity (Figure 11a). The microstructure of Al$_2$O$_3$-10 wt% TCP composites sintered at 1550°C shows a continuous phase relative to β-TCP phases and small-sized grains relative to the alumina phases (Figure 11b). Furthermore, at 1600°C, the boundaries between grains are evident in the micrographs (marked with arrows in Figure

11c), confirming the best mechanical resistance of Al_2O_3-10 wt% TCP composites in this temperature and with the addition of 10 wt% β-TCP (Figure 11c). In fact, the continuous phases
in addition to the formed spherical pores prove that a liquid phase has appeared at 1600°C
relative probably to the allotropic transformation of the β-TCP. This similar result was observed by Bouslama and colleagues [25].

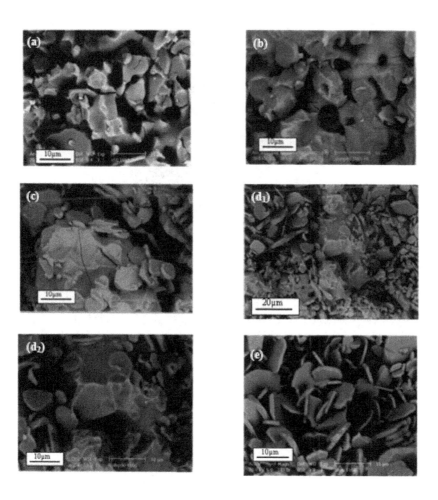

Figure 10. The SEM micrographs of the Al_2O_3 - TCP composites sintered at 1550°C for 1 hour with different percentages of β-TCP: (a) 50 wt%, (b) 40 wt%, (c) 20 wt%, (d₁-d₂) 10 wt% and (e) 0 wt%.

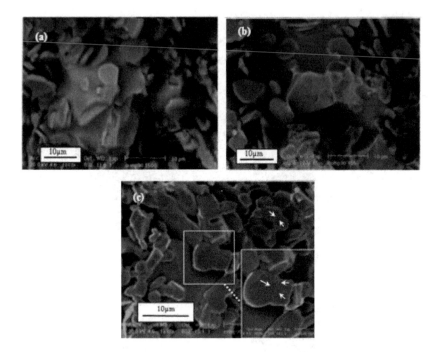

Figure 11. The SEM micrographs of the Al₂O₃-10 wt% TCP composites sintered for 1 hour at: (a) 1500°C, (b) 1550°C and (c) 1600°C.

The results of the microstructural investigations of Al$_2$O$_3$-10 wt% TCP composites sintered at 1600°C for different lengths of time (0 min, 30 min, 60 min and 90 min) are shown in Figure 12. These micrographs reveal the influence of different lengths of time on the microstructural developments during the sintering process at 1600°C. The microstructure of the samples leads to the formation of important cracks of different sizes with composites sintered for 0 min, 30 min and 90 min (Figure 12 ba-b and 12d). The continuous phases are relative to the β-TCP phase while the grains of a small size are relative to the alumina phase (Figure 12 ba-b and 12d). In Figure 12c, we notice the coalescence between the grains after the sintering process for 60 min confirming the best mechanical resistance in these conditions.

Furthermore, the sintering behavior of the Al$_2$O$_3$-TCP composites has been studied relative to the β-TCP content. It has been shown that alumina should be used in order to prevent the β-α transition of the tricalcium phosphate during the sintering process. At any rate, the results obtained in the present work would be valuable in the performance of Al$_2$O$_3$ - TCP composites resembling bone tissue engineering (Table 3). In fact, our preliminary tests indicated that the rupture strength of Al$_2$O$_3$-TCP composites is from 2 to 14 MPa. The optimum value of the Al$_2$O$_3$ - 10 wt% TCP composites sintered at 1600°C for one hour reached 13.5

MPa. This is true for the values of calcium phosphates fabricated by conventional techniques [116] and is close to a cancellous bone (2-12 MPa) [1-2, 117].

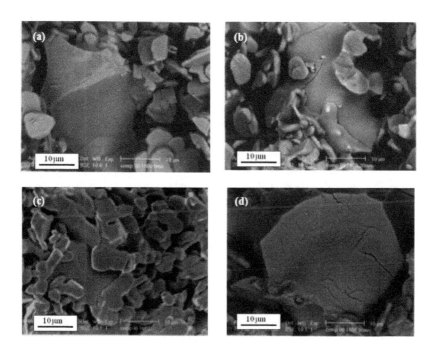

Figure 12. SEM micrographs of the Al$_2$O$_3$ - 10 wt% TCP composites sintered at 1600°C for: (a) 0 min, (b) 30 min, (c) 60 min and (d) 90 min.

According to the authors' best knowledge, the highest values of the mechanical characteristics for different samples are detailed in Table 3. As it can be seen from this table, the various techniques used to prepare dense sintered bioceramics affect the final density, as well as the composition of the phase and, consequently, the final mechanical properties of samples. The Al$_2$O$_3$ - 10 wt% TCP composites show high rupture strength, which is in concordance with the other results [10, 15, 21, 25-27, 29]. The rupture strength obtained for TCP-Al$_2$O$_3$ composites is from 2 to 14 MPa, within the values reported in the literature (Table 3). Moreover, the wide variation in the reported rupture strength of the composites is due to the synthesis route of the β-TCP powder, the size of its particle as well as to its density; it is also due to the application of different processing parameters.

At first, the objective of this work was to characterize the mechanical properties of alumina – TCP composites produced after the sintering process. A sintering stage appears to be of great importance to produce biomaterials with the required properties. Several processes occur during the sintering process of tricalcium phosphate and bioinert oxide. Firstly, the TCP powders are synthesized by solid reaction. Secondly, alumina – TCP powders are sintered for production of dense bioceramics with subsequent shrinkage of the samples. Thirdly, the mechanical properties of alumina–TCP composites are accompanied by a concurrent increase in grain size and a formation of cracks in the alumina sintered with different percentages of TCP (20 wt%, 40 wt% and 50 wt%). Besides, sintering causes the toughening and the increase of the mechanical strength of alumina–10 wt% TCP composites. An extensive study on the effect of the sintering temperature and time on the properties of alumina–TCP composites revealed a correlation between these parameters and density, porosity, grain size, chemical composition and strength of different composites. The degree of densification and mechanical properties of alumina–TCP composites appeared to depend on the sintering temperature and the duration of sintering. Alumina–TCP powders can be pressed and sintered up to theoretical density at 1400°C–1600°C. Processing them with higher percentage of TCP (20 wt%, 40 wt% and 50 wt%) may lead to exaggerated grain growth and formation of cracks because of the formation of α-TCP at higher temperatures. Indeed, the allotropic transformation of TCP is a function of the sintering temperature. The presence of cracks in the alumina–TCP composites is reported to inhibit the mechanical properties. A definite correlation between mechanical strength and grain size in sintered alumina–TCP composites was found: the strength started to decrease at lower sintering temperature and with higher percentage of TCP (20 wt%, 40 wt% and 50 wt%). The sintering process of alumina – 10 wt% TCP composites makes it possible to decrease the grain size and achieve higher densities. This leads to finer microstructures, higher thermal stability of alumina–10 wt% TCP composites and subsequently better mechanical properties of the prepared bioceramics composites. The mechanical properties of alumina – TCP composites is from 2 to 14 MPa. Generally, the mechanical properties of samples increase with the decrease in grain size. In fact, the mechanical strength of alumina–10 wt% TCP composites reaches a maximum value with the decrease in the size of the grains of composites. The optimum measured value of the strength of the alumina–10 wt% TCP composites was 13.5 MPa. This value is compared to those of cancellous bone. Similar values for porous HAp are in the ranges of 2-10 MPa [118]. Generally, variations of mechanical properties of samples are caused by a statistical nature of the strength distribution, influence of remaining microporosity, grain size, presence of impurities and Ca/P ratio [118].

In conclusion, an interfacial reaction between β-TCP and alumina has been studied in the nanocomposites of Al_2O_3-TCP. It was found that the alumina did not completely react with the β-TCP and did not form calcium aluminates. Moreover, it has been shown that the alumina prevents the formation of cracks in the microstructure of composites containing 10 wt % of β-TCP. The mechanical characteristics should be taken into consideration in order to better assess the relationship between the processing conditions, the microstructural design as well as the mechanical response.

4. Conclusions

The biomaterials of alumina-tricalcium phosphate composites have been characterized by using MAS NMR, XRD and SEM analysis after the sintering process. The effect of β-TCP additive on the alumina matrix was observed in different thermal analyses: dilatometry analysis and DTA analysis. The mechanical properties have been investigated by the Brazilian test. This investigation has allowed us to define the sintering temperature and the percentage of added alumina for which β-TCP should have an optimal densification and better mechanical properties. This study has also allowed us to summarize the effect of the sintering temperature and the length of sintering time on the mechanical properties of the Al₂O₃-TCP composites. The produced Al₂O₃-TCP composites with different percentages of β-TCP (50 wt%; 40 wt%; 20 wt% and 10 wt%) exhibited much better mechanical properties than the reported values of β-TCP without alumina. The Al₂O₃-TCP composites showed a higher rupture strength at 1600°C, which certainly increased with the alumina content and reached the optimum value with 90 wt%. However, no cracks were observed in the microstructure of the composites which contained this percentage of alumina. This is due to the allotropic transformation of the tricalcium phosphate. The partial or reversal transformation of tricalcium phosphate (β to α or α to α′) during the cooling period could induce a residual stress within the dense bioceramics, marking it much more brittle. Accordingly, the optimum performance of alumina-tricalcium phosphate composites achieved 13.5 MPa. Furthermore, the best mechanical properties of the composites were obtained after the sintering process at 1600°C for 1 hour. With different weight rations of tricalcium phosphate: alumina (50:50, 40:60 and 20:80), the performance of the composites was hindered by the formation of both cracks and intragranular porosity.

Acknowledgements

The authors thank Mr Ahmed BAHLOUL for his assistance in this work.

Author details

Siwar Sakka, Jamel Bouaziz and Foued Ben Ayed*

*Address all correspondence to: benayedfoued@yahoo.fr

Laboratory of Industrial Chemistry, National School of Engineering, Sfax University, Sfax, Tunisia

References

[1] Hench L L. Bioceramics: From Concept to clinic. J. Am. Ceram. Soc. 1991; 74 (7) 1487.

[2] Hench L L. An Introduction to Bioceramics. J. Wilson (ed.). Vol. 1. World Scientific, Singapore; 1993.

[3] Elliott J C. Structure and Chemistry of the Apatite and Other Calcium Orthophosphates. Amsterdam : Elsevier Science B.V.; 1994.

[4] Landi E, Tampieri A, Celotti G, Sprio S. Densification behaviour and mechanisms of synthetic hydroxyapatites. J. Eur. Ceram. Soc. 2000; 20, 2377.

[5] Ben Ayed F, Bouaziz J, Bouzouita K. Pressureless sintering of fluorapatite under oxygen atmosphere. J. Eur. Ceram. Soc. 2000; 20 (8) 1069.

[6] Ben Ayed F, Bouaziz J, Khattech I, Bouzouita K. Produit de solubilité apparent de la fluorapatite frittée. Ann. Chim. Sci. Mater. 2001; 26 (6) 75.

[7] Ben Ayed F, Bouaziz J, Bouzouita K. Calcination and sintering of fluorapatite under argon atmosphere. J. Alloys Compd. 2001; 322 (1-2) 238.

[8] Varma H K, Sureshbabu S. Oriented growth of surface grains in sintered b tricalcium phosphate bioceramics. Materials letters 2001; 49, 83.

[9] Destainville A, Champion E, Bernache – Assolant D. Synthesis. Characterization and thermal behavior of apatitic tricalcium phosphate. Mater. Chem. Phys. 2003; 80, 269.

[10] Wang C X, Zhou X, Wang M. Influence of sintering temperatures on hardness and Young's modulus of tricalcium phosphate bioceramic by nanoindentation technique. Materials Characterization 2004; 52, 301.

[11] Hoell S, Suttmoeller J, Stoll V, Fuchs S, Gosheger G. The high tibial osteotomy, open versus closed wedge, a comparison of methods in 108 patients. Arch.Trauma Surg. 2005; 125, 638–43.

[12] Gaasbeek R D, Toonen H G, Van Heerwaarden R J, Buma P. Mechanism of bone incorporation of β-TCP bone substitute in open wedge tibial osteotomy in patients. Biomaterials 2005; 26, 6713–6719.

[13] Jensen S S, Broggini N, Hjorting-Hansen E, Schenk R, Buser D. Bone healing and graft resorption of autograft, anorganic bovine bone and beta-tricalcium phosphate. A histologic and histomorphometric study in the mandibles of minipigs.. Clin. Oral. Implants Res. 2006; 17, 237–243.

[14] Ben Ayed F, Chaari K, Bouaziz J, Bouzouita K. Frittage du phosphate tricalcique. C. R. Physique, 2006; 7 (7) 825.

[15] Ben Ayed F, Bouaziz J, Bouzouita K. Résistance mécanique de la fluorapatite. Ann. Chim. Sci. Mater. 2006; 31 (4) 393.

[16] Gutierres M, Dias A G, Lopes M A, Hussain N S, Cabral A T, Almeid L. Opening wedge high tibial osteotomy using 3D biomodelling Bone like macroporous structures: case report. J. Mater. Sci. Mater. Med. 2007; 7 (18) 2377–2382.

[17] DeSilva G L, Fritzler A, DeSilva S P. Antibiotic-impregnated cement spacer for bone defects of the forearm and hand. Tech. Hand Up Extrem Surg. 2007; 11, 163–7

[18] Ben Ayed F, Bouaziz J. Élaboration et caractérisation d'un biomatériau à base de phosphates de calcium. C. R. Physique, 2007; 8 (1) 101-108.

[19] Ben Ayed F, Bouaziz J. Sintering of tricalcium phosphate–fluorapatite composites by addition of alumina. Ceramics Int. 2008; 34 (8) 1885-1892.

[20] Ben Ayed F, Bouaziz J. Sintering of tricalcium phosphate–fluorapatite composites with zirconia. J. Eur. Ceram. Soc., 2008; 28 (10) 1995-2002.

[21] Bouslama N, Ben Ayed F, Bouaziz J. Sintering and mechanical properties of tricalcium phosphate–fluorapatite composites. Ceramics Int. 2009; 35, 1909-1917.

[22] Bouslama N, Ben Ayed F, Bouaziz J. Mechanical properties of tricalcium phosphate-fluorapatite-alumina composites. Physics Procedia 2009; 2, 1441-1448.

[23] Chaari K, Ben Ayed F, Bouaziz J, Bouzouita K. Elaboration and characterization of fluorapatite ceramic with controlled porosity. Materials Chemistry and Physics 2009; 113, 219-226.

[24] Guha A K, Singh S, Kumarresan R, Nayar S, Sinha A. Mesenchymal cell response to nanosized biphasic calcium phosphate composites. Coll. Surf. B biointerface 2009; 73, 146-51.

[25] Bouslama N, Ben Ayed F, Bouaziz J. Effect of fluorapatite additive on densification and mechanical properties of tricalcium phosphate. J. Mechanical Behaviour of Biomedical Materials 2010; 3, 2-13.

[26] Ben Ayed F. Biomaterials - Physics and Chemistry, Chapter 18: Elaboration and characterisation of calcium phosphate biomaterial for biomedical application, ISBN 978-953-307-418-4. Croatia: In Tech; 2011. p 357 – 374.

[27] Sakka S, Ben Ayed F, Bouaziz J. Mechanical properties of tricalcium phosphate–alumina composites. IOP Conf. Series : Materials Science and Engineering, 2012. 28, 012028

[28] Sellami I, Ben Ayed F, Bouaziz J. Effect of fluorapatite additive on the mechanical properties of tricalcium phosphate-zirconia composites. IOP Conf. Series : Materials Science and Engineering, 2012. 28, 012029.

[29] Ben Ayed F. Current microscopy contributions to advances in science and technology, Chapter: The effect of the sintering process on the microstructure and the mechanical properties of biomaterials. published by Formatex Research Center Spain; to be published in 2012.

[30] Levin I, Brandon D. Metastable Alumina Polymorphs: Crystal Structures and Transition. Sequences. J. Am. Ceram. Soc. 1998, 81.

[31] Guidera A, Chaari K, Bouaziz J. Elaboration and Characterization of Alumina-Fluorapatite Composites. J. Biomat. Nano. 2011; 2, 103-113.

[32] Doremus RH. Bioceramics. J Mater Sci 1992; 27, 285–97.

[33] Vallet-Regı́ M. Ceramics for medical applications. J Chem Soc Dalton Trans 2001, 97–108.

[34] Rahaman MN, Yao A, Bal BS, Garino JP, Ries MD. Ceramics for prosthetic hip and knee joint replacement. J Am Ceram Soc 2007; 90, 1965–88.

[35] Best SM, Porter AE, Thian ES, Huang J. Bioceramics: past, present and for the future. J Eur Ceram Soc 2008; 28, 1319–27.

[36] Lowenstam HA, Weiner S. On biomineralization. Oxford University Press, 1989; pp 324.

[37] LeGeros RZ. Calcium phosphates in oral biology and medicine. Basel: Karger; 1991, 201.

[38] Weiner S, Wagner HD. Material bone: structure-mechanical function relations. Ann Rev Mater Sci 1998; 28, 271–98.

[39] Weiner S, Traub W, Wagner HD. Lamellar bone: structure-function relations. J Struct Biol 1999; 126, 241–55.

[40] Weiner S, Dove PM. An overview of biomineralization processes and the problem of the vital effect. In: Dove PM, de Yoreo JJ, Weiner S, editors. Biomineralization, series: reviews in mineralogy and geochemistry, vol. 54. Washington, D.C., USA: Mineralogical Society of America; 2003. p 1–29.

[41] Albee FH. Studies in bone growth – triple calcium phosphate as stimulus to osteogenesis. Ann Surg 1920; 71, 32–9.

[42] Nery EB, Lynch KL, Hirthe WM, Mueller KH. Bioceramic implants in surgically produced infrabony defects. J Periodontol 1975; 46, 328–47.

[43] Denissen HW, de Groot K. Immediate dental root implants from synthetic dense calcium hydroxylapatite. J Prosthet Dent 1979; 42, 551–6.

[44] Levitt GE, Crayton PH, Monroe EA, Condrate RA. Forming methods for apatite prosthesis. J Biomed Mater Res 1969; 3, 683–5.

[45] Blakeslee KC, Condrate Sr RA. Vibrational spectra of hydrothermally prepared hydroxyapatites. J Am Ceram Soc 1971; 54, 559–63.

[46] Garrington GE, Lightbody PM. Bioceramics and dentistry. J Biomed Mater Res 1972; 6, 333–43.

[47] Cini L, Sandrolini S, Paltrinieri M, Pizzoferrato A, Trentani C. Materiali bioceramici in funzione sostitutiva. Nota preventiva. (Bioceramic materials for replacement purposes. Preliminary note.). La Chirurgia Degli Organi Di Movimento 1972; 60, 423–30.

[48] Hulbert SF, Young FA, Mathews RS, Klawitter JJ, Talbert CD, Stelling FH. Potential of ceramic materials as permanently implantable skeletal prostheses. J Biomed Mater Res 1970; 4, 433–56.

[49] Hench LL, Splinter RJ, Allen WC, Greenlee TK. Bonding mechanisms at the interface of ceramic prosthetic materials. J Biomed Mater Res 1971; 2, 117–41.

[50] Hulbert SF, Hench LL, Forces D, Bowman L. History of bioceramics. In: Vincenzini P, editor. Ceramics in surgery. Amsterdam, The Netherlands: Elsevier, 1983; p 3–29.

[51] Jarcho M. Calcium phosphate ceramics as hard tissue prosthetics. Clin Orthop Relat Res 1981; 157, 259–78.

[52] de Groot K. Bioceramics consisting of calcium phosphate salts. Biomaterials 1980; 1 (1) 47–50.

[53] Aoki H, Kato KM, Ogiso M, Tabata T. Studies on the application of apatite to dental materials. J Dent Eng 1977; 18, 86–9.

[54] Roy DM, Linnehan SK. Hydroxyapatite formed from coral skeletal carbonate by hydrothermal exchange. Nature 1974; 247, 220–2.

[55] Holmes RE. Bone regeneration within a coralline hydroxyapatite implant. Plast Reconstr Surg 1979; 63, 626–33.

[56] Elsinger EC, Leal L. Coralline hydroxyapatite bone graft substitutes. J Foot Ankle Surg 1996; 35, 396–9.

[57] LeGeros RZ, LeGeros JP. Calcium phosphate bioceramics: past, present, future. Key Eng Mater 2003; 240–242, 3–10.

[58] Durucan C, Brown PW. Low temperature formation of calcium-deficient hydroxyapatite-PLA/PLGA composites. J Biomed Mater Res 2000; 51A, 717–25.

[59] Ginebra MP, Rilliard A, Ferna´ndez E, Elvira C, Roma´n JS, Planell JA. Mechanical and rheological improvement of a calcium phosphate cement by the addition of a polymeric drug. J Biomed Mater Res 2001; 57, 113–8.

[60] Yokoyama A, Yamamoto S, Kawasaki T, Kohgo T, Nakasu M. Development of calcium phosphate cement using chitosan and citric acid for bone substitute materials. Biomaterials 2002; 23, 1091–101.

[61] Barralet JE, Gaunt T, Wright AJ, Gibson IR, Knowles JC. Effect of porosity reduction by compaction on compressive strength and microstructure of calcium phosphate cement. J Biomed Mater Res 2002; 63B, 1–9.

[62] Bohner M, Gbureck U, Barralet JE. Technological issues for the development of more efficient calcium phosphate bone cements: a critical assessment. Biomaterials 2005; 26, 6423–9.

[63] Bohner M, Baroud G. Injectability of calcium phosphate pastes. Biomaterials 2005; 26, 1553–63.

[64] Link DP, van den Dolder J, van den Beucken JJ, Wolke JG, Mikos AG, Jansen JA. Bone response and mechanical strength of rabbit femoral defects filled with injectable CaP cements containing TGF-b1 loaded gelatin microspheres. Biomaterials 2008; 29, 675–82.

[65] Friedman CD, Costantino PD, Takagi S, Chow LC. Bone source hydroxyapatite cement: a novel biomaterial for craniofacial skeletal tissue engineering and reconstruction. J Biomed Mater Res 1998; 43B, 428–32.

[66] Shindo ML, Costantino PD, Friedman CD, Chow LC. Facial skeletal augmentation using hydroxyapatite cement. Arch Otolaryngol Head Neck Surg 1993; 119, 185–90.

[67] Chow LC. Calcium phosphate cements: chemistry, properties, and applications. Mat Res Soc Symp Proc 2000; 599, 27–37.

[68] Muzzarelli RAA, Biagini G, Bellardini M, Simonelli L, Castaldini C, Fraatto G. Osteoconduction exerted by methylpyrolidinone chitosan in dental surgery. Biomaterials 1993; 14, 39–43.

[69] Hing KA, Best SM, Bonfield W. Characterization of porous hydroxyapatite. J Mater Sci Mater Med 1999; 10, 135–45.

[70] Jordan DR, Gilberg S, Bawazeer A. Coralline hydroxyapatite orbital implant (Bio-Eye): experience with 158 patients. Ophthal Plast Reconstr Surg 2004; 20, 69–74.

[71] Yoon JS, Lew H, Kim SJ, Lee SY. Exposure rate of hydroxyapatite orbital implants a 15-year experience of 802 cases. Ophthalmology 2008; 115, 566–72.

[72] Schnettler R, Stahl JP, Alt V, Pavlidis T, Dingeldein E, Wenisch S. Calcium phosphate-based bone substitutes. Eur J Trauma 2004; 4, 219–29.

[73] Zyman ZZ, Glushko V, Dedukh N, Malyshkina S, Ashukina N. Porous calcium phosphate ceramic granules and their behaviour in differently loaded areas of skeleton. J Mater Sci Mater Med 2008; 19, 2197–205.

[74] Larsson S, Hannink G. Injectable boneegraft substitutes: current products, their characteristics and indications, and new developments. Injury 2011; 42, 30e4.

[75] Dorozhkin SV. Calcium orthophosphate cements for biomedical application. J Mater Sci 2008; 43, 3028e57.

[76] Dorozhkin SV. Calcium orthophosphate-based biocomposites and hybrid biomaterials. J Mater Sci 2009; 44, 2343e87.

[77] Bohner M, Gbureck U, Barralet JE. Technological issues for the development of more efficient calcium phosphate bone cements: a critical assessment. Biomaterials 2005; 26, 6423e9.

[78] Von Gonten AS, Kelly JR, Antonucci JM. Load-bearing behavior of a simulated craniofacial structure fabricated from a hydroxyapatite cement and bioresorbable fiber mesh. J Mater Sci Mater Med 2000; 11, 95e100.

[79] Canal C, Ginebra MP. Fibre-reinforced calcium phosphate cements: a review. J Mech Behav Biomed Mater 2011; 4, 1658e71.

[80] Callister Jr WD, Rethwisch DG. Materials science and engineering: an introduction. Hoboken: John Wiley Sons Inc; 2009.

[81] LeGeros RZ. Biodegradation and bioresorption of calcium phosphate ceramics. Clin Mater 1993;14, 65–88.

[82] Suchanek W, Yoshimura M. Processing and properties of hydroxyapatitebased biomaterials for use as hard tissue replacement implants. J Mater Res 1998; 13, 94–117.

[83] Hing KA, Best SM, Bonfield W. Characterization of porous hydroxyapatite. J Mater Sci Mater Med 1999; 10, 135–45.

[84] Ducheyne P, Qiu Q. Bioactive ceramics: the effect of surface reactivity on bone formation and bone cell function. Biomaterials 1999; 20, 2287–303.

[85] Pilliar RM, Filiaggi MJ, Wells JD, Grynpas MD, Kandel RA. Porous calcium polyphosphate scaffolds for bone substitute applications – in vitro characterization. Biomaterials 2001; 22, 963–72.

[86] Chu TMG, Orton DG, Hollister SJ, Feinberg SE, Halloran JW. Mechanical and in vivo performance of hydroxyapatite implants with controlled architectures. Biomaterials 2002; 23, 1283–93.

[87] Hench LL, Polak JM. Third-generation biomedical materials. Science 2002; 295, 1014–7.

[88] Tamai N, Myoui A, Tomita T, Nakase T, Tanaka J, Ochi T, et al. Novel hydroxyapatite ceramics with an interconnective porous structure exhibit superior osteoconduction in vivo. J Biomed Mater Res 2002; 59, 110–7.

[89] Simon JL, Roy TD, Parsons JR, Rekow ED, Thompson VP, Kemnitzer J, et al. Engineered cellular response to scaffold architecture in a rabbit trephine defect. J Biomed Mater Res 2003; 66A, 275–82.

[90] Deville S, Saiz E, Nalla RK, Tomsia AP. Freezing as a path to build complex composites. Science 2006; 311, 515–8.

[91] Miranda P, Pajares A, Saiz E, Tomsia AP, Guiberteau F. Fracture modes under uniaxial compression in hydroxyapatite scaffolds fabricated by robocasting. J Biomed Mater Res 2007; 83A, 646–55.

[92] Miranda P, Pajares A, Saiz E, Tomsia AP, Guiberteau F. Mechanical properties of cal-
      cium phosphate scaffolds fabricated by robocasting. J Biomed Mater Res 2008; 85A,
      218–27.

[93] Brown WE, Chow LC. A new calcium phosphate water setting cement. In: Brown
      PW, editor. Cements research progress. Westerville, OH: Am Ceram Soc; 1986. p
      352–79.

[94] Daculsi G, Weiss P, Bouler JM, Gauthier O, Millot F, Aguado E. Biphasic calcium
      phosphate/hydrosoluble polymer composites: a new concept for bone and dental
      substitution biomaterials. Bone 1999; 25 (Suppl. 2), 59S–61S.

[95] Alam I, Asahina I, Ohmamiuda K, Enomoto S. Comparative study of biphasic calci-
      um phosphate ceramics impregnated with rhBMP-2 as bone substitutes. J Biomed
      Mater Res 2001; 54, 129–38.

[96] Daculsi G, Laboux O, Malard O, Weiss P. Current state of the art of biphasic calcium
      phosphate bioceramics. J Mater Sci Mater Med 2003; 14, 195–200.

[97] Daculsi G. Biphasic calcium phosphate granules concept for injectable and moulda-
      ble bone substitute. Adv Sci Technol 2006; 49, 9–13.

[98] LeGeros RZ, Lin S, Rohanizadeh R, Mijares D, LeGeros JP. Biphasic calcium phos-
      phate bioceramics: preparation, properties and applications. J Mater Sci Mater Med
      2003;14, 201–9.

[99] Lecomte A, Gautier H, Bouler JM, Gouyette A, Pegon Y, Daculsi G, et al. Biphasic cal-
      cium phosphate: a comparative study of interconnected porosity in two ceramics. J
      Biomed Mater Res B (Appl Biomater) 2008; 84B, 1–6.

[100] Tancret F, Bouler JM, Chamousset J, Minois LM. Modelling the mechanical proper-
      ties of microporous and macroporous biphasic calcium phosphate bioceramics. J Eur
      Ceram Soc 2006; 26, 3647–56.

[101] Langstaff SD, Sayer M, Smith TJN, Pugh SM. Resorbable bioceramics based on stabi-
      lized calcium phosphates. Part II: evaluation of biological response. Biomaterials
      2001; 22, 135–50.

[102] Sayer M, Stratilatov AD, Reid JW, Calderin L, Stott MJ, Yin X, et al. Structure and
      composition of silicon-stabilized tricalcium phosphate. Biomaterials 2003; 24, 369–82.

[103] Yin X, Stott MJ, Rubio A. a- and b-tricalcium phosphate: a density functional study.
      Phys Rev B 2003; 68, 205205.

[104] Yin X, Stott MJ. Theoretical insights into bone grafting Si-stabilized a-tricalcium
      phosphate. J Chem Phys 2005; 122, 024709.

[105] Reid JW, Pietak AM, Sayer M, Dunfield D, Smith TJN. Phase formation and evolu-
      tion in the silicon substituted tricalcium phosphate/apatite system. Biomaterials 2005;
      26, 2887–97.

[106] Yin X, Stott MJ. Surface and adsorption properties of a-tricalcium phosphate. J Chem Phys 2006;124, 124701.

[107] Ruan JM, Zou JP, Zhou JN, Hu JZ. Porous hydroxyapatite – tricalcium phosphate bioceramics. Powder Metall 2006; 49, 66–9.

[108] Reid JW, Tuck L, Sayer M, Fargo K, Hendry JA. Synthesis and characterization of single-phase silicon substituted a-tricalcium phosphate. Biomaterials 2006; 27, 2916–25.

[109] da Silva RV, Bertran CA, Kawachi EY, Camilli JA. Repair of cranial bone defects with calcium phosphate ceramic implant or autogenous bone graft. J Craniofac Surg 2007; 18, 281–6.

[110] O'Neill WC. The fallacy of the calcium – phosphorus product. Kidney Int 2007; 72, 792–6.

[111] Sanchez-Sa′ lcedo S, Arcos D, Vallet-Regı′ M. Upgrading calcium phosphate scaffolds for tissue engineering applications. Key Eng Mater 2008; 377, 19–42.

[112] Brunauer S, Emmet P H, Teller. Adsorption of Gases in Multimolecular Layers. J. Amer. Chem. Soc. J. 1938; 60, 310.

[113] ISRM. Suggested methods for determining tensile strength of rock materials, Int. J. Rock Mech. Min. Sci. Geomech. Abstr. 1978; 15, 99.

[114] ASTM C496, Standard test method for splitting tensile strength of cylindrical concrete specimens Annual Book of ASTM, Standards, vol. 0.042, ASTM, Philadelphia, 1984; p 336.

[115] Balcik C, Tokdemir T, Senkoylo A, Koc N, Timucin M, Akin S, Korkusuz P, Korkusuz F. Early weight bearing of porous HA/TCP (60/40) ceramics in vivo: a longitudinal study in a segmental bone defect model of rabbit. Acta Biomaterialia 2007; 3, 985-996.

[116] Deville S, Saiz E, Nalla RK, Tomsia A P. Freezing as a path to build complex composites. Science. 2006; 311 (5760) 515-518.

[117] Murugan R, Ramakrishna S. Development of nanocomposites for bone grafting. Compos Sci Technol. 2005; 65 (15-16) 2385-2406.

[118] Suchanek WL, Yoshimura M. Processing and properties of hydroxyapatite based biomaterials for use as hard tissue replacement implants. J Mater Res 1998; 13, 94–117.

Chapter 4

Substrates with Changing Properties for Extracellular Matrix Mimicry

Frank Xue Jiang

Additional information is available at the end of the chapter

1. Introduction

Cell-ECM interactions Fundamental to the success of using biomaterials in medical and health care applications, is the understanding of their interactions with biological tissues and systems. First step towards this end is the elucidation of cell-ECM interactions, which has attracted considerable interest in recent decade. Cellular decision-making process is driven by the internal genetic program and external factors comprising primarily other cells and extracellular matrix (ECM) via soluble factors and direct physical connections such as focal adhesion [1, 2]. Three key features of ECM have been identified of great significance in affecting cells, namely, chemical and biological composition, dimensionality (two- vs. three-dimensional), and physical properties [3-6]. These features can be sensed by cells via cell-ECM linkages, and the resulting signals subsequently follow intracellular pathways and trigger a cascade of events leading to alterations in gene expression and manifestation in phenotype. In contrast to the long recognized chemical composition and adhesive character-istics of the ECM, physical cues including topography, pore size, geometric patterns, and mechanical stiffness and their significance has just started being appreciated [7-10]. Whilst characteristics of ECM have profound effect on cells, cells may also actively exert impact on ECM by secretion of soluble factors or modify properties of ECM, or contribute to maintain-ing integrity or properties of ECM. At a larger scale, biological systems may actively interact with biomaterials to maintain or re-establish homeostasis.

Dynamic aspect of ECM To date, the majority of the substrates employed in cellular studies and other biological investigations have been of fixed mechanical stiffness and/or adhesive properties throughout cell culture. There is an increasing realization that a cell's microenvir-onment is dynamic and changing with time [11-13]. It is the case in both pathologic and nor-mal tissues, at the tissue-implant interfaces, and during development and aging [14], especially for load-bearing and mechanically active tissues (e.g., heart, cartilage, lung) [15]. Not only do these changes naturally occur, but there are also benefits associated with them from a tissue engineering viewpoint, as highlighted in the series of discussions in the March 2005 issue of MRS (Materials Research Society) Bulletin [16, 17] and later studies. Whitesides [18] and Mrksich [19] and their coworkers among a number of investigators pioneered the work on engineering cell growth by using dynamic substrates. Their work and later reports on differential cell responses to materials with different properties suggest that it is beneficial for biomaterials to have controlled changing properties [20]. These facts make it very desirable for the bio-mimetic materials to have the capability of undergoing controlled remodeling with respect to time. They also raised caution in interpretation of the observations made from the majority of the biological studies, where properties of the substrates (e.g., culture flask, Petri dish, and hydrogels) remain unchanged throughout the process.

The scope of this work A significant number of reviews are available on the changes in soluble factors of ECM that may affect cellular behavior (e.g., [21]) and particularly on the changing environment in bioreactors [22] (e.g., nutrients concentration, oxygen level, temperature). Thus, they are not covered in this review. Moreover, flow conditions and the resulting traction forces, and their effect on certain cell types including blood cells (i.e., endothelial cells and red blood cells) have also been intensively reviewed and hence are not discussed here. This is also the case for mechanical forces, strain and stress applied directly to the cells (e.g., [23, 24]) in load-bearing tissues such as bone, cartilage and lung (for reference, see, e.g., [25-27]).

Therefore, this review is focused on the latest studies and current knowledge of two- or three- dimensional substrates with changing or dynamic mechanical and adhesive properties, design and conditions to trigger and achieve designed dynamics, and the impact of in-situ change of these properties on cell behavior, which provides guideline for design of biomaterials for their applications in medical and healthcare applications. Note that mechanical stiffness and elastic modulus were used interchangeably in this work.

2. Dynamic nature of the cell microenvironment

Normal tissues The micro-environment within which cells reside in natural tissues undergoes constant synthesis and degradation [16, 17], and has long been recognized as dynamic and changing [25, 28]. Although the composition of tissues generally remain tightly controlled in maturation, ECM remodeling constantly takes place [25, 29, 30], particularly when under hormonal stimulation or stress responses (e.g., [31]). Cells actively participate in tissue remodeling by secreting and mobilizing ECM molecules [32]. Alterations in ECM composition may result in changes in cell adhesion and /or tissue stiffness [33, 34] which further stimulates cellular responses. For instance, laminin component involved in cell adhesion to ECM is variant due to dynamics in exogenous factors [35]; normal cartilage shows elevated stiffness [36]; and vocal fold tissue exhibits dynamic viscoelastic properties [37]. Some specialized cell types can experience fast adhesion and detachment from ECM [38]. Changing ECM can also modify cell-cell interactions, further affecting cell behavior [39].

Pathological tissues Diseased tissue may possess properties such as mechanical stiffness different from those of the normal tissue [40, 41]. As a typical example, it has been found that tumor cells display enhanced movement towards ECM with lower mechanical rigidity, which is interesting considering the general stiffening phenomenon of tumor tissues [42], and biomechanical characteristics of tissues play a crucial role in tumor development [41]. It has also been shown that during the surgical procedures such as radio-frequency (RF) ablation, tissue properties can be modified [43]. Moreover, changes in ECM composition and relative quantity of ECM molecules can be correlated to pathology. For instance, ECM composition change that occurs during sub-epithelial tissue remodeling proved associated with asthma [33]. ECM remodeling in diseased heart valves is correlated to myofibroblast contractility [44], and certain cell types such as valvular interstitial cells can be activated and contribute to further tissue remodeling [45]. Additionally, ECM remodeling affects tissue mechanical properties in addition to inflammatory responses [46]. Moreover, mechanical forces, as experienced in traumatic brain injury or even under normal conditions, could potentially cause protein aggregation, giving rise to various diseases including neurodegenerative diseases [47]. Furthermore, early investigation of properties of central nervous (CNS) tissue under impact yielded modulus values with considerable variation. As an example, Fallenstein and coworker reported storage modulus of human brain tissue of 0.6 ~ 1.1 kPa under sinusoidal shear stress input mimicking head impact [48].

Development and aging During development, synthesis and degradation of ECM is a controlled process (e.g., [8, 49]), and mis-regulation contributes to many forms of diseases [30] Particularly, the microenvironment for embryonic and adult stem cells is regulated both temporally and spatially [2, 34], and is involved in various developmental processes including responses to soluble factors, cell differentiation, and morphogenesis [12]. ECM in musculoskeletal and other tissues adapts to increasing mechanical requirements by altering the size of tissue components [50] during development. Structural dynamics of ECM components such as collagen, laminin, and fibronectin coincides with estrous cycle and developmental progression [51]. Besides development, aging is also accompanied by changing ECM composition and structures. For example, in connective tissues, aging has been reported to be associated with increase in type I collagen content and decrease in both type III collagen and proteoglycans content, and with collagen fiber disruption and unraveling [50].

Tissue-implant interfaces With the growing interest in developing biomimetic materials for tissue engineering applications, tissue-implant interfaces have been subject to considerable research effort. Previous reports showed that cells can actively modify ECM at the interfaces, and cause drastic changes in tissue or construct mechanics using fibroblast-populated construct and other biomaterials [52, 53]. The study by Lee and co-workers suggested that dynamic moduli of an alginate material may be due to the bioactivities of the chondrocytes encapsulated in the scaffold [54]. In a similar study, different substrate composition and architecture gave rise to distinct levels of modulus increase owing to chondrocytes responses [55]. To take another example, smooth muscle cells (SMCs) in contact with engineered arterial construct displayed distinctive responses in protein synthesis and consequently the mechanical properties of ECM were significantly different [56]. Additionally, biodegradable materials used in various tissue engineering applications possess changing properties associated with specific degradation profiles.

Engineering advantages It has been suggested that temporal control over substrate or scaffold properties may entail great benefits in engineering cell growth. Among the notable examples is the stem cell differentiation and proliferation. A recent work showed enhanced hepatic functions from differentiated stem cells on softer substrates and improved expansion of undifferentiated cells on stiffer ones [57]. Therefore, it is promising to use stiffer substrates for optimal proliferations and subsequently soften them to gain better hepatic functions once differentiation completes. Langrana group also found that different neurite properties (e.g., axonal length and primary dendrite number) show differential preference towards substrate stiffness [58], suggesting the strategy of promoting nerve regeneration with scaffold of varying properties. Similar approach can be adopted to take advantage of differential cell responses (e.g., migration and functions) to adhesive properties.

The recurring indication from the above discussions is that *in vivo* ECM interacts with cells in many ways, and that the alteration in ECM composition or structures leads to changes in adhesive properties (hence cell adhesion) and/or mechanical properties. This potentially affects a variety of cell types and their properties and functioning, at different developmental stages, under normal or pathological conditions, or upon impact or injury. It also holds promises in offering novel approaches to tissue engineering applications. As a result, it is imperative to understand cellular responses to *changing substrate properties* for basic biology and biomimetic material (including biodegradable materials) design.

3. Types of dynamic substrates and stimuli

Here we consider two major classes of dynamic substrates that are based on self-assembled monolayer, or SAM, and hydrogels, as well as other types of substrates with surface or structural modifications. Since the focus of this work is on mimicking dynamic nature of ECM to examine cellular responses, those dynamic materials that are developed for other specific applications such as drug delivery [59] and do not involve changes that mimic dynamic ECM are beyond the scope of the review.

3.1. Self-assembled monolayer (SAM)

SAMs are formed by adsorption of molecules in solution or gas phase onto substrates in a spontaneous and organized fashion [60], and have emerged as an important candidate of materials in studying cellular responses to dynamic substrates [60, 61] where modifications could be made *in situ*. One of the major research focuses in this direction is to examine the effect of dynamic adhesive property of the substrate on cells, particularly by leveraging the ability to selectively capture or release cells upon application of a variety of stimuli (Table 1).

Type	Substrates	Properties changed and stimuli	Cell model	Observations and notes	Ref.
SAM	SAM incorporating O-silyl hydroquinone moiety	Adhesion on/off *Stimulus: electric potential*	3T3 fibroblasts	Modulation of cell adhesion and migration	[17, 61, 65]
	Electro-active quinine monolayer on Au	Adhesion on/off *Stimulus: electric potential*	3T3 fibroblasts	Selective release of adherent cells	[68]
	Azobenzene containing SAM on Au	Adhesion on/off *Stimulus: UV/visible light*	3T3 fibroblasts	Attachment and release of adherent cells Potential to control part of a single cell or groups of cells	[69]
Polymeric Hydrogel	MMP responsive polymer hydrogel network	Degradation of hydrogel *Stimulus: cell secreted MMP*	Human foreskin fibroblasts (HFFs)	Cell infiltration into the gel network with time	[74]
	Thermo-responsive polymer with photosensitive surface	Adhesion on/off *Stimulus: UV radiation and temperature*	CHO-K1 cells	Reversible control over cell adhesion Ability to control a population of cells	[72]
	poly(NIPAM-co-sodium acrylate) hydrogel films on rigid substrates.	Topographic change (swelling/de-swelling of gels) *Stimulus: temperature*	Porcine epithelial cells	Dynamic patterned substrates Reversible encapsulation of adherent cells	[73]
	DNA crosslinked PAM gels	Crosslinking density↑è Mechanical stiffness ↑, vice versa *Stimulus: ssDNA*	L929 & GFP fibroblasts	On dynamic substrate, L929 cells spread more than those on static stiff substrates (~23 kPa), while GFP fibroblasts respond differently to stiffening and softening of substrates Cell spreading and polarity (aspect ratio) respond differently to stiffness dynamics The range, starting point, and end point of change matter	[81, 83]
	DNA crosslinked PAM gels	Crosslinking density↓èstiffness ↓ *Stimulus: ssDNA*	Primary spinal cord cells	Neurite outgrowth respond to dynamic stiffness The trend in the response match that to the static stiffness except for primary dendrite length	[20]
	HA hydrogel	Crosslinking density change and ECM deposition è Mechanical stiffness change *Stimulus: hydrolysis or enzyme*	human mesenchym al stem cells (hMSCs)	Mechanical properties can be engineered with degradation Stiffness ↑ when degradation equals ECM deposition, and Stiffness ↓ at rapid degradtion Cellular responses to dynamic stiffness are different from static gels with the same initial or ending conditions	[78]

Type	Substrates	Properties changed and stimuli	Cell model	Observations and notes	Ref.
	Methacrylated HA hydrogel	UV exposure è stiffness ↑ *Stimulus: UV radiation and addition of reactive groups for*	hMSCs	Fate of hMSCs differentiate depends on the dynamics of stiffness change of substrates Adipogenic differentiation favored when cells is on the softer substrate long (stiffening at later times) Osteogenic differentiation when cells are on the stiffer substrate (stiffening at early times).	[79]
	Hydrogel based on PAM crosslinked by photosensitive reagent	Mechanical Stiffness (global or local)↓ *Stimulus: UV radiation*	3T3 fibroblasts	Stiffness decrease of 20-30% upon propose UV radiation Global stiffness decrease results in less spreading Localized softening to anterior and posterior area gives to differential responses	[76]
	PEG based hydrogel with photosensitive crosslinker	Mechanical Stiffness↓ Adhesive property change *Stimulus: UV radiation*	hMSCs and Valvular inter-stitial cells (VICs)	Valvular cell differentiation into myo-fibroblasts is inhibited by softening Good viability of hMSCs	[77]
Other types of substrates	Piezo-controlled substrate and AFM cantilever	Mechanical stiffness with cycling changes *Stimulus: stiffness clamp on AFM*	NIH 3T3	Apparent stiffness↑ leads to cells contraction rate↑ and contraction velocity↓ Changes took place instantaneously, and so did responses Responses were reversible, and consistent for same cell.	[84]
	Photo-active glass substrate with modifications	Adhesion on/off *Stimulus: UV radiation & pro- adhesive molecules*	HEK293, COS, NIH 3T3	Spatio-temporal control over cell adhesion Single cell control	[62]
	Substrates with photo-responsive caged peptides	Adhesion on/off *Stimulus: UV*	3T3 fibroblasts	Modifications of non-adhesive surfaces to adhesive ones	[63]
	PEG-modified ITO microelectrodes on glass substrates	Adhesion on/off *Stimulus: electric potential*	HepG2 (hepatic) and 3T3 cells, co-culture	Micro-patterned co-culture made possible	[85]
Promising materials*	Photo-crosslinked alginate hydrogel	Stiffness change; *Stimulus: light or hydrolysis*	Primary bovine chondrocytes	High survival rate for primary bovine chondrocytes Cellular responses to dynamic changes to be studied	[92]
	Gellan Gum hydrogel with both ionic crosslinking and	Stiffness, swelling, and degradation change *Stimulus: light or ion exchange*	NIH 3T3	Swelling and hydrolytic degradation vary with respect to crosslinking mechanism Stiffness may be changed quickly during photo-crosslinking process	[88]

Type	Substrates	Properties changed and stimuli	Cell model	Observations and notes	Ref.
	Methacrylated HA hydrogel with photo-crosslinker	Stiffening *Stimulus: UV radiation*	NIH3T3L HeLa Primary osteoblast	Good cell viability Cellular responses to dynamic changes to be studied	[80]
	PEG-based hydrogel incorporating CMP*	Softening *Stimulus: temperature or free CMP*	N/A	Cellular responses to dynamic changes to be studied	[90]
	PEG hydrogel (PEG vinyl sulfone crosslinked with PEG-diester-dithiol)	Softening *Stimulus: hydrolysis*	3T3 balb fibroblasts	Good cell viability in 3D gels Cellular responses to dynamic changes to be studied	[91]
	Resilin-like polypeptide (RLP) network crosslinked by THPP	Dynamic stiffness *Stimulus: oscillation*	N/A	Cellular responses to dynamic changes to be studied	[86]
	Thermo-reversible hydro-ferrogels (FGs)	Mechanical stiffness change *Stimulus: temperature change*	N/A	Cellular responses to dynamic changes to be studied	[89]

Note: ssDNA: single-stranded DNA; ↑ increase; ↓ decrease. *For 'Promising materials', most provides in vitro cyto-toxicity study, and cellular responses to dynamic properties remain to be investigated. N/A: not available

Table 1. A partial list dynamic substrates currently used in studying cell responses.

These stimuli, applied to initiate substrate dynamic, include light [62, 63], electricity [16, 17], pH, temperature, and others [16, 64] (Fig. 1). These approaches generally involve photo-chemical or electrochemical conversion, redox reactions, or stimulated configuration change of surface proteins, which leads to the attachment, detachment, shielding, or exposing of cell adhesion molecules, among which a popular choice is RGD peptide.

Mrksich group has been actively engaged in the development of SAM-based dynamic substrates by integrating surface chemistry, micro-patterning, and cell microenvironment engineering [17, 19, 61, 65, 66]. Based on an elegant design of SAM with electrochemically responsive group on a micro-patterned substrate, they first applied electrical stimulation to release 3T3 fibroblasts from designed areas on the substrate, and subsequently encouraged migration of neighboring cells to those areas with newly added adhesion molecules [65]. Refining this design by adding responsiveness to both negative and positive electric potentials, they demonstrated selective control over cell release [67] (Fig. 1C). Other groups have also engaged in the effort along this direction. By employing a hydroquinone terminated SAM based on redox reactions, Chan and colleagues proposed a SAM on gold surface that enables attachment and release of cell adhesion molecules such as those with RGD motif [68], and selectively released adherent 3T3 fibroblasts bound through RGD motifs but not those adherent based on hydro-phobic interactions (Fig. 1A). Reversibility of cell adhesion is attractive in studying cellular responses and cell-ECM interactions [60]. As an example, a surface chemistry involving azobenzene capable of switching between two configurations was utilized to expose or hide adhesion sites (e.g., RGD motif) upon photochemical stimulation[69] (Fig. 1B). While the finding is interesting, the long exposure of cells to UV may be problematic despite the reported negligible impact of light with wavelength over 320 nm on cells [63].

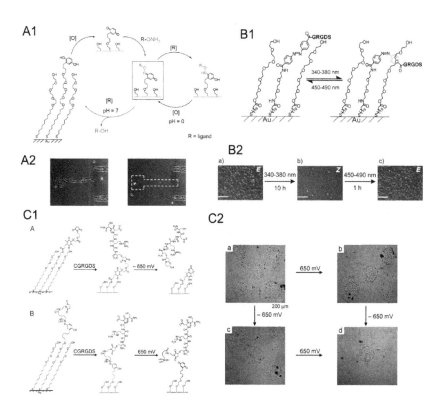

Figure 1. SAM-based dynamic substrates. (A) Schematic of the approach based on redox reaction (A1) by adjusting electrochemical potential, and cell detachment upon application of electric potential (A2). Extracted from [68]. (B) Schematic of altering configuration of azobenzene group under light of different ranges of wave length (B1) [69] and application to cell culture (B2) where NIH 3T3 fibroblasts initially adhere to adhesive surface (a) which was inhibited upon surface modification (b) followed by recovery of adhesion due to azobenzene configuration change (c). Extracted from [69]. (C) Illustration of a SAM that allows different modifications with positive and negative electric potential (C1) and its application in selective release of Swiss 3T3 cells (C2). Extracted from [67]. All with permission from publishers.

The above surveys part of the key advancement using SAM in modifying adhesion properties of the substrates mimicking those of natural cellular microenvironment. For a complete analysis of SAMs and their various applications, readers are referred to other reviews (e.g., [60, 70]). It suffices to point out that SAMs possess advantages in the precision (down to molecular level) of the control that can be applied in mechanistic studies [60, 66] of cell-ECM interactions, and are potentially useful for cell-based diagnostics among many applications. However, this approach has certain limitations. First, it mostly relies on coupling between electrical, chemical (including pH), mechanical, thermal, optical and biochemical (e.g., protein conformation) cues whose applicability under *in vivo* conditions is problematic. Next, the resulting changes in these studies are mostly of surface biochemical properties or of the presentation and biological activities of the surface ligands. Nevertheless, SAMs have greatly facilitated the probe and understanding of cell-ECM interactions and particular interplay between cells and ECM with dynamics in adhesive properties.

3.2. Polymeric hydrogels

Hydrogel materials are gaining popularity in the development of biomimetic materials, primarily due to the hydrated nature of natural ECM [14, 71]. Implantable hydrogel materials are increasingly being used in cardiovascular disease, nerve regeneration, and other conditions [59]. With careful design, hydrogel materials can have tunable materials properties, which have been demonstrated in a myriad of examples (Table 1). For instance, different than SAM-based approach, a polymer with both thermo- and photo-sensitivity was used to reversibly control adhesion of a group of cells [72]. Kim and colleagues took advantages of the thermo-responsive swelling behavior of copolymer between NIPAM and sodium acrylate, and created a hydrogel film that can be used to control cell encapsulation with surface topography [73]. Moreover, biomaterials responsive to the natural stimuli such as those experienced by biodegradable materials were found useful in mimicking biological events under physiological conditions, as illustrated in cell invasion to a MMP-responsive hydrogel scaffold [74]. This finding, among others, exemplifies the strategy of triggering material dynamic from bio-responsiveness to potential site- or disease-specific cues. The information from these studies is instrumental to the design of biodegradable materials in optimizing degradation profile for target cellular responses [75]. Naturally, in order to achieve desired outcome in adopting these strategies, it is important to gain thorough understanding of the natural environment, and minimize risks associate with biodegradable materials such as premature degradation, and potential toxicity of intermediate products from degradation.

Using a popular polyacrylamide hydrogel culture system with modifications that impart it with photo-sensitivity, Wang and colleagues [76] showed that upon UV induced substrates softening, spreading of 3T3 fibroblasts was hindered in contrast to that under static conditions (Fig. 2A). More interestingly, localized softening at anterior and posterior of cells yielded differential cellular morphology and migration responses [76]. Meanwhile, a PEG based polymer (PEGA) crosslinked by photosensitive crosslinker (PEGdiPDA) has been developed by Kloxin et al. [77], and used to lower gel stiffness upon UV exposure, which resulted in de-activation of myofibroblasts (Fig. 2B). Although UV radiation is preferentially avoided, these methods made possible high precision in applying changes of cellular mechanical microenvironment, and potentially allow creation of dynamic stiffness gradient.

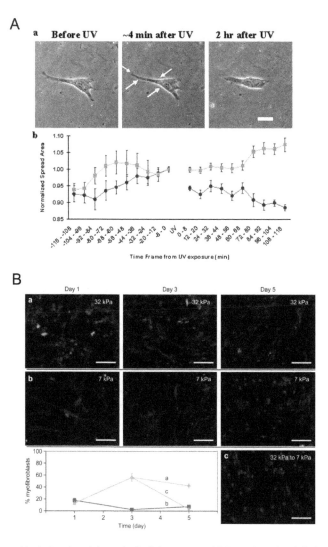

Figure 2. Photosensitive hydrogels and the study of cellular responses. (A) On a polyacrylamide hydrogel with photosensitive crosslinker, NIH 3T3 cells contract as indicated by projection area in response to UV-induced substrate softening. Extracted from [76]. (B) Valvular interstitial cells (VICs) on a PEG based hydrogel with photosensitive crosslinker displayed de-activation when UV radiation triggered substrate stiffness decrease. Extracted from [77]. Both with permission from publishers.

Similar observations were made by Burdick group for human mesenchymal stem cells (hMSCs) by using hyaluronic acid (HA) hydrogel degradable from hydrolytic and enzymatic reactions [78] (Fig. 3A). Very recently, a new material platform has been constructed by this group [79] and others [80] where the stiffness of a methacrylated hyaluronic acid hydrogel is increased via addition of photo-initiator and UV light exposure. In response to elevated stiffness, human mesenchymal stem cells (hMSCs) spread more and exert greater traction forces in hours (almost one magnitude of difference), and the rate of stiffness elevation dictates fate of cell differentiation towards adipogenic (slower) or osteogenic (faster) lineage. Their work highlighted that cellular behavior on dynamic gels is not the same as that on static gels with same initial or final properties, underlining the significance of dynamics in gel properties. This has been echoed in the concurrent work [81], where, for instance, the fibroblasts on 100% crosslinked hydrogels demonstrated different morphology from that on 100% crosslinked gels modified from 50% gels. Therefore, it is conceivable that the previous state of the cells and their ECM is also among the determinants of their current state, and that time dimension of ECM is of great importance.

Factors other than environmental conditions (e.g., light, pH, temperature) can also be delivered to stimulate dynamics in substrate properties. Incorporating DNA as crosslinker, Jiang and colleagues have developed a hydrogel system for cell attachment where mechanical properties of the substrates can be altered *in situ* in a controlled fashion when the cell culture is present [20, 81]. These DNA crosslinked hydrogels may also be designed to be potentially responsive to bio-stimuli, such as temperature or enzymes. Two representative cell types were chosen for the study of cell responses to dynamic substrate: fibroblasts whose sensitivity to mechanical cues is well documented, and neurons whose mechanosensing capability has recently just started being appreciated. The reports [20, 81] offered evidence that both cell types do respond to dynamic alternations in the mechanical characteristics of ECM, and suggest that the *alternations* in the mechanical stiffness may be involved in disease progression (Fig. 3B). It has been shown that the stiffness change resulting from pathological processes, may also aid in further progression of diseases [82].

The same material system was employed by Previera and co-workers, and they firstly proved the dual mechanical stimuli, namely strain and stiffness drop, during the dynamic processes, and secondly contrasted cell behavior to stiffness decrease with that for hardening of the substrates [83]. On hardening gels (from 12 kPa to 22 kPa), cells spread more than those on static substrates of higher stiffness (22 kPa), whereas on softening ones, they have greater spreading area than that on either starting or ending stiffnesses. In these studies, cell responses are determined by the range of rigidity change (due to crosslinking density), starting and ending rigidity, and specific cell properties (e.g., projection area vs. aspect ratio and protrusion for fibroblasts). The stress generation may also be involved in affecting cell behavior [83].

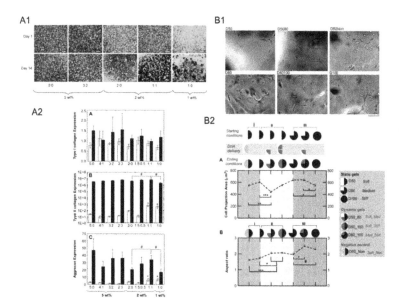

Figure 3. Substrates with dynamic mechanical stiffness and their application in cell culture studies. (A) Live/deal cell staining of human mesenchymal stem cells (hMSCs) in a hyaluronic acid hydrogel (A1) and the analysis of gene expression of type I/II collagen and aggrecan revealed that aside from type I collagen, both type II collagen and aggrecan exhibited an elevated level of expression on dynamic gels from the static ones. Extracted from [78]. With permission from publisher. (B) L929 fibroblast growth in a DNA crosslinked hydrogel with dynamic stiffness from crosslinking density change (B1) and the quantification of spreading area and aspect ratio (B2) showed that dynamic gels are significantly different from their static counterparts. Extracted from [81].

3.3. Other types of materials

The approach of employing polymeric hydrogel to study dynamic changes has certain limitations, one of which is the coupling of mechanical stiffness and forces (e.g., [83]). To address this concern and others, different from the approach by using SAM or polymeric hydrogel, AFM based method put forth by Webster and co-workers [84] probed cellular response to instant step change in stiffness excluding influence from stress or strain in the substrates (Table 1). It has been confirmed that indeed individual 3T3 fibroblasts are able to sense and respond to the stiffness in a scale of seconds as demonstrated in traction rate and contraction velocity [84]. However, this approach is most likely with inherent limitation in mimicking natural cell environment while remains an interesting tool in probing cellular responses to instantaneously change in stiffness. Additionally, this approach is applicable mostly to cells with dynamic morphology.

Common cell culture substrates (e.g., glass coverslip) modified with common photo-cleavable agents (NPE-TCSP) were shown to be useful for controlling cell adhesion selectively and temporally [62]. In this method, target areas were first irradiated to remove BSA known to prevent cell adhesion, and then pro-adhesive molecules (e.g., fibronectin) were added, followed by cell seeding. It is useful to study dynamics in interactions between single cells. Petersen et al. [63] used light to stimulate photosensitive surface modification resulting in uncovering of the RGD motif upon release of a caging group (Fig. 4A). In doing so, adhesion of 3T3 fibroblasts was first inhibited and then encouraged, although this process is not reversible. With a sequential activation of adhesive sites upon application of electric potential, a recent study [85] demonstrated the utility of substrates with ITO (indium tin oxide) microelectrodes modified with poly(ethylene glycol), or PEG, in co-culture of two cell types (hepatic cells and fibroblasts) in a controlled manner (Fig. 4B).

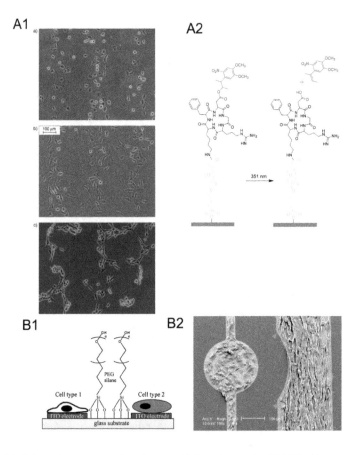

Figure 4. Cellular behavior in responses to other substrates with dynamic properties. (A) 3T3 fibroblasts grown in areas of patterned stripes (A1) generated from UV radiation based on the surface chemistry involving a caging group (A2). Extracted from [63]. (B) With PEG-modified ITO microelectrodes on glass substrates (B1), co-culture of two different cell types, HepG2 (hepatic) and 3T3 cells, was made possible. Extracted from [85]. Both with permission from publishers.

3.4. Promising substrates

By applying an oscillation to a resilin-like polypeptide network crosslinked by THPP (β-[Tris(hydroxymethyl) phosphino] propionic acid (betaine), Li and colleagues were able to observe dynamic mechanical stiffness of the gels varying with regard to oscillatory frequency mimicking the load from human vocal tissues [86] Oscillatory shear induced stiffening and softening of the collagen network might also serve as good substrates for mimicking cellular microenvironment particularly that in mechanically active tissues [87]. Ion concentration may be another stimulus to allow for temporal modification of hydrogel properties as exchange of ions between monovalent and divalant cations [88], and further work is needed to confirm it. Temperature-dependent substrate softening has been demonstrated by Krekhova et al. [89] and 3D complex with temperature-mediated crosslinking hence mechanical properties has been proposed by Stahl et al. [90], while applicability of these systems in mimicking cellular microenvironment remains to be seen. Zustiak et al. [91] reported mechanical stiffness drop, from approximately 1 kPa and at different rate, along with degradation of a poly(ethylene glycol), or PEG, hydrogel which might serve as not only drug delivery vehicle but also biomaterial construct, and they have offered preliminary evidence of good viability of 3T3 balb fibroblasts on the hydrogel substrate. Similarly, rigidity change from ~180 kPa to tens of kPa in 3-week period of degradation from a photo-crosslinked alginate hydrogels based on alginate methacrylation were presented by Jeon et al [92], and cyto-toxicity has been found to be low. In summary, these substrates holds promises as substrates with modifiable properties *in situ*, and need to be carefully tuned and evaluated for use as substrates with dynamic properties (Table 1). Other materials responsive to various stimuli including pH, temperature, and biochemical factors for a variety of applications, including can be found in the earlier reviews [64, 70, 93], and thus are not discussed in detail here due to the focus of the current analysis.

4. Design considerations and outlook

4.1. Dynamic properties of the substrates

As indicated in the discussions in Background and Motivation, the progression in changes of ECM properties is also critical in addition to changes *per se* in light of the observations in normal and pathological tissues, development and aging, and potential engineering benefits. Towards this end, rate of change (e.g., gradual vs. abrupt), range of change (e.g., small perturbation vs. drastic modifications), and change profile (e.g., monotonic increase vs. fluctuation) characterizing the nature of changes and their impact on cellular processes are subject to research effort, apparently adding to the complexity of the problem (Table 1). Take biodegradable material (e.g., [94]) as an example. It would be relevant to understand how mechanical and adhesive characteristics evolve with degradation and how the degradation profile affects the changes in the cellular micro-environment. Experimental design along this line may include, for example, different rates of release of RGD motif decreasing adhesiveness while keeping the same range of change (e.g., half of the total RGD presenting sites), or altering the range of change while maintaining the same rate of change. Furthermore, it is not clear at this point whether cellular responses to opposite changes (e.g., increase vs. decrease in adhesiveness or rigidity) of substrate properties are symmetric, thus their behavior to one direction of dynamic alterations may not be a reliable predictor of that to the opposite changes.

4.2. Potential effect on cell-cell interactions

Changes in adhesive or mechanical properties of ECM can stimulate cells, which, in response, secrete soluble factors and ECM molecules, and this further impacts neighboring cell types. Additionally, some cell types such as neurons may use other cells (e.g., astroglia) as substrate [95], and stiffness change of 'underlying' cells per se due to ECM stimulation may give rise to further alternations thanks to cell-cell interactions. For instance, during asthma, ECM stiffening contributes to stiffness increase of airway smooth muscle (ASM) cells, which potentially affects other cell types in the close proximity [33].

4.3. Design parameters for biomaterials and outlook

The design parameters of dynamic substrates from current studies are summarized in Table 2, which includes, but are not limited to, material system to consider (e.g., SAM or polymeric hydrogel materials), nature of change (mechanical stiffness or adhesion), rate of change (e.g., transient or gradual change, controllability of the rate of change), range of change (e.g., at different stiffness range) as well as potential issues in further investigations and applications to medical and healthcare applications. If the interest is in understanding the cellular behavior to mechanical stiffness alone, then an AFM based approach might be more attractive [84] as others will involve stress or strain as part of the stiffening or softening process. If precise control over stiffness range is desired, the DNA crosslinked PAM hydrogel system will serve the purpose better [20, 58, 81]. Polymeric hydrogel materials with controllable degradation profile and hence mechanical stiffness dynamics during degradation (e.g., [88]) will serve the purpose best when biodegradable materials are applied. Some of the material systems do offer unique benefits such as reversible property change or without using environmental factors (by applying oscillation, crosslinker, or ssDNA).

Meanwhile, there are inherent limitations to each of the material system under discussion (Table 2). UV exposure generally causes concern to its impact on cellular activities despite the findings of little impact from a number of studies based on a range of biological assays. Under physiological conditions, application of certain cues (e.g., ssDNA, light, or ion) might be too difficult or it might be greatly limited (e.g., temperature triggered changes). However, it is still possible to find ways to apply these cues with careful design. For instance, ssDNA design based on pre-screening using BLAST search against targeted specie or tissue type may minimize the chance of interfering with normal biological activities. Local heating/cooling may be carefully applied to induce dynamic changes to achieve cellular responses. Three dimensional system may better mimic natural cellular micro-environment than their 2D counter parts.

Stimuli	Material system	Nature of change	Range of change	Rate of change	Invasiveness of stimulus and potential issues	Ref.
Ion	Ion-crosslinked GC hydrogel	Stiffness	~22 to ~17 kPa (with chemical crosslinking)	N/A	Under physiological conditions, divalent ions exchanged by mono-valent ones	[88]
Light	Hydrogels based on PAM crosslinked by photosensitive agents	Softening	Stiffness: 5.5~7.2 kPa	Approximately 0.5~0.6 kPa/ min	UV exposure for 3 min UV radiation with low energy density Depth of penetration and limit on dose	[76]
	Methacrylated HA hydrogel	Stiffening Irreversible change	Stiffness: ~3 to ~30 kPa	Approximately 9 kPa/hr (short term); 2 kPa/day (long-term)	UV exposure for a few min Potential toxicity of photoinitiator Depth of penetration and limit on dose	[79]
	Photo-crosslinked methacrylated Gellan Gum hydrogel	Stiffness; Swelling Hydrolytic degradation	Stiffness: a few kPa to 22 kPa (by physical crosslinking)	Approximately 20 kPa/ min	UV exposure for one min Depth of penetration and limit on dose	[88]
	Methacrylated HA hydrogel with photo-crosslinker	Stiffness; Irreversible change	Stiffness: 1.6 to 3.8 kPa; 3-12 kPa	Approximately 0.1 or 0.3 kPa/min (during gelation)	UV exposure for a few min Potential toxicity of photo-initiator Depth of penetration and limit on dose	[80]
	PEG based hydrogel with photosensitive crosslinker	Stiffness↓ Adhesive property Irreversible change	N/A	N/A	Depth of penetration and limit on dose	[77]
DNA	DNA crosslinked PAM system	Stiffening & softening, potentially coupled with strain/stress Reversible change	Stiffness: ~5.9 to 22.9 kPa Stress > 0.5 Pa	Up to 8.5 kPa/ day	No differentiation in cellular responses between forces, stress, and stiffness Potentially interference from DNA with bio-activity (e.g., as anti-sense DNAs), and potential issue with DNase BLAST search against target specie & tissue type	[20, 81, 83]
AFM/ stiffness clamp	Piezo-controlled substrates and AFM stiffness clamp	Instantaneous change in stiffness Unidirectional	Stiffness: 3.6 to 90 nN/μm	Step change (instantane-ously)	Applicable only to cells with dynamic morphology	[84]
Hydro-lysis	Photo-crosslinked alginate hydrogel	Softening due to degradation	Stiffness: ~25 to ~180 kPa	7-8 kPa/ day	In sample preparation (with cells), UV exposure for 10 mins	[92]
	HA hydrogel	Stiffening & structure change	Stiffness: e.g., ~5 to 30 kPa for one case	0.7 kPa/ day	Dense crosslinking may impede cellular growth limited by diffusion& concentration of radicals	[78]
	PEG hydrogel (PEG vinyl sulfone	Softening due to degradation	Stiffness: from ~1 kPa-3 kPa to very low	From ~900 Pa/day to 500 Pa/day	Good cell viability Hydrogel degraded in 16 hours	[91]

Stimuli	Material system	Nature of change	Range of change	Rate of change	Invasiveness of stimulus and potential issues	Ref.
	crosslinked with PEG-diester-dithiol)					
Temperature	Thermo-reversible hydro-ferrogels (FGs)	Stiffening due to structural transition	Stiffness: ~28-24 kPa for 2ºC change at 37ºC	A few kPa for 1ºC of temperature change	Temperature change needs to be defined to be relevant to cell culture	[89]
	PEG-based hydrogel incorporating CMP*	Stiffness change Due to temperature and free CMP	Stiffness (indirect measurement)	N/A	Temperature change needs to be defined to be relevant to cell culture Bio-compatibility of free CMP	[90]
Oscillation	Resilin-like polypeptide based elastomer	Stiffness change due to oscillation	Storage modulus between 0.5 and 10 kPa	Highly dynamic	Strain/stress that is associated with oscillation	[86]

Note: N/A: not available; This is a partial list of the current work under examination.

Table 2. Design considerations in constructing dynamic substrates mimicking extra-cellular matrix (ECM).

A few new material system have been identified with the potential as dynamic cell culture platform as well as choice of biomaterials (Table 1). Many of them have demonstrated good cyto-compatibility, and investigation of impact of *in situ* changes to cells will be desired.

5. Concluding remarks

There is an increasing recognition of the discrepancy between static nature of the current cell culture substrates or scaffolds and the dynamics in ECM in natural or diseased tissue, during development and aging, or at tissue-scaffold interfaces. This has motivated the development of materials with controlled changing properties that mimic those of ECM. An array of stimuli, including environmental factors (temperature, pH, light, electrical potential) and non-environmental cues including enzyme and DNA, have been implemented to trigger dynamics in a number of material platform such as SAMs, polymeric hydrogels and other substrates with surface chemistry and modifications.

To date, most of the effort along this line has been devoted to *in vitro* models, and *in vivo* studies of the effect of dynamic tissue properties on cellular behavior are still rather limited, which awaits further development in cell biology and proper tools such as imaging techniques [12, 14, 29].

Understanding the interplay between cells and the extracellular matrix (ECM) including its dynamic aspect is fundamental to biology, development, aging and pathology, and can aid in the design of biomaterials. Ultimately, the system enabling both spatial and temporal control [96] of cells would be most relevant in terms of bio-mimicry and tissue engineering applications. Some of the potential directions include creating dynamic adhesive gradient to guide cell migration or neurite outgrowth at desired time point, constructing scaffolds with suitable mechanical rigidity to inhibit glia cell growth (thus hinder scar formation) while promoting nerve regeneration with compliance gradient, and developing dynamic platform for stem cell harvesting and differentiation for cell-based therapies.

Acknowledgments

The helpful discussions and advice from Langrana group at Rutgers University, New Jersey, USA as well as previous collaborators are greatly appreciated.

Author details

Frank Xue Jiang

Address all correspondence to: Frank.Jiang@unilever.com

Unilever Research & Development, Shanghai, P.R. China

Any opinions, findings, and conclusions or recommendations expressed in this material are those of the authors and do not necessarily reflect the views of the Unilever, its management or employees. The authors have no financial interest in this publication and receive nothing in exchange for providing this review.

References

[1] Keatch RP, Schor AM, Vorstius JB, Schor SL. Biomaterials in regenerative medicine: engineering to recapitulate the natural. Curr Opin Biotechnol 2012;23:579-582.

[2] Brizzi MF, Tarone G, Defilippi P. Extracellular matrix, integrins, and growth factors as tailors of the stem cell niche. Curr Opin Cell Biol 2012;(Epub).

[3] Cukierman E, Pankov R, Stevens DR, Yamada KM. Taking cell-matrix adhesions to the third dimension. Science 2001;294:1708-1712.

[4] Geiger B. Cell biology. Encounters in space. Science 2001;294:1661-1663.

[5] Discher DE, Mooney DJ, Zandstra PW. Growth factors, matrices, and forces combine and control stem cells. Science 2009;324:1673-1677.

[6]   Page H, Flood P, Reynaud EG. Three-dimensional tissue cultures: current trends and beyond. Cell Tissue Res 2012;(Epub).

[7]   Benjamin M, Hillen B. Mechanical influences on cells, tissues and organs - 'Mechanical Morphogenesis'. Eur J Morphol 2003;41:3-7.

[8]   Mammoto T, Ingber DE. Mechanical control of tissue and organ development. Development 2010;137:1407-1420.

[9]   Tee SY, Bausch AR, Janmey PA. The mechanical cell. Curr Biol 2009;19:R745-748.

[10] Zhu C, Bao G, Wang N. Cell mechanics: mechanical response, cell adhesion, and molecular deformation. Annu Rev Biomed Eng 2000;2:189-226.

[11] Lu P, Takai K, Weaver VM, Werb Z. Extracellular matrix degradation and remodeling in development and disease. Cold Spring Harb Perspect Biol 2011;3.

[12] Rozario T, Desimone DW. The extracellular matrix in development and morphogenesis: A dynamic view. Dev Biol 2010;341:126-140.

[13] Xu R, Boudreau A, Bissell MJ. Tissue architecture and function: dynamic reciprocity via extra- and intra-cellular matrices. Cancer Metastasis Rev 2009;28:167-176.

[14] Goody MF, Henry CA. Dynamic interactions between cells and their extracellular matrix mediate embryonic development. Mol Reprod Dev 2010;77:475–488.

[15] Godier AF, Marolt D, Gerecht S, Tajnsek U, Martens TP, Vunjak-Novakovic G. Engineered microenvironments for human stem cells. Birth Defects Res C Embryo Today 2008;84:335-347.

[16] Lahann J, Langer R. Smart Materials with Dynamically Controllable Surfaces. MRS Bulletin 2005;30:185-188.

[17] Mrksich M. Dynamic Substrates for Cell Biology. MRS BULLETIN 2005;30:180-184.

[18] Abbott NL, Gorman CB, Whitesides GM. Active Control of Wetting Using Applied Electrical Potentials and Self-Assembled Monolayers. Langmuir 1995;11:16-18.

[19] Yousaf MN, Houseman BT, Mrksich M. Using electroactive substrates to pattern the attachment of two different cell populations. Proc Natl Acad Sci U S A 2001;98:5992-5996.

[20] Jiang FX, Yurke B, Schloss RS, Firestein BL, Langrana NA. Effect of dynamic stiffness of the substrates on neurite outgrowth by using a DNA-crosslinked hydrogel. Tissue Eng Part A 2010;16:1873-1889.

[21] Peerani R, Zandstra PW. Enabling stem cell therapies through synthetic stem cell-niche engineering. J Clin Invest 2010;120:60-70.

[22] Dawson E, Mapili G, Erickson K, Taqvi S, Roy K. Biomaterials for stem cell differentiation. Adv Drug Deliv Rev 2008;60:215-228.

[23] Haq F, Keith C, Zhang G. Neurite development in PC12 cells on flexible micro-textured substrates under cyclic stretch. Biotechnol Prog 2006;22:133-140.

[24] Nicodemus GD, Bryant SJ. Mechanical loading regimes affect the anabolic and catabolic activities by chondrocytes encapsulated in PEG hydrogels. Osteoarthritis Cartilage 2010;18:126-137.

[25] Brown L. Cardiac extracellular matrix: a dynamic entity. Am J Physiol Heart Circ Physiol 2005;289:H973-974.

[26] Jung Y, Kim SH, Kim YH. The effects of dynamic and three-dimensional environments on chondrogenic differentiation of bone marrow stromal cells. Biomed Mater 2009;4:055009.

[27] Tschumperlin DJ, Boudreault F, Liu F. Recent advances and new opportunities in lung mechanobiology. J Biomech 2010;43:99-107.

[28] Gorstein F. The dynamic extracellular matrix. Hum Pathol 1988;19:751-752.

[29] Dallas SL, Chen Q, Sivakumar P. Dynamics of assembly and reorganization of extracellular matrix proteins. Curr Top Dev Biol 2006;75:1-24.

[30] Daley WP, Peters SB, Larsen M. Extracellular matrix dynamics in development and regenerative medicine. J Cell Sci 2008;121:255-264.

[31] Shi YB, Fu L, Hsia SC, Tomita A, Buchholz D. Thyroid hormone regulation of apoptotic tissue remodeling during anuran metamorphosis. Cell Res 2001;11:245-252.

[32] Sivakumar P, Czirok A, Rongish BJ, Divakara VP, Wang YP, Dallas SL. New insights into extracellular matrix assembly and reorganization from dynamic imaging of extracellular matrix proteins in living osteoblasts. J Cell Sci 2006;119:1350-1360.

[33] An SS, Kim J, Ahn K, Trepat X, Drake KJ, Kumar S, et al. Cell stiffness, contractile stress and the role of extracellular matrix. Biochem Biophys Res Commun 2009;382:697-703.

[34] Reilly GC, Engler AJ. Intrinsic extracellular matrix properties regulate stem cell differentiation. J Biomech 2010;43:55-62.

[35] Chen ZL, Indyk JA, Strickland S. The hippocampal laminin matrix is dynamic and critical for neuronal survival. Mol Biol Cell 2003;14:2665-2676.

[36] Coles JM, Zhang L, Blum JJ, Warman ML, Jay GD, Guilak F, et al. Loss of cartilage structure, stiffness, and frictional properties in mice lacking Prg4. Arthritis Rheum 2010;62:1666-1674.

[37] Kutty JK, Webb K. Tissue engineering therapies for the vocal fold lamina propria. Tissue Eng Part B Rev 2009;15:249-262.

[38] Siu MK, Cheng CY. Dynamic cross-talk between cells and the extracellular matrix in the testis. Bioessays 2004;26:978-992.

[39] Hui EE, Bhatia SN. Micromechanical control of cell-cell interactions. Proc Natl Acad Sci U S A 2007;104:5722-5726.

[40] Discher DE, Janmey P, Wang YL. Tissue cells feel and respond to the stiffness of their substrate. Science 2005;310:1139-1143.

[41] Yu H, Mouw JK, Weaver VM. Forcing form and function: biomechanical regulation of tumor evolution. Trends Cell Biol 2011;21:47-56.

[42] Zaman MH, Trapani LM, Sieminski AL, Mackellar D, Gong H, Kamm RD, et al. Migration of tumor cells in 3D matrices is governed by matrix stiffness along with cell-matrix adhesion and proteolysis. Proc Natl Acad Sci U S A 2006;103:10889-10894.

[43] Bharat S, Techavipoo U, Kiss MZ, Liu W, Varghese T. Monitoring stiffness changes in lesions after radiofrequency ablation at different temperatures and durations of ablation. Ultrasound Med Biol 2005;31:415-422.

[44] Walker GA, Masters KS, Shah DN, Anseth KS, Leinwand LA. Valvular myofibroblast activation by transforming growth factor-beta: implications for pathological extracellular matrix remodeling in heart valve disease. Circ Res 2004;95:253-260.

[45] Rabkin-Aikawa E, Farber M, Aikawa M, Schoen FJ. Dynamic and reversible changes of interstitial cell phenotype during remodeling of cardiac valves. J Heart Valve Dis 2004;13:841-847.

[46] Dobaczewski M, Gonzalez-Quesada C, Frangogiannis NG. The extracellular matrix as a modulator of the inflammatory and reparative response following myocardial infarction. J Mol Cell Cardiol 2010;48:504-511.

[47] Hachiya NS, Kozuka Y, Kaneko K. Mechanical stress and formation of protein aggregates in neurodegenerative disorders. Med Hypotheses 2008;70:1034-1037.

[48] Fallenstein GT, Hulce VD, Melvin JW. Dynamic mechanical properties of human brain tissue. J Biomech 1969;2:217-226.

[49] Latimer A, Jessen JR. Extracellular matrix assembly and organization during zebrafish gastrulation. Matrix Biol 2010;29:89-96.

[50] Silver FH, DeVore D, Siperko LM. Invited Review: Role of mechanophysiology in aging of ECM: effects of changes in mechanochemical transduction. J Appl Physiol 2003;95:2134-2141.

[51] Yamada O, Todoroki J, Takahashi T, Hashizume K. The dynamic expression of extracellular matrix in the bovine endometrium at implantation. J Vet Med Sci 2002;64:207-214.

[52] Marquez JP, Genin GM, Pryse KM, Elson EL. Cellular and matrix contributions to tissue construct stiffness increase with cellular concentration. Ann Biomed Eng 2006;34:1475-1482.

[53] Bellows CG, Melcher AH, Aubin JE. Contraction and organization of collagen gels by cells cultured from periodontal ligament, gingiva and bone suggest functional differences between cell types. J Cell Sci 1981;50:299-314.

[54] Lee B, Han L, Frank EH, Chubinskaya S, Ortiz C, Grodzinsky AJ. Dynamic mechanical properties of the tissue-engineered matrix associated with individual chondrocytes. J Biomech 2010;43:469-476.

[55] Appelman TP, Mizrahi J, Elisseeff JH, Seliktar D. The differential effect of scaffold composition and architecture on chondrocyte response to mechanical stimulation. Biomaterials 2009;30:518-525.

[56] Crapo PM, Wang Y. Physiologic compliance in engineered small-diameter arterial constructs based on an elastomeric substrate. Biomaterials 2010;31:1626-1635.

[57] Li L, Sharma N, Chippada U, Jiang X, Schloss R, Yarmush ML, et al. Functional modulation of ES-derived hepatocyte lineage cells via substrate compliance alteration. Ann Biomed Eng 2008;36:865-876.

[58] Jiang FX, Yurke B, Firestein BL, Langrana NA. Neurite outgrowth on a DNA cross-linked hydrogel with tunable stiffnesses. Ann Biomed Eng 2008;36:1565-1579.

[59] Ulijn RV, Bibi N, Jayawarna V, Thornton PD, Todd SJ, Mart RJ, et al. Bioresponsive hydrogels. Materials Today 2007;10:40-48.

[60] Robertus J, Browne WR, Feringa BL. Dynamic control over cell adhesive properties using molecular-based surface engineering strategies. Chem Soc Rev 2010;39:354-378.

[61] Mrksich M. Using self-assembled monolayers to model the extracellular matrix. Acta Biomater 2009;5:832-841.

[62] Nakanishi J, Kikuchi Y, Takarada T, Nakayama H, Yamaguchi K, Maeda M. Photoactivation of a substrate for cell adhesion under standard fluorescence microscopes. J Am Chem Soc 2004;126:16314-16315.

[63] Petersen S, Alonso JM, Specht A, Duodu P, Goeldner M, del Campo A. Phototriggering of cell adhesion by caged cyclic RGD peptides. Angew Chem Int Ed Engl 2008;47:3192-3195.

[64] Mendes PM. Stimuli-responsive surfaces for bio-applications. Chem Soc Rev 2008;37:2512-2529.

[65] Yeo WS, Yousaf MN, Mrksich M. Dynamic interfaces between cells and surfaces: electroactive substrates that sequentially release and attach cells. J Am Chem Soc 2003;125:14994-14995.

[66] Mrksich M. A surface chemistry approach to studying cell adhesion. Chem Soc Rev 2000;29:267 - 273.

[67] Yeo WS, Mrksich M. Electroactive self-assembled monolayers that permit orthogonal control over the adhesion of cells to patterned substrates. Langmuir 2006;22:10816-10820.

[68] Chan EW, Park S, Yousaf MN. An electroactive catalytic dynamic substrate that immobilizes and releases patterned ligands, proteins, and cells. Angew Chem Int Ed Engl 2008;47:6267-6271.

[69] Liu D, Xie Y, Shao H, Jiang X. Using azobenzene-embedded self-assembled monolayers to photochemically control cell adhesion reversibly. Angew Chem Int Ed Engl 2009;48:4406-4408.

[70] Nandivada H, Ross AM, Lahann J. Stimuli-responsive monolayers for biotechnology. Progress in Polymer Science 2010;35:141-154.

[71] Gillette BM, Jensen JA, Wang M, Tchao J, Sia SK. Dynamic hydrogels: switching of 3D microenvironments using two-component naturally derived extracellular matrices. Adv Mater 2010;22:686-691.

[72] Edahiro J, Sumaru K, Tada Y, Ohi K, Takagi T, Kameda M, et al. In situ control of cell adhesion using photoresponsive culture surface. Biomacromolecules 2005;6:970-974.

[73] Kim J, Yoon J, Hayward RC. Dynamic display of biomolecular patterns through an elastic creasing instability of stimuli-responsive hydrogels. Nat Mater 2010;9:159-164.

[74] Lutolf MP, Lauer-Fields JL, Schmoekel HG, Metters AT, Weber FE, Fields GB, et al. Synthetic matrix metalloproteinase-sensitive hydrogels for the conduction of tissue regeneration: engineering cell-invasion characteristics. Proc Natl Acad Sci U S A 2003;100:5413-5418.

[75] Baker BM, Nerurkar NL, Burdick JA, Elliott DM, Mauck RL. Fabrication and modeling of dynamic multipolymer nanofibrous scaffolds. J Biomech Eng 2009;131:101012.

[76] Frey MT, Wang YL. A photo-modulatable material for probing cellular responses to substrate rigidity. Soft Matter 2009;5:1918-1924.

[77] Kloxin AM, Benton JA, Anseth KS. In situ elasticity modulation with dynamic substrates to direct cell phenotype. Biomaterials 2010;31:1-8.

[78] Chung C, Beecham M, Mauck RL, Burdick JA. The influence of degradation characteristics of hyaluronic acid hydrogels on in vitro neocartilage formation by mesenchymal stem cells. Biomaterials 2009;30:4287-4296.

[79] Guvendiren M, Burdick JA. Stiffening hydrogels to probe short- and long-term cellular responses to dynamic mechanics. Nat Commun 2012;3:792.

[80] Hachet E, Van Den Berghe H, Bayma E, Block MR, Auzely-Velty R. Design of Biomimetic Cell-Interactive Substrates Using Hyaluronic Acid Hydrogels with Tunable Mechanical Properties. Biomacromolecules 2012;(Epub).

[81] Jiang FX, Yurke B, Schloss RS, Firestein BL, Langrana NA. The relationship between fibroblast growth and the dynamic stiffnesses of a DNA crosslinked hydrogel. Biomaterials 2010;31:1199-1212.

[82] Huang S, Ingber DE. Cell tension, matrix mechanics, and cancer development. Cancer Cell 2005;8:175-176.

[83] Previtera ML, Trout KL, Verma D, Chippada U, Schloss RS, Langrana NA. Fibroblast morphology on dynamic softening of hydrogels. Ann Biomed Eng 2012;40:1061-1072.

[84] Webster KD, Crow A, Fletcher DA. An AFM-based stiffness clamp for dynamic control of rigidity. PLoS One 2011;6:e17807.

[85] Shah S, Lee JY, Verkhoturov S, Tuleuova N, Schweikert EA, Ramanculov E, et al. Exercising spatiotemporal control of cell attachment with optically transparent microelectrodes. Langmuir 2008;24:6837-6844.

[86] Li L, Teller S, Clifton RJ, Jia X, Kiick KL. Tunable mechanical stability and deformation response of a resilin-based elastomer. Biomacromolecules 2011;12:2302-2310.

[87] Kurniawan NA, Wong LH, Rajagopalan R. Early stiffening and softening of collagen: interplay of deformation mechanisms in biopolymer networks. Biomacromolecules 2012;13:691-698.

[88] Coutinho DF, Sant SV, Shin H, Oliveira JT, Gomes ME, Neves NM, et al. Modified Gellan Gum hydrogels with tunable physical and mechanical properties. Biomaterials 2010;31:7494-7502.

[89] Krekhova M, Lang T, Richter R, Schmalz H. Thermoreversible hydroferrogels with tunable mechanical properties utilizing block copolymer mesophases as template. Langmuir 2010;26:19181-19190.

[90] Stahl PJ, Romano NH, Wirtz D, Yu SM. PEG-based hydrogels with collagen mimetic peptide-mediated and tunable physical cross-links. Biomacromolecules 2011;11:2336-2344.

[91] Zustiak SP, Leach JB. Hydrolytically degradable poly(ethylene glycol) hydrogel scaffolds with tunable degradation and mechanical properties. Biomacromolecules 2010;11:1348-1357.

[92] Jeon O, Bouhadir KH, Mansour JM, Alsberg E. Photocrosslinked alginate hydrogels with tunable biodegradation rates and mechanical properties. Biomaterials 2009;30:2724-2734.

[93] Mano JF. Stimuli-Responsive Polymeric Systems for Biomedical Applications. Advanced Engineering Materials 2008;10:515-527.

[94] Kim S, Chung EH, Gilbert M, Healy KE. Synthetic MMP-13 degradable ECMs based on poly(N-isopropylacrylamide-co-acrylic acid) semi-interpenetrating polymer networks. I. Degradation and cell migration. J Biomed Mater Res A 2005;75:73-88.

[95] Lu YB, Franze K, Seifert G, Steinhauser C, Kirchhoff F, Wolburg H, et al. Viscoelastic properties of individual glial cells and neurons in the CNS. Proc Natl Acad Sci U S A 2006;103:17759-17764.

[96] Yousaf MN. Model substrates for studies of cell mobility. Curr Opin Chem Biol 2009;13:697-704.

Biocompatibility Studies

Chapter 5

Overview on Biocompatibilities of Implantable Biomaterials

Xiaohong Wang

Additional information is available at the end of the chapter

1. Introduction

A biomaterial is any material that comprises whole or part of a living structure or biomedical device which performs, augments, or replaces a natural function to improve the quality of life of the patients [1]. Over the past fifty years biomaterials has been developed as a science with various forms of implants/medical devices, and have been widely used to replace and/or restore the function of traumatized or degenerated tissues or organs. As a life-saving and life-improving option for countless patients, biomaterials have been paid more and more attention during the last decade. Only in the United States, more than 13 million implant/medical devices implanted annually. As a result, the impact factor of the journal of "Biomaterials" has boomed from 2.489 to 7.404 from the year 2001 to 2012.

The implant/medical device scope of biomaterials ranges from simple implants like intraocular lenses (which restore sight to millions of cataract patients every year), sutures, wound dressings, decellular matrices, bone plates, joint replacements to more complex materials like biosensors, catheters, pacemakers, blood vessels, artificial heart (that provide both mechanical and biological functions in a body), left ventricular assist devices and prosthetic arterial grafts. According to the resources and properties biomaterials can be assorted into autografts, allografts, organic polymers, such as natural collagen, fibrin, chitosan, hyaluronan, heparin, cellulose, and synthetic polyurethane (PU), polyester, metal, such as aluminium, steel, titanium, inorganic salts, such as calcium phosphate, hydroxyapatite, and their compounds or derivatives. There are more than one hundred different biomaterials which have been applied *in vivo*. All biomaterials when implanted into a body initiate a host response that reflects the first steps of tissue repair. The host/biomaterial interactions which follow implantation of any prosthesis or device are a series of complex events that have not been well defined. Generally, host reactions following implantation of biomaterials include injury, blood–material interactions, provisional matrix formation, acute inflammation, chronic inflammation, granulation tissue development, foreign body reaction, and fibrosis/fibrous capsule development [2]. There are numerous types of host responses to a broad spectrum of biomaterials.

When considering a biomaterial for implantation or medical use, the first and most important requirement is nontoxic, nonimmunogenic, chemically inert/active, and acceptable by the human body. Biocompatible in most cases means that the biomaterials must not form thrombi in the blood system, result in tumors in the surround tissues, or be immediately attacked, encapsulated, or rejected by the body [3]. According to the host responses to implantable biomaterials, there are many different kinds of biocompatibilities, including local tissue responses, such as necrosis, repulsion, infection, inflammation, calcification, scar, cyst, amalgamation, thrombus, tumor, cancer, and whole body responses, such as fever, toxicity, circulation impediment, nerve anesthesia, malformation, etc. The overall biocompatibilities including cyto-compatibility, hemo-compatibility, and tissue-compatibility, are often evaluated using histological sections, cell markers, and metabolite measurements. Sometimes, polymers with similar chemical characteristics behave differently in certain situations. For example, polyethylene and ultrahigh molecular weight polyethylene behave differently as orthopedic biomaterials for knee and hip replacement [4]. Until present, most of the implantable biomaterials trigger acute or/and chronic inflammatory responses in the body. These reactions can totally black a biomaterial and even lead to huge disasters or personal misfortunes. Among the numerous types of host responses, early interactions between implants and inflammatory cells are probably mediated by a layer of host proteins on the biomaterial surface. Franz and coworkers have described several typical host responses of implantable biomaterials (Figure 1) [5]. This model can be used as a reference for evaluation of an implantable biomaterial when it is implanted shortly *in vivo*.

In this chapter, I will focus on the *in vivo* host responses about twenty common used biomaterials which cover nearly every tissue and organ in human body. Advanced biologic techniques have been employed in determining the mechanisms behind observed macroscopic or microscopic responses. An understanding of the molecular and cellular events which occur in response to implantable biomaterials may allow us to manipulate responses and design more biocompatible, bioactive and functional biomaterials for clinical applications, such as regenerative medicine and controlled releasing drugs.

2. Allografts

Allograft (also called homograft) is a tissue/organ graft from one individual to another of the same species with a different genotype [6]. It has been successfully used in various medical procedures for more than 150 years. Approximately 1500000 allografts are transplanted each year for a variety of life-saving and life-enhancing surgeries. For example, skeletal grafts for patients with bone defects from cancer or traffic accidents; cornea transplants to help restore sight; heart valves to replace damaged heart tissues; skin grafts to save the lives of burn victims, and tendon replacements to help people with more active lives [7].

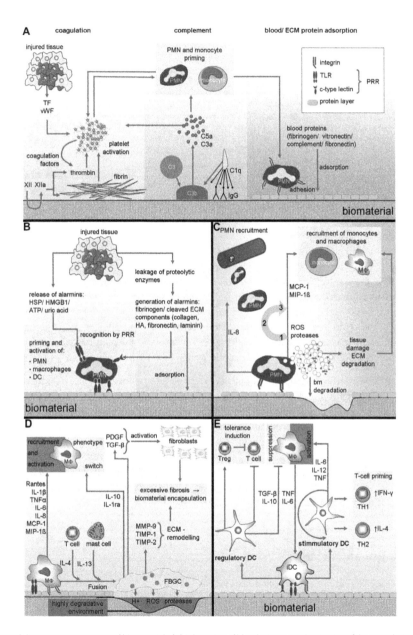

Figure 1. Immune response toward biomaterials. (A) Adsorption of blood proteins and activation of the coagulation cascade, complement and platelets result in the priming and activation of polymorphonuclear leukocytes (PMNs), monocytes and resident macrophages. (B) Danger signals (alarmins) released from damaged tissue additionally prime the immune

cells for enhanced function via pattern recognition receptor (PRR) engagement. (C) The acute inflammatory response is dominated by the action of PMNs. PMNs secrete proteolytic enzymes and reactive oxygen species (ROS), corroding the biomaterial surface. Interleukin (IL)-8 released from PMNs enhances PMN influx and priming. In the transition from acute to chronic inflammation, PMNs stop secreting IL-8 in favor of cytokines promoting immigration and activation of monocytes and macrophages. (D) Macrophages are the driving force of chronic inflammation. Constant release of inflammatory mediators like tumor-nekrose-faktor alpha (TNFα), IL-6, and monocyte chemotactic protein (MCP)-1 results in permanent activation of macrophages. Fusion-inducing stimuli like IL-4 and IL-13 promote the fusion of macrophages to foreign body giant cells (FBGCs,) which form a highly degradable environment on the biomaterial surface. Furthermore, FBGC promote extracellular matrix (ECM) remodeling and fibroblast activation resulting in excessive fibrosis and biomaterial encapsulation. (E) Macrophage-derived cytokines and pattern recognition receptor engagement activate dendritic cells (DCs) on the biomaterial surface. Depending on the nature of the stimulus, DCs mature to either immunogenic or tolerogenic subtypes, amplifying or suppressing the inflammatory response [5].

Compared with autografts which come from the same bodies and are only available in limited amounts, allografts are more readily available and accompany with less risk and postoperative morbidity. The healing times is therefore shorter and less painful for a patient with no second surgical site is required (as there is when an autograft is utilised). Currently, the use of allograft tissues is increasingly popular all over the world, with widespread orthopaedic surgeons and debilitating musculoskeletal conditions. Nearly one tissue/organ donor can save or improve the lives of up to 60 people. Especially, Musculoskeletal Transplant Foundation, the world's largest tissue bank, provides allograft tissue and biologic solutions for ligament reconstruction [8]. Meanwhile bone and soft tissue allografts from the Steri-Graft™ line has been in existence for over 13 years and has helped doctors and their patients with over one hundred thousand successful transplantations. Before transplantation, a blood sample from the donor is normally tested in case any infected diseases, such as human immunodeficiency virus (HIV), Hepatitis, and Syphilis [9].

Specially, decellularized tissue/organ matrices derived from allografts have been used since the 1940s to support tissue repair and replacement. Their popularity has grown sharply during the last decade with the advent of tissue engineering [10]. At present, decellularized tissues/organs have been successfully used in a variety of tissue/organ regenerative medicines. The efficiency of cell removal from a tissue/organ is dependent on the origin of the tissue/organ and the specific physical, chemical, and enzymatic methods that are used. Each of these treatments affects the biochemical composition, tissue ultrastructure, and mechanical behavior of the remaining extracellular matrix (ECM) scaffold, which in turn, affect the host response to the material [11].

3. Collagen and gelatin

Collagen is one of the most prevalent proteins in the connective tissue of animals and constitutes approximately 25% of total body protein in vertebrates. It therefore is an important biomaterial in medical, dental, and pharmacological fields. After the immunogens in the collagen molecules are dislodged, collagen has excellent biocompatibilities either *in vitro* or *in vivo*. Collagen is capable of being cross-linked into solid or lattice-like gels. Resorbable forms of collagen have been used to dress oral, skin or some of the other soft tissue wounds, for closure of graft and extraction sites, and to promote healing [12]. During *in vivo* implantation, collagen irritates slight inflammation accompanying with some scar tissues.

A collagen sponge obtained from Beijing Yierkang Biengineering Development Center China was implanted subcutaneously in rats for time periods up to 8 weeks (Figure 2) [13]. One week after implantation, slight inflammation with some lymphocytes, myofibrils and fibroblasts were observed. The appearance of myofibrils and fibroblasts indicated that scar tissue was developed (Figure 2A). Two weeks after implantation, fibrous tissue was formed with scattered macrophage and lymphocyte cells in the fibrous layer. Newly formed blood vessels appeared in the implant site while the collagen sponges were completely resorbed (Figure 2B). Four weeks after implantation, the thin fiber layer had changed into wavelike scar tissue and tightly connected with the surrounding muscles. Capillaries were evident in the new fibrous scars (Figure 2C). Six weeks after implantation, scar tissue in the collagen samples was mature (Figure 2D). Eight weeks after implantation, the wave-like scar tissue in the collagen samples became thinner with some lipocytes and vacuoles (Figure 2E) [13].

Collagen compounds, such as collagen/chitosan, collagen/hyaluronan, have been investigated extensively during the past several decades. The biocompatibilities of these compounds depend largely on the incorporated constituents. For example, a corneal collagen crosslinked with riboflavin and ultraviolet radiation-A has been used for keratoconus repair of a 29-year-old woman with some good results [14]. In some instances, it is more competing to use a compound to improve the mechanical properties of the collagen based biomaterials. For example, a porous implantable dexamethasone-loaded polylactide-co-glycolide (PLGA) microspheres/collagen glucose sensors [15] and a mitomycin C (MMC) delivery system (MMC-film), incorporating polylactide (PLA)–MMC nanoparticles in a composite film from blends of collagen–chitosan–soybean phosphatidylcholine (SPC) with a mass ratio of 4:1:1 have been explored with no sign of internal infection and fibrous encapsulation in any animals after 20 days of implantation [16].

Gelatin is a mixture of peptides/proteins produced by partial hydrolysis of collagen extracted from the skin, boiled crushed bones, connective tissues, organs and some intestines of animals such as domesticated cattle, chicken, horses hooves, and pigs [17]. Gelatin possesses a better biocompatibility than its ancestry collagen. Alloimplants of bone matrix gelatin are effective in the treatment of bone defects with a low risk of complication such as rejection or infection [18]. Aqueous gelatin solution is an amorphous natural hydrogel in which cells can be encapsulated, extruded and deposited at desired positions. Unlike collagen hydrogel, gelatin hydrogel holds a special gelation property around 20°C. In Tsinghua University the author's own group, this property has been explored extensively for rapid prototyping (RP) (or additive manufacturing) of three-dimensional (3D) complex geometrical structures with computer-aided design channel models [19-24]. Until now, a hybrid hierarchical 3D construct consisting both synthetic polyurethane PU and natural cell/ gelatin-based hydrogel with interconnected macro-channels has been produced via a double nozzle RP technique at a low temperature (-28°C). These constructs have demonstrated excellent in vivo biocompatibilities [23,25]. This technique holds the potential to be widely used in the future complex tissue/organ manufacturing areas.

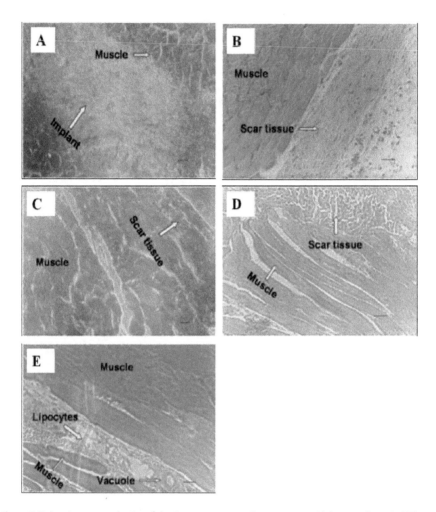

Figure 2. Light-microscope evaluation of the tissue response to collagen sponges with hamatoxylin-eosin (HE) staining: (A) 1 week after implantation; (B) 2 weeks after implantation; (C) 4 weeks after implantation; (D) 6 weeks after implantation; (E) 8 weeks after implantation. The scale bar indicates a distance of 50μm in (A), (C), and (D), and a 25μm in (B) and (E) [13].

Combination of gelatin microspheres/scaffolds with other biomaterials, such as collagen, alginate, chitosan, hyaluronan, and fibrin has also been explored extensively. For example, a gelatin microsphere containing basic fibroblast growth factor and preadipocytes, is essential to achieve a engineered fat tissue [26]. A PLGA microparticles containing an anticancer agent paclitaxel was formulated for the treatment of lung cancers [27]. Gelatin hydrogel incorporating hepatocyte growth factor induced angiogenic change around the implanted hydrogel [28]. A silk fibroin/gelatin composite scaffold was implanted into subcutaneous pockets on male Sprague-Dawley rats with a slight inflammation reaction. By day 30, the scaffold had been completely infiltrated and organized by fibroblasts and inflamed cells. The greater the gelatin concentration in the scaffold, the faster the degradation rate [29].

4. Fibrin

Fibrin (also called Factor Ia) is a fibrous, non-globular protein involved in the clotting of blood. It is formed from fibrinogen by the protease thrombin, and is then polymerised to form a hemostatic plug or clot (in conjunction with platelets) over a wound site [30]. The clot fibrin can be naturally degraded by proteolytic enzymes from the fibrinolytic system, such as plasmin [31,32]. *In vivo*, fibrin(ogen) plays an important role in hemostasis, inflammation, signal transduction, platelet activation, wound healing, osteoinductive and angiogenesis [33-36]. The food and drug administration (FDA) in American has approved commercially made fibrin sealants in 1998 [37].

During the last decade, autologous fibrin-based matrices have demonstrated great potential as being used as tissue engineered replacements, such as heart valves [38-40], cartilages [41], and blood vessels [42]. Immunohistochemistry and ECM assay demonstrated that the fibrin scaffolds can be completely absorbed *in vivo* in about 3 months with low granulomatous inflammation (Figure 3) [43-46]. Farhat and coworkers have evaluated whether a fibrin glue spray technique enhances cell seeded acellular matrix (ACM) repopulation in a porcine bladder model. The *in vivo* central fibrosis results indicated that while fibrin glue enhanced cellular organization on ACM *in vitro*, factors supporting seeded cell survival are lacking [47].

On the other hand, spatio-temporal controlled delivery of bioactive molecules within fibrin has been expanded rapidly. Various states of fibrin, such as scaffold, sheets, microparticles and fibrin-coated drug particles have been used as drug delivery systems [48,49]. Growth factors, such as vascular endothelial growth factor (VEGF) and transforming growth factor-β (TGF-β) can easily bind to the fibrin molecules and be controlled released subsequently by diffusion [50-56]. In the future, autologous fibrin may play an important role in customized clinical applications, such as anti-immune drug delivery systems and human tissue/organ constructions to avoid any negative host reactions [57].

5. Dextran and its derivatives

Dextran, a high-molecular-weight polymer of d-glucose, formed by sucrose enzymes on the cell surface of certain lactic acid bacteria in the mouth adhere to the tooth surfaces and produce dental plaque. Uniform molecular weight dextrans (named for their average molecular weight) from Leuconostoc mesenteroides with specific preparations has been used for over 50 years in plasma volume expansion, thrombosis prophylaxis, peripheral blood flow enhancement and for the rheological improvement of, for instance, artificial tears [30,58]. Dextrans with an average molecular weight of 1000 to 2 million g/mol are commercially available for research purposes [59]. Two preparations of dextran with lower fractions (40000 and 70000 g/mol) are suitable for nontoxic clinical use [60]. However, high fractions of dextrans can produce erythrocyte aggregation, impaired microcirculation, and a clinical picture akin to shock and certain other diseases.

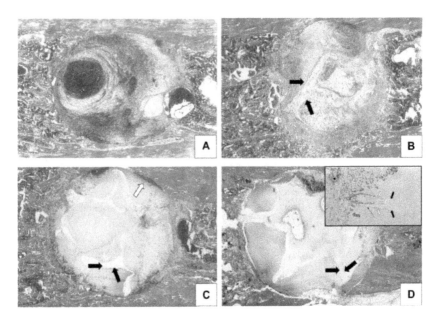

Figure 3. Eleven-day Masson's trichrome (MT) staining sections of a fibrin scaffold. (A) Untreated defects and (B) defects containing empty scaffolds were filled with new bone tissue. However, no reparative bone was observed in the center of defects containing (C) scaffolds filled with fibrin (low T) and (D) scaffolds filled with fibrin (high T). (Inset) Patches of multinucleated giant cells (striped arrow) were observed at the scaffold interface in all scaffold-containing groups. Black arrows point to areas occupied by the scaffold, whereas white arrows point to the advancing bone front. Field width 5.2 mm, inset field width 0.2 mm [46].

During 1990-1994, extensive toxicologic evaluations indicate that small-volume infusions of 7.5% NaCl/6% dextran 70 (HSD) at the proposed therapeutic dose of 4 mL/kg, present little risk as implantable biomaterials [61,62]. Dextran hydrogels have offered good opportunities as protein delivery systems or tissue engineering scaffolds because of an inherent biocompatibility [63]. The hydrophilic, soft and rubbery properties of the dextran hydrogels ensure minimal tissue irritation and a low tendency of cells and proteins to adhere to the hydrogel surface [59]. Althogh dextran itself is not toxic, some of the methods used for crosslinking the polymer may result in toxic byproducts. For example, the toxicity of dialdehyde crosslinked dextran/gelatin hydrogel can be detected in fibroblast and endothelial cell cultures. Subcutaneous implantation studies in mice showed that the foreign body reaction seen around the implanted hydrogel samples was moderate and became minimal upon increasing implantation time [64]. A methacrylate-derivatized dextran hydrogel also shows good *in vitro* biocompatibilities [65].

More recently another effect of dextran, namely that of antithrombogenesis, has been recognized [66]. Dextran sulfate, a dextran derivative, its effects on coagulation has already been proven [67]. It has been reported that dextran sulfate has been found to activate the polymerization of fibrin monomer, ATIII, conversion of prekallikrein to kallikreinand fibrinolysis. Kallikrein, the conversion of fibrinogen to fibrin appears to be inhibited by dextran sulfate. These effects are, *inter alia*, concentration dependent [67,68]. Meanwhile, a dextran sulphate sodium model of colitis has demonstrated several correlations of this biomaterial with human inflammatory bowel disease [69]. Furthermore, a lauric acid modified dextran-agmatine bioconjugate (Dex-L-Agm) was prepared by 1,1'-carbonyldiimidazole activation and the nucleophilic reaction between tosyl of tosylated dextran and primary amine of agmatine was found to be highly cytocompatible without causing hemolysis and red blood cell aggregation [70].

6. Hyaluronan

Hyaluronan (also called hyaluronic acid or hyaluronate, HA) is a natural anionic, viscoelastic and hygroscopic glycosaminoglycan, discovered in 1934, by Karl Meyer and his assistant, John Palmer in the vitreous of bovine eyes [71]. As one of the chief components of the ECM, hyaluronan distributes widely throughout connective, epithelial, and neural tissues. It is unique among glycosaminoglycans in that it is nonsulfated, forms in the plasma membrane instead of the Golgi, and can be very large in molecular weight (often reaching the millions) [72]. HA plays several important organizational roles in the ECM by binding with cells and other protein components through specific and nonspecific interactions [73] and is responsible for various functions within the ECM such as cell growth, proliferation, differentiation, migration [74], and even some malignant tumors [76].

Basically hyaluronan is a highly non-toxic, non-antigenic and non-immunogenic polysaccharide, owing to its high structural homology across species, and poor interaction with blood components [77,78]. The FDA in American has approved the use of hyaluronic acid for certain eye surgeries, such as cataract removal, corneal transplantation, and detached retina [79]. People take hyaluronic acid for various joint disorders (lubricant agents), lip fillers, "youth fountains", and even wound healing catalysts [80]. Nowadays various hyaluronan hydrogels have been used to delivery drugs and cell growth factors [81,82]. There are some evidence show that fragmented hyaluronan stimulates the expression of inflammatory genes by a variety of immune cells at the injury site. With the protein-bonding abilities, hyaluronan fragments signal through both Toll-like receptor (TLR) 4 and TLR2 as well as CD44 to stimulate inflammatory genes in inflammatory cells. Hyaluronan presents on the epithelial cell surface can provide protection against tissue damage from the environment by interacting with TLR2 and TLR4 [83-85]. It is well known that accumulation and turnover of ECM components are the hallmarks of tissue injury. Current model of hyaluronic acid appear in the early stages of wound healing is to physically make room for white blood cells, which mediate the immune response and at least in part, reduce collagen deposition and therefore lead to reduced scarring [86]. This hypothesis is in agreement with the research of West and coworkers, who have showed that in adult and late gestation fetal wound healing process, removal of HA results in fibrotic scarring [87].

HA can be modified through several different ways, such as chemically esterify its carboxylic groups with some types of alcohol. The physico-chemical properties of the new biopolymers allow the preparation of many biomaterials with different biocompatibilities for various medical applications [88]. Shen and coworkers implanted hyaluronan hydrogel and periodate oxidated hyaluronan hydrogel in ischemic myocardium and found rapid degradation rates, low quantity of inflammation-mediating cells, thin fibrous capsules with dense blood vessels around the hydrogels at week 2 [89]. Praveen and coworkers used HA/polyvinyl alcohol (PVA) coating membrane to minimize the problems related to protein deposition and fibrous tissue formation on an implanted glucose sensor [90]. HA hydrogels modified with laminin could support cell infiltration, angiogenesis, and simultaneously inhibit the formation of glial scar after being implanted into the lesion of the cortex [91]. Compared with pure gelatin hydrogen, HA/gelatin composite has a better compatibility and contiguity with the surrounding brain tissue with no inflammatory reaction and fibrous encapsulation [92]. Intravitreal implants of hyaluronic acid esters represent useful biocompatible and biodegradable properties for a potential drug delivery system in the treatment of posterior segment ocular diseases [93]. A crosslinked HA hydrogel that contained a covalently bound derivative of the anti-proliferative drug MMC was synthesized and evaluated *in vitro* and *in vivo*. This hydrogel has strong potential as anti-fibrotic barriers for the prevention of post-surgical adhesions [94]. Two injectable thiolated HA derivatives were coupled to four alpha, beta-unsaturated ester and amide derivatives of poly(ethylene glycol) (PEG) 3400 and were found that the encapsulated cells can retained their original fibroblast phenotype and secreted ECM in vivo [95]. A fibrin/HA composite gel with autologous chondrocytes has been synthesized for tracheal reconstruction. Histologically, the grafts showed no signs of inflammatory reaction and were covered with ciliated epithelium [96].

7. Heparin

Heparin (from Ancient Greek ηπαρ (hepar), liver), a highly sulfated glycosaminoglycan, is widely used as an injectable anticoagulant, and has the highest negative charge density of any known biological molecule [97]. Heparins are involved in different pathways of the coagulation cascade with anticoagulant, antithrombotic, profibrinolytic, anti-aggregative, as well as anti-inflammatory effects [98]. As stated in the fibrin section, the primary anticoagulant effect of heparin is through the suppression of thrombin-dependent amplification of the coagulation cascade, and inhibition of thrombin-mediated conversion of fibrinogen to fibrin [99].

Heparin holds the ability to relieve pain, inhibit clotting and inflammation, restore blood flow, enhance healing, and can be a useful addition to a range of available treatments for burn wounds [100]. Unfractioned heparin exhibits a broad spectrum of immunomodulating and anti-inflammatory properties, by inhibiting the recruitment of neutrophils and reducing pro-inflammatory cytokines in the treatment of inflammatory bowel disease [101]. Low-molecular-weight heparin can reduce or prevent development of signs/symptoms associated with post-thrombotic syndrome [102]. Heparin has been widely used to form an inner anti-coagulant surface on various experimental and medical devices such as membranes [103,104], tubes and renal dialysis machines [105,106].

Although heparin is used principally in medicine for anticoagulation, its true physiological role in the body remains unclear. Blood anti-coagulation is usually achieved by heparan sulfate proteoglycans which derive from endothelial cells stored within the secretory granules of mast cells and only released into the vasculature at sites of tissue injury [107]. Rather than anticoagulation, the main role of heparin may be defense at such sites against invading bacteria and other foreign materials [108]. A thiol-modified heparin in the Extracel-HP® mimics heparan sulfate proteoglycans also normally presents in the ECM and regulates the *in vivo* growth factor release for a functional microvessel network development [109]. A well-known adverse effect of heparin therapy is thrombocytopenia, a serious, immune system-mediated complication with significant mortality (Figure 4) [110-112].

8. Alginate

Alginate, is a salt of alginic acid (medical-dictionary.thefreedictionary.com), and an anionic polysaccharide distributed widely in the cell walls of brown algae, where it, through binding water, forms a viscous gum (Wikipedia, the free encyclopedia). Sodium alginate (composed of mannuronic and guluronic (G) dimmers) is a biocompatible and biodegradable polymer, and has been widely used in cell encapsulation technology, though the biocompatibility of the alginates in relation to their composition is a matter of debate [113]. In the molecules of sodium alginate the primary block guluronic acid contains available carboxylic acid groups that allow the alginate to be reversibly crosslinked by divalent cations, such as Ca^{+2} and Mg^{+2}, to form a relatively stable hydrogel [114,115]. Clinically, water-soluble alginates are useful as materials for dental impressions. Calcium alginates have been widely used as a base material to encapsulate glucose-sensing pancreatic islets that secrete insulin into the lymphatic system to reverse the effects of insulin-dependent diabetics [116]. Some investigators have utilized alginates to promote the viability of encapsulated cells [117]. Alginate-poly-L-lysine-alginate (APA) microcapsules continue to be the most widely studied device for the immuno-protection of transplanted therapeutic cells [118]. Alginate-chitosan-alginate (ACA) microcapsules have been developed as a device for the transplantation of living cells with protein adsorption onto the surface of microcapsules immediately upon implantation [119].

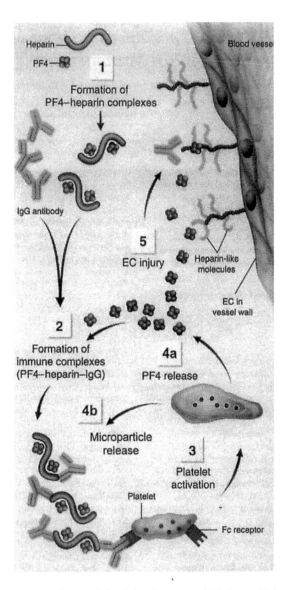

Figure 4. Model of pathogenesis of heparin-induced thrombocytopenia (HIT). Heparin binds with Platelet factor 4 (PF4), which exposes neoepitopes on PF4 and leads to antibody production (1). Heparin-PF4-IgG immune complexes form (2), and IgG in multimolecular complex triggers platelet activation via binding to Fc receptors (3). Activated platelet releases additional PF4 (4a) and prothrombotic platelet microparticles (4b). Thrombotic risk is further promoted by binding of PF4 to heparin-like molecules on endothelial cells (EC), contributing to immune system–mediated endothelial damage (5) [112].

9. Chitin, chitosan and their derivatives

Chitosan is a naturally occurring linear polysaccharide, consisting of glucosamine and N-acetyl-glucosamine, normally made of deacetylated chitin which is the structural polymer found in the shells of crabs and shrimp (lobster, squid, some yeast and mould), by N-deacetylation using strong alkali [120]. More than 40 years have lapsed since this biomaterial had aroused the interest of the scientific community around the world for its potential biomedical applications [121]. Until now chitosan possess a number of commercial and biomedical applications in wound dressing, drug delivery and tissue engineering. For example, chitosan based scaffold biomaterials have demonstrated versatile properties to promote the epithelial and soft tissue regeneration in the body [122,123]. Chitosan patches in various sizes that have been cleared by the FDA are a topical hemostat for moderating severe bleeding. Nevertheless, an obvious disadvantage of this implantable, absorbable biomaterial is that chitosan initiates serious host inflammation reactions (Figure 5) [13,124]. Additionally, chitosan is bioadhesive and has the ability to transiently open tight junctions in the nasal epithelia, thereby permitting drugs to diffuse through this barrier. Advantages of this nasal route of administration include: a higher permeability of the nasal mucosa than in the gastrointestinal tract; a low degree of pre-systemic metabolism; and a high level of patient compliance, compared to injectable systems [125].

It is very interesting that when the number of N-acetyl-glucosamine units in a chitin/chitosan mixture is higher than 50%, the biopolymer is termed chitin. 50% deacetylated chitosan has a less inflammation reaction than the others when they are implanted *in vivo* [126]. Cross-linking of chitosan membrane using genipin and some other chemical agents can increase the membrane's ultimate tensile strength but significantly reduced its strain-at-fracture and swelling ratio [127]. In the author's own group, an ammonia treated chitosan sponge was implanted subcutaneously in rats for 8 weeks (Figure 5). One week after implantation, the chitosan sponges were entirely retained and wrapped with a layer of purulent cells. The purulent cells had infiltrated the outside chitosan sponges (Figure 5A). Two weeks after implantation, the encapsulated purulent layer was enlarged at the periphery of chitosan sponges. More acute inflammatory cells had infiltrated the chitosan sponges and there was no sign of biodegradation of the chitosan sponges (Figure 5B). Four weeks after implantation, the chitosan sponges still maintained their porous structure. A much thicker purulent layer and more acute inflammatory cells were found around or in the chitosan sponges (Figure 5C). Six weeks after implantation, most of the chitosan still maintained their scaffold integrity with numerous interspersed purulent cells. Some purulent cells even formed large channels throughout the chitosan sponges (Figure 5D). Eight weeks after implantation, purulent cell infiltrations had further increased in the chitosan sponges. Some collapsed matrix structures were detected at the outer margins of the implants and more channel structures were found between the remnants of chitosan lamellae (Figure 5E).

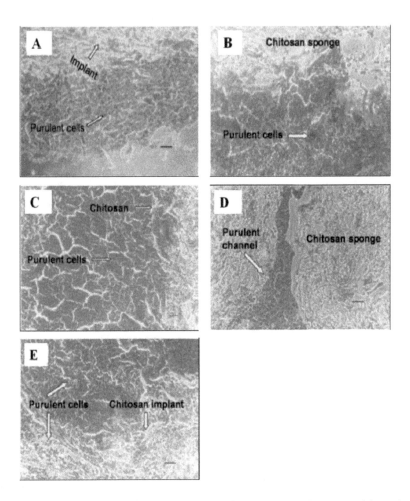

Figure 5. Light-microscope evaluation of the tissue response to chitosan sponges with HE staining: (A) 1 week after implantation; (B) 2 weeks after implantation; (C) 4 weeks after implantation; (D) 6 weeks after implantation; (E) 8 weeks after implantation. The scale bar indicates a distance of 50 μm in (A), (C), and (D), and a 25 μm in (B) and (E) [13].

Also in this author's own group, a series of bone repair materials were fabricated by adding three chitosan derivatives, such as phosphorylated chitin (P-chitin), phosphorylated chitosan (P-chitosan), and disodium (1→4)-2-deoxy-2-sulfoamino-β-D-glucopyranuronan (S-chitosan) into two kinds of biodegradable calcium phosphate cements (CPCs). All the chitosan derivatives can greatly improve the mechanical properties and reduce the biodegradation rates of the CPCs. At least six totally different tissue responses were detected when the implants were examined in tibial and radial defects of rabbits. Large bone defect (9 mm in length for radii and 3 mm in depth and diameter for tibias) repair in rabbits with the P-chitosan incorporated CPCs exhibits excellent tissue compatibilities with no any adverse or negative effects, such as fibrous encapsulation, osteolysis, hyperplasia, and inflammation, no matter the concentrations of P-chitosan is high or low (Figure 6) [128,129]. Tissue responses to P-chitin are highly sensitive (Figure 7) [130,131]. Three different bone formation types in the resorption lacuna of the P-chitin incorporated CPCs due to the P-chitin concentrations were found during the 22 weeks implantation. The first is that with low P-chitin content trabeculae formed directly from the implant (Figure 7A). The second is that with middle P-chitin content cartilages formed from the outside of fibers before they turned into trabeculae (Figure 7B, 7C). The third is that with high P-chitin content callous formed from the outside of fibers before they turned into trabeculae (Figure 7D, 7E). P-chitin content has a negative relationship with the biodegradation rate of the cements. However, the degradation rates are compatible with the ingrowth of trabeculae. A mild foreign-body reaction in the high P-chitin content sample during the first three time spans did not impair its placement by a newly formed bone. The generally properties of these biomaterials have met the main requirements for bone repair (Figure 7) [130,131]. Different from the above mentioned bone repair types, tissue responses to water-soluble S-chitosan, prepared from chitin by successive N-deacetylation, specific carboxylation at C-6 and sulfonation, was rather obtuse. No inflammation or other negative response was found in the S-chitosan containing samples (S-CPCs). After 4 weeks implantation, newly formed trabeculae contacted with the implant directly in the lower S-chitosan sample, while a thin layer of fibers formed between the newly formed bone and the implant in the higher S-chitosan samples [132,133]. These results indicate that the concentrations and functional groups in a linear polysaccharide play a key role in determining the ultimate biocompatibilities of an implantable biomaterial. In addition, as a derivative of chitin, chitosan initiates blood coagulation while S-chitosan inhibits blood coagulation when they are used as hemo-contact biomaterials.

Recently, chitosan and its derivatives have been widely used in skin wound, burn and disease treatments. For instance, a chitosan-gelatin-hyaluronic acid scaffold was found flexible with good mechanical properties when it was used as artificial skin substitutes [134]. A bacterial cellulose synthesized by Acetobacter xylinum and modified by chitosan was found to be optimal in providing wound dresses with a moist environment for wound healing [135]. When an artificial chitosan skin regenerating template was implanted subcutaneously it showed a similar inflammatory pattern as Integra, a two-layer skin regeneration system, constructed of a matrix of crosslinked fibers [136,137].

With the combination with other natural polymers, such as collagen, gelatin, hyaluronan, fibrin, the strong host inflammation reactions of chitosan can be reduced to a certain degree. It was found that a bioactive glass-chitosan composite containing 17% (wt%) chitosan produced by a freeze-drying process and implanted in the femoral condyl of an ovariectomised rat can promote a highly significant bioactive and osteoinductive property [138-140]. The ultimate biocompatibility of a chitosan compound depends largely on the ratio of the different components. Host tissues, such as smooth muscle and hepatic tissue have a similar response to the chitosan containing collagen/chitosan mixtures [141]. A collagen/chitosan matrix

crosslinked by agent 1-ethyl-3-(3-dimethylaminopropyl)-carbodiimide in a N-hydroxysucci-
nimide and 2-morpholinoethane sulfonic acid buffer system has exhibited improved blood
and cell compatibilities than the pure chitosan samples [142,143].

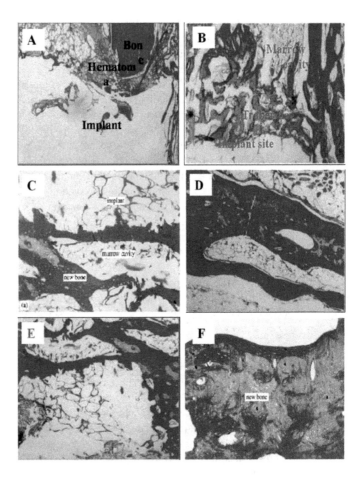

Figure 6. Tissue responses to the P-chitosan incorporated CPC specimen at different time points with MT staining. (A)
1 week after implantation in the high P-chitosan content (0.12 g/mL) sample with very little hematoma. (B) 4 weeks
after implantation in the high P-chitosan content (0.12 g/mL) sample newly formed woven bone clearly appeared
with tightly bonding between the implant and host bone. No macrophage was found around the implant. The implant was directly changed into new trabeculae after degradation. (C) 12 weeks after implantation newly formed long
bone in the low P-chitosan content (0.02 g/mL) sample. (D) 12 weeks after implantation newly formed long bone in
the middle P-chitosan content (0.07 g/mL) sample. (E) 12 weeks after implantation newly formed long bone in the
high P-chitosan content (0.12 g/mL) sample. Trabeculae formed after the implant was gobbled up (infiltrated) by
body fluid. Clear evidence of remodeling around the implant surface was displayed. (F) 22 weeks after implantation
the newly formed dense trabeculae in the high P-chitosan content (0.12 g/mL) sample [129].

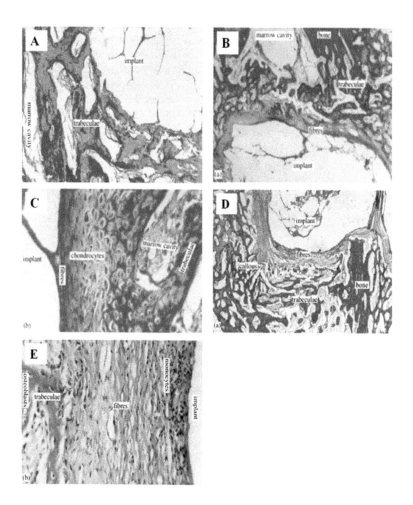

Figure 7. Tissue responses to the P-chitin incorporated CPC specimen 4 weeks after implantation. (A) P-chitin: 0.02 g/mL with MT staining. Magnification ×100. (B) P-chitin: 0.08 g/mL with MT staining. Magnification ×40. (C) A magnification of (B) with MT staining. Magnification ×400. (D) P-chitin: 0.14 g/mL with MT staining. Magnification ×40. (E) A magnification of (D) with HE staining. Magnification ×400 [131].

Current advances in some drug delivery systems make it possible to improve the therapeutic efficacy and minimized the side effects associated with toxicity of the drug. Chitosan has shown promise in the development of non-parenteral delivery systems for challenging drugs. For example, a 5-Fluorouracil (5-FU) loaded scaffold composed of chitosan fibers were prepared by a modified wet spinning technique [144]. Thermosensitive hydrogel composed of chitosan and glycerophosphate is proposed to be the potential candidate of *in situ* gel-forming implant for long-term drug delivery [145]. However, unpredictable body responses to the chitosan systems as stated above can complicate their applications to some degree. The composite chitosan-collagen-soybean phosphatidylcholine film impregnated with MMC-PLA-nanoparticles for treatment of hepatocellular carcinoma in mice has exhibited some special characteristics compared with pure chitosan delivery systems. In vivo, the growth of the tumors were inhibited considerably and dose-dependently by the MMC-film ($P<0.05$) with no any signs of vice reactions, such as inflammation, infection, and fibrous encapsulation after 20d of implantation [16,146,147]. Thus a careful balance between the immune reaction and drug effectiveness is needed when a chitosan pertaining template is used for biomedical applications.

10. Polyglycolide (PGA), Polylactide (PLA) and poly(Lactic-co-Glycolic Acid) (PLGA)

Polyglycolide also named polyglycolic acid (PGA) is a biodegradable, thermoplastic polymer and the simplest linear, aliphatic polyester which contains the ester functional group in it's main chain [148]. It can be prepared starting from glycolic acid by means of polycondensation or ring-opening polymerization. PGA has been known since 1954 as a tough fiber-forming polymer. Owing to its hydrolytic instability, its use has initially been limited [149]. *In vivo*, PGA initiates a marked host reaction around the implantations. This leads to the development of a foreign body response that comprises an initial acute inflammatory phase and a subsequent chronic inflammatory phase. For example, when a synthetic PGA scaffold seeding with adult-derived or somatic lung progenitor cells from mammalian lung tissue was implanted in an immunocompetent host, a serious foreign body response totally altered the integrity of the developing lung tissue [150].

Polylactic acid or polylactide (PLA) is another thermoplastic aliphatic polyester derived from renewable resources, such as corn starch, tapioca products, and sugarcanes [30]. A poly(L-lactide) (PLLA) coil stent has ever been implanted in pigs with no stent thrombosis and late restenosis [151]. However, PLA, as well as PLLA, and poly(D,L-lactide) (PDLA), induces a strong inflammatory response when they are implanted in the body due to their acidic products [152]. Aframian and coworkers implanted tubular PLLA, PGA coated with PLLA (PGA/PLLA), or nothing (sham-operated controls) in Balb/c mice either beneath the skin on the back, and found that inflammatory reactions were shorter and without epithelioid and giant cells in the sham-operated controls. Tissue responses to PLLA and PGA/PLLA scaffolds are generally similar in areas subjacent to skin in the back and oral cavity. Biodegradation proceeded more slowly with the PLLA tubules than with the PGA/PLLA tubules. No significant changes in clinical chemistry and hematology were seen due to the implantation of tubular scaffolds. [153]. It was reported that, after the PLLA segments were swallowed *in vivo* by phagocytes, cell damage and cell death were obvious. The highest numbers of necrotic cells were observed on day 2 [154]. These reactions can result in an unexpected risk for patients and have strongly limited in clinical applications of this kind of biomaterials.

To date, numerous strategies have been investigated to overcome body reactions induced by this kind of biomedical devices [155]. As a result, most of the PLA, PLLA, and PDLA have been used as a composite or compound with some other biomaterials. For example, a PLLA and poly(ethylene oxide) (PEO) blend has been prepared by mechanical mixture and fusion of homopolymers [156]. A biodegradable star-shaped 8 arms PEG-b-PLLA block copolymer was synthesized by Nagahama and coworkers to create a novel implantable soft material with drastically lowered crystallinity, increased swelling ability, and desirable mechanical properties [157,158].

Currently PGA, PLA and their copolymers, such as poly(lactide-co-caprolactone) (PLCA), poly(glycolide-co-caprolactone) (PGC), and poly (glycolide-co-trimethylene carbonate) are widely used as biomaterials for the synthesis of absorbable sutures and tissue engineering scaffolds in the biomedical field [159,160]. For example, a resorbable PLGA bone fixation implanted in craniofacial patients in 1996 resulted in 0.2 percent significant infectious complications, 0.3 percent device instability, and 0.7 percent self-limiting local foreign-body reactions [161]. As long-term implants, the toxicity of the accumulated acidate products made the situations even worse [162]. Until the present, most of the implanted PGA, PLA and PLGA related biomaterials still encounter an immune tissue response due to tissue trauma during implantation and the presence of foreign body reactions [163]. Surface coating has become one of the research hot points for the implantable devices with poor biocompatibilities. For instance, the biocompatibilities of some artificial polymer devices, such as heart valves, stents and vascular prosthesis that come into contact with bodily tissues or fluids particularly blood, have been improved by Venkatraman and coworkers with endothelialization surface layers [164,165].

Similarly, when a polyvinyl acetate (PVA)/PLGA microsphere was implanted into the subcutaneous tissue of rats, acute inflammation with neutrophils was found at day 3. Chronic inflammation with multinucleate giant cells, fibrosis, and mixed inflammatory cells was found at day 30. Mineralization around the implant was found at day 60 [166]. On the contrary, a dexamethasone/PLGA microsphere system can suppress the inflammation reaction by a fast releasing of dexamethasone [167]. A highly monodisperse and smooth PLGA-paclitaxel microspheres against malignant brain tumors were fabricated using an electrohydrodynamic atomization (EHDA) process [168]. In addition, PLA, PGA and PLGA can be tailored to meet mechanical performance and resorption rates required for applications ranging from non-structural drug delivery applications, nanoparticles (nanofibers), to resorbable screws and anchors [169,170].

11. Polycaprolactone (PCL)

Polycaprolactone (PCL) is a biodegradable polyester with a low melting point of around 60°C and a glass transition temperature of about −60°C. It is commonly used as an additive for resins or starch to improve their processing characteristics, lower their costs, and change their properties (e.g. impact resistance), or as a plasticizer in the manufacture of special polymers (e.g. Pus) [30]. PCL has been approved by the FDA for specific applications, such as a drug delivery devices, sutures, or adhesion barriers. It has been widely used as a scaffold material for tissue engineering with mismatched mechanical properties and slow degradation rate [171,172]. In rats the *in vivo* degradation of PCL is about 3 years [173].

Various categories of drugs have been encapsulated in PCL, in microsphere, nanosphere or bulk states, for targeted drug delivery and for controlled drug release [174-176]. For example, a PCL scaffold modified by grafting nerve growth factor (NGF) and Tirofiban (TF) has been used as nerve conduits to promote the regeneration of sciatic nerves [177]. Low molecular weight PCL pieces can be ingested and digested ultimately by phagocyte and giant cell without any cumulate vice-products (Figure 8) [178-180].

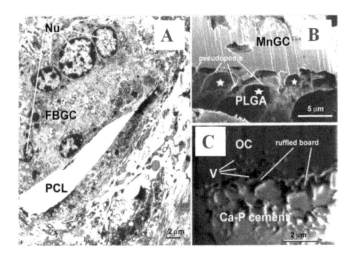

Figure 8. Micrographs illustrating extracellular degradation of biomaterials by macrophage fused multinuclear giant cells. (A) A foreign body giant cell (FBGC) engulfed a fragment of poly(epsilon-caprolactone), PCL polymer *in vivo*. Nu, nuclei of FBGC. The PCL polymer was dissolved during sample preparation. Transmission electron microscopy (TEM), bar = 2 μm. (B) *In situ* cross-section of the interface between a multinuclear giant cell (MnGC) and PLGA film. Note the pseudopodia of the MnGC penetrated deep inside the surface of PLGA film and formed sealed compartments. PLGA polymers are eroded within the compartments. Focused ion beam (FIB) microscopy, bar = 5 μm. (C) *In situ* cross-section of the interface between an osteoclasts-like cell (OC) and calcium phosphate cement. Note the typical ruffled board of OC and vesicles (V) secreting from OC to the sealed extracellular space. FIB microscopy, bar = 2 μm [162].

12. Polyurethane (PU)

PU is a series of biomaterials that contains urethane radical and offers the greatest versatility in compositions and properties of any family of polymers. Especially, a few specific elastomeric PU compositions have demonstrated a combination of toughness, durability, biocompatibility and biostability for being used as implantable medical devices, which is not achieved by any other available materials [181]. Because urethane is available in a very broad hardness range (e.g. eraser-soft to bowling-ball-hard), it allows the engineer to replace rubber, plastic and metal with the ultimate goals in abrasion resistance and physical properties. During the last half century, PUs have become and remained the most valuable implantable elastomers for uses requiring toughness, durability, biocompatibility and biostability [182]. With their inherently stable in the body environment, some of the PUs have been widely used in medical applications such as synthetic heart valves, vascular grafts, and pacemaker electrodes. However, these usages of PUs have been limited by three major complications: calcification, thrombosis, and chemical degradation [183].

In the 1970s and 1980s as the PUs became recognized as the blood contacting material and were used in a wide range of cardiovascular devices in long-term implants, they fell under scrutiny with the failure of pacemaker leads and breast implant coatings in the late 1980s. According to the manufacturer's report, high voltage coil fracture and PU defects were the predominant causes of lead failure [184,185]. During the next decade PUs had been extensively researched for their relative sensitivity to biodegradation and the desire to further understand the biological mechanisms for *in vivo* implantation [186,187]. Some investors have seeded autologous sheep blood outgrowth endothelial cells (BOECs) on a cholesterol (Chol)-modified PU (PU-Chol) heart valve leaflet to result in an intact, shear-resistant endothelium that would promote resistance to thrombosis [188]. Because of the complex behavior of implantable PUs in the body environment, special attention to the choice of the constituted components must be paid for designing and manufacturing the PU-containing devices. Subsequent treatment during sterilization, storage, implantation, *in vivo* operation and explantation also determine the performance and provide the means for assessing the efficacy of the PUs implants [189].

The most prominent disadvantages of PUs being used as artificial heart valves include mineralization, environmental stress-cracking and oxidation. While the mechanisms of these forms of degradation are not fully understood, an awareness of their causes and effects that leads to all of the long-term functionality is required for the sophisticated PU-based devices of today and tomorrow [190-191]. Over the last half century, extremely efforts have been paid in the biomedical research field to improve the biocompatibilities and biodurability of the PU implants, but only resulted in very little clinical effects [192-194].

In the later 1990s a number of new bioresorbable materials with all the versatility of PUs in terms of physical properties and biocompatibility have been yielded. AorTech Biomaterials was set up in 1997 to commercialise a range of medical grade PUs developed by the Australian research group (Commonwealth Scientific and Industrial Research Organization, CSIRO). The company estimates that the worldwide market for surgical heart valve products is worth more than $1bn (€705 m) and to be growing at a rate of 8% a year. Meanwhile, the market for catheter-delivered heart valves is worth around $200 m (€141 mm) [195]. In the authors' own group in Tsinghua University, China, a novel PU made of PCL, PEG, and 1,6-hexmethyldiisocyanate has been synthesized. The hydrolytic degradation property of the PU can be highly tuned by changing the composition and structure of copolymers, such as PEG and PCL. When this kind of PU was used as a small-caliber (1.2 mm inner diameter) vein and nerve repair grafts it demonstrated excellent antithrombogenicity and superior bio-compatibility (Figure 9) [196,197].

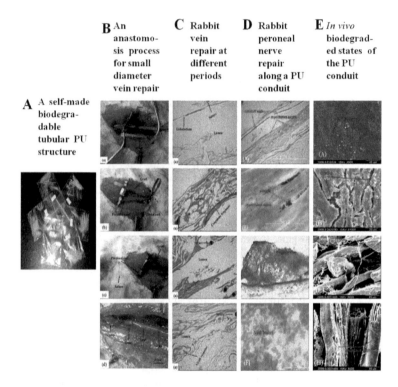

B An anastomo-sis process for small diameter vein repair

C Rabbit vein repair at different periods

D Rabbit peroneal nerve repair along a PU conduit

E *In vivo* biodegrad-ed states of the PU conduit

A A self-made biodegra-dable tubular PU structure

Figure 9. An implantable small-diameter nerve and blood vessel repair PU conduit. (A) PU conduits with different in-ner diameters. (B) The PU conduit was connected to the vein of a rabbit. (C) The vein defect repair processes with a very thin layer of fibrin-platelet deposition. (D) The nerve repair processes in rabbits with growing myelinated axons. (E) The PU conduits degraded gradually *in vivo* in 12 weeks [196, 197].

13. Polytetrafluoroethylene (PTFE)

Polytetrafluoroethylene (PTFE), Discovered in 1938 by Roy J. Plunkett, is a synthetic high-molecular-weight compound consisting wholly of carbon and fluorine with numerous ap-plications [198]. The best known brand name of PTFE is Teflon made by DuPont Co. It is insoluble in all normally used organic solvents, not biodegradable *in vivo* and can suffer high temperatures as 260 ℃ permanently. Clinically, PTFE has been widely used as a large blood vessels repair materials.

A 5 year research using PTFE-Gore-Tex grafts mainly for superficial femoral occlusion has been conducted. The majority of the grafts were inserted in an elderly poor risk group of patients with critical ischaemia of the lower limb. The overall cumulative patency at 2 years was 29% falling to 18% at 5 years. Perioperative angiographic indicated that inflammatory reaction is the only risk factor significantly affecting the cumulative graft patency. The presence of diabetes was found to have a significant detrimental effect on limb salvage [199]. A permanently implantable left ventricular assist device, made of Dacron velour, Teflon felt, and Teflon-coated polyester fiber sutures, has been tested in chronic animal experiments. *In vivo* experiments demonstrated that all components elicited mild to moderate inflammatory reactions. Tissue responses to PTFE are rather passivated. Hematocele occurred only when the components were implanted in the aorta with direct blood contact and exposed to arterial blood pressures [200]. An 8 cm long PTFE prosthesis was implanted into defects of the abdominal aorta of dogs, and the following changes were found: the blood flow through the vascular prosthesis induced a shortening of the blood clotting time and a slight increase in the prothrombin consumption. It has a favourable effect of the sealing of pores in the prosthesis and covering its internal surface with a fibrin membrane [201].

14. Silicone

Silicon is a metal in the same column as carbon in the periodic table with the symbol Si and atomic number 14 [30]. It is the most abundant element on earth and does not occur naturally in its pure metallic state. Dimethylsiloxane is the building block for most medical-grade silicone products, including breast implants. This FDA Grade Silicone sheeting is commonly used in applications where food or consumables are present. For more than 20 years silicone miami breast implants have gone through a lot of changes since their first uses. After the mid-1980s many reports concerns the rupture rate of the thinner-shell products, the risk of subsequent breast cancer, and the connective-tissue diseases or symptoms in women with silicone gel-filled breast implants appeared. In the United States a moratorium (in place since 1992) on the use of these prostheses has been maintained by the pressure of overwhelming litigation. At the same time, Australian authorities also restricted the availability of silicone breast implants. Huge damages awarded by United States courts forced Dow Corning, manufacturer of a large percentage of breast prostheses, to file for Chapter 11 bankruptcy in May 1995 [202].

As with any implantable medical devices or drugs, the risk of possible adverse effects must always be weighed against the ability to provide benefits. A great deal of safety research combined with more than 40 years of clinical experience has proven the efficacy and relative safety of the silicone gel breast implants. A rough estimate of implant shell rupture rate is ~10% at 10 years with both biocompatibility and biodurability problems [203]. A fibroconnective tissue capsule was found around all the samples [204]. The capsule formed around implanted mammary prosthesis is highly differentiated and organized, consisting of three layers: interface layer in three variations, intermediate fibrous layer of dense rough collagen fibers and light elongated cells with oval nucleus between them and adventitious layer. Between the fibers of the interface and the middle strata intra- and extracellular silicone drop-lets and bulks were observed, representing the location where further pathological processes can take place [205]. It is said by Dr. Sidney Wolfe, director of Public Citizen's Health Research Group, in a statement that: "Public Citizen continues to oppose the FDA's 2006 decision to return silicone breast implants to the market for cosmetic use in women for augmentation. The agency's newer information about the risk of implant-associated lym-phoma and the previously known risks are serious enough to warrant advising women against having these implanted."

On March 9, 2012 a new silicone breast implant, which joins the two other silicone breast implants on the market - one made by Allergan and the other by Mentor, was approved by the FDA of the United States of America. Recommended monitoring after initially silicone breast implantation is 3 years and then every two years thereafter. In a review Roach and coworkers concern the importance of length and time on physicochemical interactions be-tween living tissue and biomaterials that occur on implantation. The review provides de-tailed information on material host interactions, dynamic material/cell surface states, surface chemistry and topological roles during the first stage of implant integration, namely protein adsorption. Generally, after the first contact of material with host tissue a state of flux due to protein adsorption, cell adhesion and physical and chemical alteration of the implanted ma-terial is followed (Figure 10) [206]. This model can answer many questions concerning the conformational form and bound proteins and therefore has instruction meanings in new im-plantable biomaterial design field.

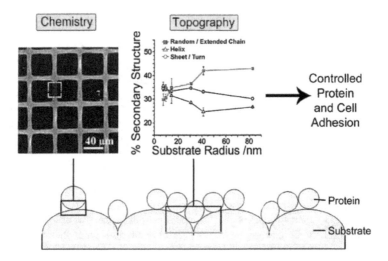

Figure 10. Schematic of protein–surface interactions: Chemistry—adsorption onto biotinylated stripes which appear white, whilst adsorption is hindered on square oligoethylene-glycol regions, the white box shows an intentionally bleached area Topography—albumin adsorption onto hydrophilic silica spheres of varying dimensions as a model of surface curvature [206].

Beside the breast implants a silicon-silk transistor about one millimeter long and 250 nanometers was created. So far the technique has been tested on mice with no adverse effects. Electrical, bending, water dissolution, and animal toxicity studies suggest that this approach might provide many opportunities for future biomedical devices and clinical applications [207]. A silicone catheter attached to a 2-5 x 1-3 cm stainless steel chamber with a self sealing injection port had been intravenously for antimicrobial chemotherapy. Peripheral venous access had become unsatisfactory in all of patients, and six had required central venous catheterisation [208]. More recently, a silicon-based neural probe with microfluidic channels was developed [209].

Origins of controlled release of implantable drug delivery dates back to 1964 when silicone implants were used to prolong a drug effect. Over 40 years, the progress to a safe, effective and acceptable implant system has been slow. The critical factors in implant research which need to be addressed include: erodibility, reproducibility, lack of irritation and carcinogenicity, lack of dose dumping, duration and pulses. While it is possible to surgically implant and remove drug-containing devices or polymeric matrices, the requirement for such intervention could have a significant negative impact on the acceptability of a product candidate. In recent years, two implant systems have been approved for human use; (a) a silicone-based device (Norplant^R), and (b) a system based on lactide/glycolide copolymers to release a luteinizing hormone - releasing hormone (LHRH) agonist for treatment of male reproductive tract tumours. This drug delivery approach is very appealing for a number of classes of drugs, particularly those that cannot be given via the oral route, and drug candidates whose therapeutic index is relatively large [210].

15. Aluminium (or aluminum) and ceramics

Aluminium (or aluminum) is the third most abundant chemical element (after oxygen and silicon in the boron group) with symbol Al and atomic number 13. It is one of the typical metals which has been widely used as hard tissue repair materials with unique properties, such as strong mechanical strength, not soluble and degradable in body fluid under normal circumstances, combined in over 270 different minerals, low density (weight) and corrosion resistances [211]. It is generally accepted that metallic implant materials with higher strength/modulus ratios are more favorable for hard tissue repair due to a combined effect of high strength and reduced stress-shielding risk [212].

Al alloys, such as Al-silicon (Si), Al-platinum, and Al-titanium (Ti) are widely used in implantable engineering structures and components where light weight or corrosion resistance is required except for blood-contacting surfaces [213,214]. For example, an implantable double-sided electrode microdevices, called flexible nerve plates, with a prototype of Al layer could reduce the number of insertion sites and thereby the insertion trauma during implantation of neural prostheses [215]. A Ti-6Al-4vanadium (V) alloy was selected as the ceramic-to-metal seal because its excellent mechanical properties and favorable biocompatibility [216]. The first-generation of implantable left ventricular assist devices (LVADs) were Ti-Alvanadium alloy pulsatile, volume-displacement pumps. The modern LVAD era began with the introduction of the HeartMate X (vented electric) VE in 1998 [217]. These devices can provide excellent circulatory support and improve survival until heart transplantation. However, they have many application limitations, such as a large volume, an excessive surgical dissection, a large diameter driveline, a noisy pump operation, and particularly a limited mechanical durability. Other complications include bleeding, infections and thromboembolic events. During the succeeding decade, vast improvements in pump design resulted in a new crop of LVADs, whose attributes are transforming LVAD therapy into a kind of standard of care for end-stage heart failure [218]. LVAD therapy has now evolved into a solution which is strikingly superior to optimal medical therapy [219, 220].

It was reported that changes in the porous hydroxyapatite and Al oxide orbital implant densities may correspond to healing and maturation of soft tissues surrounding and penetrating the implants [221]. The thermal oxidation behavior of Al ion implanted Ti nitride films has been studied in dry oxygen atmosphere and found that Al implantation caused the oxidation rate of TiN films to slow down at the initial stage of oxidation [222]. Until recently, there is limited evidence regarding comparative effectiveness of various hip implant bearings, especially metal on metal or ceramic on ceramic implants compared with traditional metal on polyethylene or ceramic on polyethylene bearings [223].

For clinical applications, it is an important character that the metal devices do not cause mental or body uncomfortable reactions, such as delaminate or infiltrate ions to the surround tissues. For example, a defibrillator is a medical device that generates and delivers a shock to the heart of someone in cardiac arrest. Although this device can save lives, there are risks involved, for both the patient and the first responders. One risk associated with defibrillator use is that of burns. Certain transdermal medication patches contain aluminum backings, and when they come in contact with the defibrillator paddle, can cause minor burns to the patient. Accidental shocks to others can occur when first responders accidentally contact with the patient who is being defibrillated. The only objects that should touch the patient during treatment are the defibrillator paddles held by the administrator of the procedure. Sometimes internally implanted defibrillators discharge shocks when they are unnecessary. When this occurs, it can cause pain and promote a dangerous heart rhythm. In addition, the event can be emotionally disturbing and frightening. Doctor can recalibrate the device to minimize the risk of additional unnecessary shocks, and offer suggestions on how to manage these rare events [224].

A ceramic is an inorganic, nonmetallic solid material possessing strong mechanical properties prepared by the action of heat and subsequent cooling [30]. The uses of ceramics have been revolutionizing the biomedical field in deployment as implants for humans during the past three decades. In the search to improve the biocompatibility and mechanical strength of skeletal implant materials, attention has been directed towards the potential use of ceramic composites [225]. Since 1975 alumina ceramic has proven its bioinertness and have been accepted in biomedical applications, some alumina ceramic, such as Al_2O_3 has been characterized with high hardness and high abrasion resistance. Noiri and coworkers evaluated the biocompatibility of alumina-ceramic material histopathalogically for eight weeks by implanting in the eye sockets of albino rabbits with no signs of implant rejection or prolapse of the implanted pieces. After a period of four weeks of implantation, fibroblast proliferation and vascular invasion were noted. By the eighth week, tissue growth was observed in the pores of the implants [226].

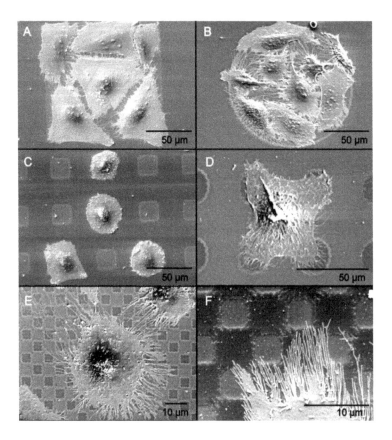

Figure 11. Scanning electron microscopy (SEM) images of SaOS-2 cells cultured for 48 h on micropatterned Ti (A-D) and diamond-like carbon (DLC) (E, F) surfaces. Large-sized (125 μm) squared (A) and circular (B) features facilitated the adhesion of several cells on one Ti island with the cells aligning themselves along the edges of the cell-friendly material. The cells adhering to mediumsized Ti islands no longer conformed strictly to the geometrical shape of the patterns (C) but particularly on circularly patterned surfaces, star-like cellular morphologies appeared (D). On small-sized inverse DLC samples, the cell bodies non-selectively covered large micro-patterned areas (E), but their filopodia clearly showed a preference for DLC trying to avoid bare Si circles (F) [222].

16. Conclusion remarks

Biocompatible is a vital important aspect for an implantable biomaterial. Among the numerous types of host responses to a broad spectrum of biomaterials, those with no adverse or negative effects, such as, fibrous encapsulation, osteolysis, hyperplasia, and inflammation are among the most expectant ones. As advances are made in biomaterial science and technology, new implants/medical devices will be continually explored, alternatives to conventional implants will become more and more effective, and hence more and more attractive. In an effort to provide the best clinical outcomes for the patients, we need to develop the best candidates with minimum invasive surgery times and unnecessary health risks. In the future, design and manufacture immuno or low-immuno implantable biomaterials according to or mimicking the patients' own ingredients, such as blood components, ECMs, tissues and organs, will be possible. For an implantable biomaterial biocompatibility should be always put into the primary importance position no matter it is used as a temporary scaffold, a permanent template, or a drug delivery vihicle.

Acknowledgment

Work in the authors' laboratory is supported by the State Key Laboratory of Materials Processing and Die & Mould Technology, Huazhong University of Science and Technology (No. 2012 - P03), the National Natural Science Foundation of China / the Research Grants Council of Hong Kong (NSFC/RGC, No. 50731160625), the National Natural Science Foundation of China (No. 81271665 & 30970748), the National High Tech 863 Grant (No. 2009AA043801), the Finland Distinguished Professor program (FiDiPro) of Tekes (No. 40041/10), and the Cross-Strait Tsinghua Cooperation Basic Research (No.2012THZ02-3).

Author details

Xiaohong Wang[1,2,3]

Address all correspondence to: wangxiaohong@tsinghua.edu.cn

1 Key Laboratory for Advanced Materials Processing Technology, Ministry of Education & Center of Organ Manufacturing, Department of Mechanical Engineering, Tsinghua University, Beijing, P.R. China

2 Business Innovation Technology (BIT) Research Centre, School of Science and Technology, Aalto University, Aalto, Finland

3 State Key Laboratory of Materials Processing and Die & Mould Technology, Huazhong University of Science and Technology, Wuhan, P.R. China

References

[1] Tathe A, Ghodke M, Nikalje AP. International Journal of Pharmacy and Pharmaceutical Sciences (Int J Pharm Pharm Sci) 2010;2(4):19-23.

[2] Anderson JM, Rodriguez A, Chang DT. Foreign body reaction to biomaterials. Seminars in Immunology 2008;20 (2): 86–100.

[3] Patel NR, Gohil PP. A review on biomaterials: scope, applications & human anatomy significance. International Journal of Emerging Technology and Advanced Engineering 2012; 2(4): 91-101.

[4] Seal BL, Otero TC, Panitch A. Polymeric biomaterials for tissue and organ regeneration. Materials Science and Engineering R 2001;34:147-230.

[5] Franz S, Rammelt S, Scharnweber D, Simon JC. Immune responses to implants - A review of the implications for the design of immunomodulatory biomaterials. Biomaterials 2011;32(28): 6692-6709

[6] Medical-dictionary.thefreedictionary.com.

[7] The American Heritage® Medical Dictionary Copyright © 2007, 2004 by Houghton Mifflin Company.

[8] www.indeed.com.

[9] www.bonebank.com/cancellous-bone.html

[10] Hodde J. Naturally occurring scaffolds for soft tissue repair and regeneration. Tissue Eng 2002;8:295-308.

[11] Thomas W. Gilbert, Tiffany L. Sellaro, Stephen F. Badylak. Decellularization of tissues and organs. Biomaterials 2006;27(19): 3675–3683.

[12] Patino MG, Neiders ME, Andreana S, Noble B, Cohen RE. Collagen as an implantable material in medicine and dentistry. J Oral Implantol. 2002;28(5):220-225.

[13] Wang XH, Yan YN, Zhang RJ. A comparison of chitosan and collagen sponges as heostatic sressings. J Bioact Compat Polym 2006;21(1)::39-54.

[14] George D. Kymionis, Michael A. Grentzelos, Alexandra E. Karavitaki, Zotta Paraskevi, Sonia H. Yoo, Ioannis G. Pallikaris. Combined corneal collagen cross-linking and posterior chamber toric implantable collamer lens implantation for keratoconus. Ophthalmic Surgery, Lasers and Imaging. DOI: 10.3928/15428877-20110210-0.

[15] Ju YM, Yu B, West L, Moussy Y, Moussy F. A dexamethasone-loaded PLGA microspheres/collagen scaffold composite for implantable glucose sensors. J Biomed Mater Res A. 2010;93(1):200-210.

[16] Hou ZQ, Sun Q, Wang Q, Han J, Wang Y, Zhang QQ. *In vitro* and *in vivo* evaluation of novel implantable collagen–chitosan–soybean phosphatidylcholine composite film for the sustained delivery of mitomycin C. Drug Dev Res 2009;70(3):169-219.

[17] Ward, A.G.; Courts, A. The Science and Technology of Gelatin. New York: Academic Press. 1977;ISBN0-12-735050-0.

[18] Kakiuchi M, Hosoya T, Takaoka K, Amitani K, Ono K. Human bone matrix gelatin as a clinical alloimplant. A retrospective review of 160 cases. Int Orthop 1985;9(3): 181-188.

[19] Wang XH, Yan YN, Zhang RJ. Gelatin-based hydrogels for controlled cell assembly. In: Ottenbrite RM, ed. Biomedical Applications of Hydrogels Handbook. New York: Springer, 2010;269-284.

[20] Wang XH, Yan YN, Zhang RJ Rapid prototyping as a tool for manufacturing bioartificial livers. Trends Biotechnol 2007;25:505-513.

[21] Wang XH, Yan YN, Zhang RJ. Recent trends and challenges in complex organ manufacturing. Tissue Eng Part B 2010;16:189-197.

[22] Wang XH, Zhang QQ. Overview on "Chinese–Finnish workshop on biomanufacturing and evaluation techniques. Artificial Organs 2011;35(10):E191- E193.

[23] Wang XH. Intelligent freeform manufacturing of complex organs. Artificial Organs. 2012; doi:10.1111/j.1525-1594.2012.01499.x.

[24] Xu W, Wang XH, Yan YN, Zhang RJ. A polyurethane-gelatin hybrid construct for manufacturing implantable bioartificial livers. J Bioact Compat Polym 2008;23(5): 409-422.

[25] He K, Wang XH. Rapid prototyping of tubular polyurethane and cell/hydrogel construct. J Bioact Compat Polym 2011;26(4):363-374.

[26] Kimura Y, Ozeki M, Inamoto T, Tabata Y. Adipose tissue engineering based on human preadipocytes combined with gelatin microspheres containing basic fibroblast growth factor. Biomaterials 24 (2003) 2513–2521.

[27] Liu J. Controlled trans-lymphatic delivery of chemotherapy for the treatment of lymphatic metastasis in lung cancer. A thesis submitted in conformity with the requirements for the degree of Doctor of Philosophy Institute of Medical Science, University of Toronto, 2008.

[28] Ozeki M, Ishii T, Hirano Y, Tabata Y. Controlled release of hepatocyte growth factor from gelatin hydrogels based on hydrogel degradation. J Drug Target. 2001;9(6): 461-471.

[29] Yang Z, Xu LS, Yin F, Shi YQ, Han Y, Zhang L, Jin HF, Nie YZ, Wang JB, Hao X, Fan DM, Zhou XM. *In vitro* and *in vivo* characterization of silk fibroin/gelatin composite scaffolds for liver tissue engineering. J Dig Dis. 2012 Mar;13(3):168-178.

[30] en.wikipedia.org/wiki, the free encyclopedia.

[31] Radosevich M, Goubran H, Burnouf T. Fibrin sealant: scientific rationale, production methods, properties and current clinical use. Vox Sang 1997;72:133-143.

[32] Dunn C, Goa K. Fibrin sealant: a review of its use in surgery and endoscopy. Drugs 1999;58:863-886.

[33] Weisel JW. Fibrinogen and fibrin. Adv Protein Chem 2005;70:247-299.

[34] Clark RA. Fibrin is a many splendored thing. J Invest Dermatol 2003;121(5):xxi-xxii.

[35] Herrick S, Blanc-Brude O, Gray A, Laurent G. Fibrinogen. Int J Biochem Cell Biol 1999;31(7):741-746.

[36] Abiraman S, Varma HK, Umashankar PR, John A. Fibrin glue as an osteoinductive protein in a mouse model. Biomaterials 23 (2002) 3023–3031.

[37] Hwang TL, Chen MF. Randomized trial of fibrin tissue glue for low output enterocutaneous fistula. Br J Surg 1996;83:112.

[38] Flanagan TC, Sachweh JS, Frese J, Schnöring H, Gronloh N, Koch S, Tolba RH, Schmitz-Rode T, Jockenhoevel S. *In vivo* Remodeling and Structural Characterization of Fibrin-Based Tissue-Engineered Heart Valves in the Adult Sheep Model. Tissue Engineering Part A. 2009;15(10):2965-2976.

[39] Mol A, Driessen NJ, Rutten MC, Hoerstrup SP, Bouten CV, and Baaijens FP. Tissue engineering of human heart valve leaflets: a novel bioreactor for a strain-based conditioning approach. Ann Biomed Eng 2005;33(12):1778-1788

[40] Barsotti MC, Felice F, Balbarini A, Di Stefano R. Fibrin as a scaffold for cardiac tissue engineering. Biotechnol Appl Biochem 2011;58(5):301-310.

[41] Peretti GM, Xu JW, Bonassar LJ, Kirchhoff CH, Yaremchuk MJ, Randolph MA. Review of injectable cartilage engineering using fibrin gel in mice and swine models. Tissue Eng. 2006;12(5):1151-1168.

[42] Daniel D. Swartz, James A. Russell, Stelios T. Andreadis. Engineering of fibrin-based functional and implantable small-diameter blood vessels. Am J Physiol Heart Circ Physiol 2005;288: H1451–H1460.

[43] Sameem M, Wood TJ, Bain JR. A systematic review on the use of fibrin glue for peripheral nerve repair. Plast Reconstr Surg. 2011;127(6):2381-2390.

[44] Koch S, Flanagan TC, Sachweh JS, Tanios F, Schnoering H, Deichmann T, Ellä V, Kellomäki M, Gronloh N, Gries T, Tolba R, Schmitz-Rode T, Jockenhoevel S. Fibrin-polylactide-based tissue-engineered vascular graft in the arterial circulation. Biomaterials 2010;31(17):4731-4739

[45] Guéhennec LL, Daculsi G. A review of bioceramics and fibrin sealant. LE.u Lroe pGeuanéh Ceenlnles ca netd aMl.aterials 2004;8: 1-11.

[46] Jeffrey M. Karp JM, Sarraf F, Shoichet MS, Davies JE. Fibrin-filled scaffolds for bone-tissue engineering: An *in vivo* study. J Biomed Mater Res 2004;71A:162–171.

[47] Farhat WA, Chen J, Sherman C, Cartwright L, Bahoric A, Yeger H. Impact of fibrin glue and urinary bladder cell spraying on the in-vivo acellular matrix cellularization: a porcine pilot study. Can J Urol 2006;13(2):3000-3008.

[48] Breen A, O'Brien T, and Pandit A. Fibrin as a Delivery System for Therapeutic Drugs and Biomolecules. Tissue Eng Part B Rev. 2009;15(2):201-214.

[49] Briganti E, Spiller D, Mirtelli C, Kull S, Counoupas C, Losi P, Senesi S, Di Stefano R, and Soldani G. A. Composite fibrin-based scaffold for controlled delivery of bioactive pro-angiogenetic growth factors. J Control Release 2010;142(1):14-21.

[50] Jockenhoevel S, Zund G, Hoerstrup SP, Chalabi K, Sachweh JS, Demircan L, Messmer BJ, Turina M. Fibrin gel -- advantages of a new scaffold in cardiovascular tissue engineering. Eur J Cardiothorac Surg 2001;19(4):424-430.

[51] Catelas I, Dwyer JF, and Helgerson S. Controlled release of bioactive transforming growth factor Beta-1 from fibrin gels *in vitro*. Tissue Eng Part C Methods 2008;14(2):119-128.

[52] Arkudas A, Pryymachuk G, Hoereth T, Beier JP, olykandriotis E, Bleiziffer O, Horch RE, and Kneser U. Dose- Finding Study of Fibrin Gel-Immobilized Vascular Endothelial Growth Factor 165 and Basic Fibroblast Growth Factor in the Arteriovenous Loop Rat Model. Tissue Eng Part A. 2009;15(9):2501-2511.

[53] Breen A, O'Brien T, and Pandit A. Fibrin as a Delivery System for Therapeutic Drugs and Biomolecules. Tissue Eng Part B Rev 2009;15(2):201-214.

[54] Sakiyama SE, Schense JC, and Hubbell JA. Incorporation of heparin-binding peptides into fibrin gels enhances neurite extension: an example of designer matrices in tissue engineering. FASEB J. 1999;13(15):2214-2224.

[55] Zisch AH, Schenk U, Schense JC, Sakiyama-Elbert SE, and Hubbell JA. Covalently conjugated VEGF—fibrin matrices for endothelialization. J Control Release 2001;72(1-3):101-113.

[56] Hara T. Bhayana B, Thompson B, Kessinger CW, McCarthy AKR, Weissleder R, Lin CP, Tearney GJ, Jaffer FA. Molecular Imaging of Fibrin Deposition in Deep Vein Thrombosis Using Fibrin-Targeted Near-Infrared Fluorescence. J Am Coll Cardiol Img 2012;5:607–1551.

[57] Ruszymah BH. Autologous human fibrin as the biomaterial for tissue engineering. Med J Malaysia 2004;59(Suppl B):30-31.

[58] Roderick P, Ferris G, Wilson K, Halls H, Jackson D, Collins R, Baigent C. Towards evidence-based guidelines for the prevention of venous thromboembolism: systematic reviews of mechanical methods, oral anticoagulation, dextran and regional anaesthesia as thromboprophylaxis. Health Technol Assess 2005;9(49):iii-iv, ix-x, 1-78.

[59] Sophie R. Tomme V, Hennink WE. Biodegradable dextran hydrogels for protein delivery applications. Expert Review of Medical Devices 2007;4:147-164.

[60] Atik M. Dextran 40 and Dextran 70. A Review. Arch Surg 1967;94(5):664-672.

[61] Dubick MA, Wade CE. A review of the efficacy and safety of 7.5% NaCl/6% dextran 70 in experimental animals and in humans. J Trauma 1994;36(3):323-330.

[62] Richardson D, Deakin CD. Hypertonic saline dextran. A review of current literature. Scand J Trauma Resusc Emerg Med. 2004;12:142-146.

[63] Sun GM, Zhang XJ, She Y-I, Sebastian R, Dickinson LE, Fox-Talbot K, Reinblatt M, Steenbergen C, Harmon JW, Gerecht S. Dextran hydrogel scaffolds enhance angiogenic responses and promote complete skin regeneration during burn wound healing. PNAS 14, 2011;108:20975-20980.

[64] Draye J-P, Delaey B, Van de Voorde A. Van Den Bulcke A, Reu BD, Schacht E. *In vitro* and *in vivo* biocompatibility of dextran dialdehyde cross-linked gelatin hydrogel films. Biomaterials 1998;19(18):1677-1687.

[65] Groot CJD, Van Luyn MJA, Van Dijk-Wolthuis WND, Cadée JA, Plantinga JA, Otter WD, Hennink WE. *In vitro* biocompatibility of biodegradable dextran-based hydrogels tested with human fibroblasts. Biomaterials 2001;22(11):1197-1203.

[66] Dhaneshwar SS, Kandpal M, Gairola N, Kadam SS. Dextran: a promising macromolecular drug carrier. Indian Journal of Pharmaceutical Sciences 2006;68(6):705-714.

[67] de Belder AN. Dextran. Hndbooks from Amersham bosciences. 18-1166-12, Edition Amersham AA. Biosciences AB 2003. (ww.amershambiosciences.com.)

[68] Roderick P, Ferris G, Wilson K, Halls H, Jackson D, Collins R, Baigent C. Towards evidence-based guidelines for the prevention of venous thromboembolism: systematic reviews of mechanical methods, oral anticoagulation, dextran and regional anaesthesia as thromboprophylaxis. Health Technology Assessment 2005;9:(49): Editor-in-Chief: Professor Tom Walley. 2005 Crown Copyright.

[69] Solomon L, Mansor S, Mallon P, Donnelly E, Hoper M, Loughrey M, Kirk S, Gardiner K. The dextran sulphate sodium (DSS) model of colitis: an overview. Comp Clin Pathol 2010;19:235–239.

[70] Yang J, Liu Y, Wang H, Liu L, Wang W, Wang C, Wang Q, Liu W. The biocompatibility of fatty acid modified dextran-agmatine bioconjugate gene delivery vector. Biomaterials 2012;33(2):604-613.

[71] Necas J, Bartosikova L, Brauner P, Kolar J. Hyaluronic acid (hyaluronan): a review. Veterinarni Medicina, 2008;53(8):397–411.

[72] Frasher JRE; Laurent TC; Laurent UBG. Hyaluronan: its nature, distribution, functions and turnover. Journal of Internal Medicine 1997;242(1):27–33.

[73] Kahmann JD, O'Brien R, Werner JM, Heinegard D, Ladbury JE, Campbell ID, Day AJ. Localization and characterization of the hyaluronan-binding site on the Link module from human TSG-6. Structure 2000;8:763–774.

[74] Jaracz S, Chen J, Kuznetsova LV, Ojima I. Recent advances in tumor-targeting anticancer drug conjugates. Bioorganic and Medicinal Chemistry 2005;13:5043–5054.

[75] Paiva P, Van Damme MP, Tellbach M, Jones RL, Jobling T, Salamonsen LA. Expression patterns of hyaluronan, hyaluronan synthases and hyaluronidases indicate a role for hyaluronan in the progression of endometrial cancer. Gynecologic Oncology 2005;3:202.

[76] Lokeshwar, VB, Lopez LE, Munoz D, Chi A, Shirodkar SP, Lokeshwar SD, Escudero DO, Dhir N, Altman N. Antitumor activity of hyaluronic acid synthesis inhibitor 4-methylumbelliferone in prostate cancer cells. Cancer Res 2010;70(7):2613–2623.

[77] Amarnath LP, Srinivas A, Ramamurthi A. *In vitro* hemocompatibility testing of UV-modified hyaluronan hydrogels. Biomaterials 2006; 27(8):1416–1424.

[78] Jansen K., van der Werff JFA, van Wachem PB, Nicolai JPA, de Leij L.F.M.H, van Luyn MJA. A hyaluronan-based nerve guide: *in vitro* cytotoxicity, subcutaneous tissue reactions, and degradation in the rat. Biomaterials 2004;25(1):483–489.

[79] Rah MJ. A review of hyaluronan and its ophthalmic applications. Optometry 2011;82(1):38-43.

[80] De Andrés Santos MI, Velasco-Martín A, Hernández-Velasco E, Martín-Gil J, Martín-Gil FJ. Thermal behaviour of aqueous solutions of sodium hyaluronate from different commercial sources". Thermochim Acta 1994;42:153-160.

[81] Peattie RA, Rieke E, Hewett E, Fisher RJ, Shu XZ, Prestwich GD. Dual growth factor-induced angiogenesis *in vivo* using hyaluronan hydrogel implants.Biomaterials 2006; 27 (9):1868-1875,

[82] Pike DB, Cai S, Pomraning KR, Firpo MA, Fisher RJ, Shu XZ, Prestwich GD, Peattie RA. Heparin-regulated release of growth factors *in vitro* and angiogenic response *in vivo* to implanted hyaluronan hydrogels containing VEGF and Bfgf. Biomaterials 2006;27(30):5242–5251.

[83] Dianhua Jiang, Jiurong Liang, Paul W. Noble. Hyaluronan as an Immune Regulator in Human Diseases. Physiol Rev January 1, 2011 vol. 91 no. 1 221-264.

[84] Jiang DH, Liang JR, Noble PW. Hyaluronan in Tissue Injury and Repair. Annual Review of Cell and Developmental Biology 2007;23:435-461.

[85] Luke R. Bucci, Amy A. Turpin. Will the real hyaluronan please stand up? Journal of applied nutrition 2004;54(1):10-33.

[86] Longaker MT, Chiu ES, Adzick NS, Stem M, Harrison MR, Stem R. Studies in fetal wound healing: V. A prolonged presence of hyaluronic acid characterizes fetal wound fluid. Annals of Surgery. Annals of Surgery 1991;213(4):292-296.

[87] Chen WYJ, Giovanni Abatangelo G. Functions of hyaluronan in wound repair. Wound Repair and Regeneration 1999;7(2):79-89.

[88] Benedetti L, Cortivo R, Berti T, Berti A, Pea F, Mazzo M, Moras M, Abatangelo G. Biocompatibility and biodegradation of different hyaluronan derivatives (Hyaff) implanted in rats. Biomaterials 1993;14(15):1154-1160.

[89] Shen X, Tanaka K, Takamori A. Coronary arteries angiogenesis in ischemic myocardium: biocompatibility and biodegradability of various hydrogels. Artificial Organs 2009;33(10):781-787.

[90] Praveen SS, Hanumantha R, Belovich JM, Davis BL. Novel hyaluronic acid coating for potential use in glucose sensor design. Diabetes Technol Ther. 2003;5(3):393-399.

[91] Hou SP, Xu QY, Tian WM, Cui FZ, Cai Q, Ma J, Lee I-S. The repair of brain lesion by implantation of hyaluronic acid hydrogels modified with laminin. Journal of Neuroscience Methods 2005;148:60–70.

[92] Zhang T, Yan YN, Wang XH, Xiong Z, Lin F, Wu RD, Zhang RJ. Three-dimensional gelatin and gelatin/hyaluronan hydrogel structures for traumatic brain injury. J Bioact Compat Polym 2007;22(1):19-29.

[93] Avitabile T, Marano F, Castiglione F, Bucolo C, Cro M, Ambrosio L, Ferrauto C, Reibaldi A. Biocompatibility and biodegradation of intravitreal hyaluronan implants in rabbits. Biomaterials 2001;22(3):195-200.

[94] Li H, Liu Y, Shu XZ, Gray SD, Prestwich GD. Synthesis and biological evaluation of a cross-linked hyaluronan-mitomycin C hydrogel. Biomacromolecules 2004;5(3):895-902.

[95] Zheng SX, Liu Y, Palumbo FS, Luo Y, Prestwich GD. In situ crosslinkable hyaluronan hydrogels for tissue engineering. Biomaterials 2004;25(7-8):1339-1348.

[96] Hong HJ, Lee JS, Choi JW, Min BH, Lee HB, Kim CH. Transplantation of Autologous Chondrocytes Seeded on a Fibrin/Hyaluronan Composite Gel Into Tracheal Cartilage Defects in Rabbits: Preliminary Results. Artif Organs 2012;30:1525-1594.

[97] Cox M; Nelson D. Lehninger, Principles of Biochemistry. Freeman 2004:1100.

[98] Jang I-K, Hursting MJ. When Heparins Promote Thrombosis : Review of Heparin-Induced Thrombocytopenia. Circulation 2005;111:2671-2683.

[99] Moore BR, Hinchcliff KW. Heparin: a review of its pharmacology and therapeutic use in horses. J Vet Intern Med. 1994;8(1):26-35.

[100] Saliba Jr MJ . Heparin in the treatment of burns: a review. Burns 2001;27(4):349-358.

[101] Papa A, Danese S, Gasbarrini A, Gasbarrini G. Review article: potential therapeutic applications and mechanisms of action of heparin in inflammatory bowel disease. Aliment Pharmacol Ther. 2000 Nov;14(11):1403-1409.

[102] Hull RD, Liang J, Townshend G. Long-term low-molecular-weight heparin and the post-thrombotic syndrome: a systematic review. Am J Med. 2011;124(8):756-765.

[103] Wang XH, Yan YN, Lin F, Xiong Z, Wu RD, Zhang RJ, Lu QP. Preparation and characterization of a collagen/chitosan/heparin matrix for an implantable bioartificial liver. J Biomater Sci.Polym Ed 2005;16(9):1063-1080.

[104] Yu X, Bichtelen A, Wang XH, Yan YN, Lin F, Xiong Z, Wu RD, Zhang RJ, Lu QP. Collagen/chitosan/heparin complex with improved biocompatibility for hepatic tissue engineering. J Bioact Compat Polym 2005;20(1):15-28.

[105] Matthew D. Mitchell, Barbara Jo Anderson, Kendal Williams & Craig A. Umscheid. Heparin flushing and other interventions to maintain patency of central venous catheters: a systematic review. Journal of Advanced Nursing 2009;65(10), 2007–2021.

[106] Ziakas PD, Pavlou M, Voulgarelis M. Heparin treatment in antiphospholipid syndrome with recurrent pregnancy loss: a systematic review and meta-analysis. Obstet Gynecol. 2010;115(6):1256-1262.

[107] Marcum JA, McKenney JB, Galli SJ, Jackman RW, Rosenberg RD. Anticoagulantly active heparin-like molecules from mast cell-deficient mice. Am J Physiol 1986;250 (5 Pt 2): H879–888.

[108] Nader HB, Chavante SF, dos-Santos EA, Oliveira FW, de-Paiva JF, Jerônimo SMB, Medeiros GF, de-Abreu LRD, Leite EL, de-Sousa-Filho JF, Castro RAB, Toma L, Tersariol ILS, Porcionatto MA, Dietrich CP. Heparan sulfates and heparins: similar compounds performing the same functions in vertebrates and invertebrates? Braz J Med Biol Res 1999;32(5):529–538.

[109] Peattie RA, Rieke E, Hewett E, Fisher RJ, Shu X Z, Prestwich G D. Dual growth factor-induced angiogenesis *in vivo* using hyaluronan hydrogel implants. Biomaterials 2006;27(9):1868-1875.

[110] Swanson JM. Heparin-induced thrombocytopenia: a general review. J Infus Nurs. 2007;30(4):232-240.

[111] Hong MS, Amanullah AM. Heparin-induced thrombocytopenia: a practical review. Rev Cardiovasc Med 2010;11(1):13-25.

[112] James L. Januzzi, Jr. and Ik-Kyung Jang. Heparin Induced Thrombocytopenia: Diagnosis and Contemporary Antithrombin Management. J Thromb Thrombolysis 1999;7:259–264.

[113] Strand BL, Ryan L, Veld PI, Kulseng B, Rokstad AM, Skjåk-Bræk G., Especik T. Cell Transplant. 2001;10:263-275.

[114] Yao R, Zhang RJ, Yan YN, Wang XH. *In vitro* angiogenesis of 3D tissue engineered adipose tissue. J Bioact Compat Polym 2009;24(1):5-24.

[115] Yao R, Zhang RJ, Wang XH. Design and evaluation of a cell microencapsulating device for cell assembly technoloty. J Bioact Compat Polym 2009;24(1):48-62.

[116] Soon-Shiong P, Heintx RE, Merideth N, Yao QX, Yao Z, Zheng T, Murphy M, Moloney MK, Schmedhl M, Harris M, Mendez R, Mendez R, Sanford PA. The Lancet 1994;16:950-951.

[117] Li RH. Materials for Immunoisolated Cell Transplantation. Advanced Drug Delivery Reviews 1998;33:87–109.

[118] Tam SK, de Haan BJ, Faas MM, Hallé JP, Yahia L, de Vos P. Adsorption of human immunoglobulin to implantable alginate-poly-L-lysine microcapsules: effect of microcapsule composition. J Biomed Mater Res A. 2009;89(3):609-615.

[119] Xie H-G, Li X-X, Lv G-J, Xie W-Y, Zhu J, Luxbacher T, Ma R, Ma X-J. Laboratory of Biomedical MaterialDevelopment of an implantable alginate scaffold for the treatment of spinal cord trauma. J Biomed Mater Res 2010;92A:1357–1365.

[120] Shahidi F, Synowiecki J. Isolation and characterization of nutrients and value-added products from snow crab (Chionoecetes opilio) and shrimp (Pandalus borealis) processing discards. Journal of Agricultural and Food Chemistry (American Chemical Society) 1991;39 (8): 1527–1532.

[121] Khor E, Lim LY. Implantable applications of chitin and chitosan. Biomaterials. 2003; 24(13):2339-2349.

[122] Yang T-L. Chitin-based Materials in tissue engineering: applications in soft tissue and epithelial organ. Int J Mol Sci 2011;12:1936-1963.

[123] Costa-Pinto AR, Reis RL, Neves NM. Scaffolds based bone tissue engineering: the role of chitosan. Tissue Engineering Part B 2011;17(5):1-17.

[124] Wang XH, Yu X, Yan YN, Zhang RJ. Liver tissue responses to gelatin and gelatin/chitosan gels. J Biomed Mater Res 2008;87A(1):62-68.

[125] Michael Dornish, VP research and development, and Dr Are Kristiansen, commercial development manager, at FMC BioPolymer.

[126] Khor E, Lim LY. Implantable applications of chitin and chitosan. Biomaterials 2003;24 (13):2339–2349.

[127] Mi FL, Tan YC, Liang HC, Huang RN, Sung HW. *In vitro* evaluation of a chitosan membrane cross-linked with genipin. J Biomater Sci Polym Ed 2001;12(8):835-850.

[128] Wang XH, Ma JB, Wang YN, He BL. Structural characterization of phosphorylated chitosan and their applications as effective additives of calcium phosphate cements. Biomaterials 2001;22(16):2247-2255.

[129] Wang XH, Ma JB, Wang YN, He BL. Skeletal repair in radii and tibias of rabbits with phosphorylated chitosan reinforced calcium phosphate cements. Biomaterials. 2002;23(21):4167-4176.

[130] Wang XH, Ma JB, Wang YN, He BL. Reinforcement of calcium phosphate cements with phosphorylated chitin. Chin J Polym Sci 2002;4:325-332.

[131] Wang XH, Ma JB, Feng QL, Cui FZ. Skeletal repair in rabbits with calcium phosphate cements incorporated phosphorylated chitin. Biomaterials 2002;23(23):4591-4600.

[132] Wang XH, Ma JB, Feng QL, Cui FZ. *in vivo* evaluation of S-chitosan enhanced calcium phosphate cements. J Bioact Compat Polym 2003;18(4):259-271.

[133] Wang XH, Feng QL, Cui FZ, Ma JB. The effects of S-chitosan on the physical properties of calcium phosphate cements. J Bioact Compat Polym 2003;18(1):45-57.

[134] Liu H, Mao J, Yao K, Yang G, Cui L, Cao Y. A study on a chitosan-gelatin-hyaluronic acid scaffold as artificial skin *in vitro* and its tissue engineering applications. J Biomater Sci Polym Ed 2004;15(1):25-40.

[135] Fu LN, Wang W, Yu LJ, Zhang SM, Yang G. Fabrication of novel cellulose/chitosan artificial skin composite. Materials Science Forum 2009;610-613:1034-1038.

[136] Yussof SJM, Halim AS, Saad AZM, Jaafar H. Evaluation of the Biocompatibility of a Bilayer Chitosan Skin Regenerating Template, Human Skin Allograft, and Integra Implants in Rats. International Scholarly Research Network (ISRN) Materials Science Volume 2011:1 -7.

[137] Schulz III JT, Tompkins RG, Burke JF. Artificial Skin. Annual Review of Medicine 2000;51:231-244.

[138] Jebahi S, Oudadesse H, Bui XV, Keskes H, Rebai T, Feki A, Feki H. Repair of bone defect using bioglass-chitosan as a pharmaceutical drug: An experimental study in an ovariectomised rat model. African Journal of Pharmacy and Pharmacology 2012; 6(16):1276-1287.

[139] Zhang Z, Cui HF. Biodegradability and Biocompatibility Study of Poly(Chitosan-g-lactic Acid) Scaffolds. Molecules 2012;17:3243-3258.

[140] Li XG, Yang ZY, Zhang AF, Wang TL, Chen WC. Repair of thoracic spinal cord injury by chitosan tube implantation in adult rats. Biomaterials 2009;30(6):1121–1132.

[141] Wang XH, Yan YN, Xiong Z, Lin F, Wu RD, Zhang RJ, Lu, QP. Preparation and Evaluation of Ammonia Treated Collagen/Chitosan matrices for Liver Tissue Engineering. J Biomed Mater Res Part B Appl. Biomater 2005;75B: 91-98.

[142] Wang XH, Li DP, Wang WJ, Feng QL,Cui FZ, Xu YX, Song XH, van der Werf M. Crosslinked collagen/chitosan matrix for artificial livers, Biomaterials 2003;24(19): 3213-3220.

[143] Wang XH, Cui FZ, Feng QL, Li JC, Zhang YH. Preparation and characterization of collagen/chitosan matrices as potential biomaterials. J Bioact Compat Polym 2003;18(6):453-467.

[144] Denkbas EB, Seyyal M, Piskin E. Implantable 5-fluorouracil loaded chitosan scaffolds prepared by wet spinning. Journal of Membrane Science 2000;172(1):33-38.

[145] Sun J, Jiang G, Qiu T, Wang Y, Zhang K, Ding F. Injectable chitosan-based hydrogel for implantable drug delivery: body response and induced variations of structure and composition. J Biomed Mater Res A. 2010;95(4):1019-1027.

[146] Feng M, Han J, Sun Q, Hou ZQ, Zhang QQ. Preparation and Evaluation of Implantable Chitosan-Collagen-Soybean Phosphatidylcholine Film Impregnated with Mitomycin C-PLA- Nanoparticles. 2009. ICBBE 2009. 3rd International Conference on Bioinformatics and Biomedical Engineering

[147] Sun JL, Jiang GQ, Wang YJ, Ding FX. Thermosensitive chitosan hydrogel for implantable drug delivery: Blending PVA to mitigate body response and promote bioavailability. Journal of Applied Polymer Science 2012;125(3):2092-2101.

[148] Rosato DV, Rosato DV; Rosato MV. Plastic product material and process selection handbook, Elsevier, 2004 p.85, ISBN 978-1-85617-431-2.

[149] Gilding DK; Reed AM. Biodegradable polymers for use in surgery - polyglycolic/poly (lactic acid) homo- and copolymers: 1. Polymer 1979;20(12):1459–1464.

[150] Cortiella J, Nichols JE, Kojima K, Bonassar LJ, Dargon P, Roy AK, Vacant MP, Niles JA, Vacanti CA. Tissue-Engineered Lung: An *In vivo* and *In Vitro* Comparison of Polyglycolic Acid and Pluronic F-127 Hydrogel/Somatic Lung Progenitor Cell Constructs to Support Tissue Growth. Tissue Engineering 2006;12(5):1213-1225.

[151] Tamai H, Igaki K, Kyo E, Kosuga K, Kawashima A, Matsui S, Komori H, Tsuji T, Motohara S, Uehata H. Initial and 6-month results of biodegradable poly-l-lactic acid coronary stents in humans. Circulation. 2000;102:399-404.

[152] Bergsma JE, Bos RRM, Rozema F R, Jong W, Boering G. Biocompatibility of intraosseously implanted predegraded poly(lactide): an animal study. Journal of Materials Science: Materials in Medicine 1996;7(1):1-7.

[153] Aframian DJ, Redman RS, Yamano S, Nikolovski J, Cukierman E, Yamada KM, Kriete MF, Swaim WD, Mooney DJ, Baum BJ. Tissue compatibility of two biodegradable tubular scaffolds implanted adjacent to skin or buccal mucosa in mice. Tissue Eng 2002;8(4):649-659.

[154] Lam KH, Schakenraad JM, Esselbrgge H, Esselbrugge H, Feijen J, Nieuwenhuis P. The effect of phagocytosis of poly(L-lactic acid) fragments on cellular morphology and viability. Journal of Biomedical Materials Research 1993;27:1569-1577.

[155] Onuki Y, Bhardwaj U, Papadimitrakopoulos F, Burgess DJ. A review of the biocompatibility of implantable devices: current challenges to overcome foreign body response. J Diabetes Sci Technol. 2008;2(6):1003–1015.

[156] Zoppi RA, Duek EAR, Coraça DC. Barros PP. Preparation and characterization of poly (L-lactic acid) and poly(ethylene oxide) blends. Materials Research 2001;4(2): 117-125.

[157] Nagahama K, Ohya Y, Ouchi T. Synthesis of Star-shaped 8 arms Poly(ethylene gly-col)-Poly(L-lactide) Block Copolymer and Physicochemical Properties of Its Solution Cast Film as Soft Biomaterial. Polymer Journal 2006;38:852–860.

[158] van der Lei B, Bartels HL, Nieuwenhuis P, Wildevuur CR. Microporous, complaint, biodegradable vascular grafts for the regeneration of the arterial wall in rat abdominal aorta. Surgery. 1985 Nov;98(5):955-963.

[159] Middleton J; Tipton A. Synthetic biodegradable polymers as medical devices". Medical Plastics and Biomaterials Magazine. 1998 Retrieved 2006-07-04.

[160] Muhonen J, Suuronen R, Oikarinen VJ, Sarkiala E, Happonen R-P. Effect of polygly-colic acid (PGA) membrane on bone regeneration around titanium implants inserted in bone sockets. Journal of Materials Science: Materials in Medicine 1994; 5(1):40-42.

[161] Taylor MS, Daniels AU, Andriano KP, Heller J. Six bioabsorbable polymers: *in vitro* acute toxicity of accumulated degradation products. J Appl Biomater 1994;5(2): 151-157.

[162] Anderson JM. Biological responses to materials. Annu Rev Mater Res. 2001;31:81–110.

[163] van der Giessen WJ, Lincoff AM, Schwartz RS, van Beusekom HM, Serruys PW, Holmes DR, Jr, Ellis SG, Topol EJ. Marked inflammatory sequelae to implantation of biodegradable and nonbiodegradable polymers in porcine coronary arteries. Circulation. 1996;94(7):1690–1697.

[164] Venkatraman S, Boey YC. Patent: Implantable article, method of forming same and method for reducing thrombogenicity. IPC8 Class: AA61F206FI, USPC Class: 623001440, Publication date: 2012-07-12, Patent application number: 20120179242.

[165] Bhardwaj U, Papadimitrakopoulos F, Burgess DJ. A review of the development of a vehicle for localized and controlled drug delivery for implantable biosensors. J Diabetes Sci Technol. 2008;2(6):1016-1029.

[166] Onuki Y, Bhardwaj U, Burgess PDJ. A Review of the Biocompatibility of Implantable Devices: Current Challenges to Overcome Foreign Body Response. J Diabetes Sci Technol 2008;2(6):1003-1015.

[167] Bhardwaj U, Sura R, Papadimitrakopoulos F, Burgess DJ. Controlling acute inflammation with fast releasing dexamethasone-PLGA microsphere/PVA hydrogel composites for implantable devices. Journal of Diabetes Science and Technology 2007;1(1):8-17.

[168] Ranganath SH, Yang A, Chan YY, Huang J, Krantz WB, Wang CH. Implantable hydrogel beads entrapping PLGA-paclitaxel microspheres: exploring the effects of near-zero order drug release for intracranial chemotherapy. AIChE Annual meeting, Philadelphia, USA, November 2008.

[169] Corey JM, Gertz CC, Wang BS, Birrell LK, Johnson SL, Martin DC, Feldman EL. The design of electrospun PLLA nanofiber scaffolds compatible with serum-free growth of primary motor and sensory neurons. Acta Biomater 2008;4(4):863-875)

[170] Leach KJ, Takahashi S, Mathiowitz E. Degradation of double-walled polymer microspheres of PLLA and P(CPP:SA)20 : 80. II. *In vivo* degradation. Biomaterials 1998;19(21):1981-1988.

[171] Liu JY, LiRen L, Wei Q, Wu JL, Liu S, Wang YJ, Li GY. Toward better bone repair. 2012 Society of Plastics Engineers (SPE).

[172] Woodruff MA, Hutmacher DW. The return of a forgetten polymer – polycaprolactone in the 21st century. Progress in Polymer Science 2010;35:1217-1256.

[173] Sun HF, Mei L, Song CX, Cui XM, Wang PY. The *in vivo* degradation, absorption and excretion of PCL-based implant. Biomaterials 2006;27(9):1735–1740.

[174] Sinha VR, Bansal K, Kaushik R, Kumria R, Trehan A. Poly- -caprolactone microspheres and nanospheres: an overview. International Journal of Pharmaceutics 2004;278(1):1-23.

[175] LaVan AD, McGuire T, Langer R. Smallscale systems for *in vivo* drug delivery. Nature Biotechnology 2003; 21:1184-1191.

[176] Orosz KE, Gupta S, Hassink M, Abdel-Rahman M, Moldovan L, Davidorf FH, Moldovan NI. Delivery of antiangiogenic and antioxidant drugs of ophthalmic interest through a nanoporous inorganic filter. Molecular Vision 2004;10:555-565.

[177] Chung TW, Yang MC, Tseng CC, Sheu SH, Wang SS, Huang YY, Chen SD. Promoting regeneration of peripheral nerves in-vivo using new PCL-NGF/Tirofiban nerve conduits. Biomaterials. 2011;32(3):734-743.

[178] Pitt CG, Schinder A. Capronor-A biodegradable delivery system for levonorgestrel. In: Zatachini GL, editor. Long-acting contraceptive systems. Philadelphia: Harpen and Row; 1984. p.63–84.

[179] Woodward SC, Brewer PS, Moatamed F, Schindler AK Pitt CG. The intracellular degradation of poly (epsilon-caprolactone). J Biomed Mater Res 1985;19(4):437–44.

[180] Xia Z, Triffitt JT. A review on macrophage responses to biomaterials. Biomed. Mater 2006;1:R1–R9.

[181] Coury AJ, Slaikeu PC, Cahalan PT, Stokes KB, Hobot CM. Factors and interactions affecting the performance of polyurethane elastomers in medical devices. J Biomater Appl 1988 Oct;3(2):130-179.

[182] Coury AJ, Stokes KB, Cahalan PT, Slaikeu PC. Biostability considerations for implantable polyurethanes. Life Support Syst 1987;5(1):25-39.

[183] Maisel WH. Increased failure rate of a polyurethane implantable cardioverter defibrillator lead. Pacing Clin Electrophysiol. 2002;25(6):877-878.

[184] Hauser RG, Cannom D, Hayes DL, Parsonnet V, Hayes J, Ratliff N 3rd, Tyers GF, Ep-
       stein AE, Vlay SC, Furman S, Gross J. Long-term structural failure of coaxial polyur-
       ethane implantable cardioverter defibrillator leads. Pacing Clin Electrophysiol.
       2002;25(6):879-882.

[185] Stokes KB, Church T. Ten-year experience with implanted polyurethane lead insula-
       tion. Pacing Clin Electrophysiol. 1986;;9(6 Pt 2):1160-1165.

[186] Santerre JP, Woodhouse K, Laroche G, Labow RS. Understanding the biodegradation
       of polyurethanes: From classical implants to tissue engineering materials. Biomateri-
       als 2005;26(35):7457-7470.

[187] Wang Y. Patent: Implantable Medical Devices Fabricated From Polyurethanes With
       Grafted Radiopaque Groups. IPC8 Class: AA61F282FI, USPC Class: 623 134, Class
       name: Prosthesis (i.e., artificial body members), parts thereof, or aids and accessories
       therefor arterial prosthesis (i.e., blood vessel) having marker (e.g., color, radiopaque,
       etc.), Publication date: 2009-10-15, Patent application number: 20090259297

[188] Stachelek SJ, Alferiev I, Connolly JM, Sacks M, Hebbel RP, Bianco R, Levy RJ. Choles-
       terol-modified polyurethane valve cusps demonstrate blood outgrowth endothelial
       cell adhesion post-seeding *in vitro* and *in vivo*. Ann Thorac Surg. 2006 Jan;81(1):47-55.

[189] Ghanbari H, Viatge H, Kidane AG, Burriesci G, Tavakoli M, Seifalian AM. Polymeri-
       ca heart valves: new materials, emerging hopes. Trends in Biotechnology 2009;27(6):
       359-367.

[190] Gwendolyn M.R. Wetzels, Leo H. Koole. Photoimmobilisation of poly(N-vinylpyrro-
       lidinone) as a means to improve haemocompatibility of polyurethane biomaterials.
       Biomaterials 1999;20(20):1879}-1887.

[191] Staniszewska-Kuś J, Paluch D, Krzemień-Dabrowska A, Zywicka B, Solski L.Tissue
       reaction to implanted polyurethane designed for parts of the artificial heart. Polym
       Med. 1995;25(3-4):3-18.

[192] Stachelek SJ, Alferiev I, Choi H, Chan CW, Zubiate B, Sacks M, Composto R, Chen I-
       W, Levy R. Prevention of oxidative degradation of polyurethane by covalent attach-
       ment of di-tert-butylphenol residues. J Biomed Mater Res A. 2006;78(4):653-661).

[193] Stachelek SJ, Alferiev I, Connolly JM, Sacks M, Hebbel RP, Bianco R, Levy RJ. Choles-
       terol-modified polyurethane valve cusps demonstrate blood outgrowth endothelial
       cell adhesion post-seeding in vitro and *in vivo* Ann Thorac Surg. 2006 Jan; 81(1):47-55.

[194] Alferiev I, Stachelek SJ, Lu ZB, Fu AL, Tiffany L. Sellaro TL, Jeanne M. Connolly JM,
       Richard W. Bianco RW, Michael S. Sacks MS, Robert J. Levy RJ. Prevention of polyur-
       ethane valve cusp calcification with covalently attached bisphosphonate diethylami-
       no moieties. J Biomed Mater Res A. 2003; 66(2):385-395.

[195] Chris Smith. Implantable PU developer wins heart valve patent. Time:2009-08-03.

[196] Yan YN, Wang XH, Yin DZ, Zhang RJ. A new polyurethane/heparin vascular graft for small-caliber vein repair. J Bioact Compat Polym 2007;22(3):323-341.

[197] Yin DZ, Wang XH, Yan YN, Zhang RJ. Preliminary studies on peripheral nerve re-generation using a new polyurethane conduit. J Bioact Compat Polym 2007;22(2): 143-159.

[198] Fluorine and health:molecular imaging, biomedical materials and pharmaceuticals. Edited by Alain Tressaud and Günter Haufe. Elsevier, UK

[199] Williams MR, Mikulin T, Lemberger J, Hopkinson BR, Makin GS. Five year experi-ence using PTFE vascular grafts for lower limb ischaemia. Ann R Coll Surg Engl. 1985; 67(3):152–155.

[200] von Recum AF, Imamura H, Freed PS, Kantrowitz A, Chen ST, Ekstrom ME, Baech-ler CA, Barnhart MI. Biocompatibility tests of components of an implantable cardiac assist device. J Biomed Mater Res. 1978 Sep;12(5):743-765.

[201] Głowiński S, Worowski K. Local activation of blood coagulation by polyester pros-theses implanted into defects of the abdominal aorta of dogs. Polim Med 1977;7(4): 241-243.

[202] Renwick SB. Silicone breast implants: implications for society and surgeons. Med J Aust 1996 Sep 16;165(6):338-341.

[203] Daniels AU. Silicone breast implant materials. Swiss Med Wkly. 2012;142:doi: 10.4414/smw.2012.13614.

[204] Dewan PA, Condron SK, Morreau PN, Byard RW, Terlet J. Plastic migration from im-planted central venous access devices. Arch Dis Child 1999;81:71–72.

[205] Pavlov St, Guidoin R, Marinov G. Histological organization of the capsulae formed around implanted silicone breast prostheses. Acta Morphologica et Anthropologica 01/2004; 9:50-57.

[206] Roach P, Eglin D, Rohde K, Perry CC. Modern biomaterials: a review—bulk proper-ties and implications of surface modifications. Journal of Materials Science: Materials in Medicine 2007;Volume 18, Number 7 , 1263-1277.

[207] Kim D-H, Kim Y-S, Amsden KJ, Panilaitis B, Kaplan DL, Omenetto FG, Zakin MR, Rogers JA. Silicon electronics on silk as a path to bioresorbable, implantable devices. Appl Hys Lett 2009;95:133701.

[208] Stead RJ, Davidson TI, Duncan FR, Hodson ME, Batien JC. Use of a totally implanta-ble system for venous access in cystic fibrosis. Thorax 1987;42:149-150.

[209] Guo K, Pei WH, Li XQ, Gui Q, Tang RY, Liu J, Chen HD. Fabrication and characteri-zation of implantable silicon neural probe with microfluidic channels. Science China Technological Sciences January 2012;55 No(1): 1–5.

[210] Danckwerts M, Fassihi A. Implantable Controlled Release Drug Delivery Systems: A Review. 1991;17(11):1465-1502.

[211] Shakhashiri BZ. Chemical of the Week: Aluminum. SciFun.org. University of Wisconsin. http://scifun.chem.wisc.edu/chemweek/PDF/Aluminum.pdf. Retrieved 2012-03-04 (17 March 2008).

[212] Takami Y, Yamane S, Makinouchi K, Niimi Y, Sueoka A, Nosé Y. Evaluation of platelet adhesion and activation on materials for an implantable centrifugal blood pump 1. Artif Organs 1998;;22(9):753-758.

[213] Polmear IJ. Light Alloys, Arnold, 1995.

[214] Tseung ACC, King WJ, Wan BYC. An encapsulated, implantable metal-oxygen cell as a long-term power source for medical and biological applications. Medical and Biological Engineering and Computing 1971;9(3):175-184.

[215] Stieglitz T. Flexible biomedical microdevices with double-sided electrode arrangements for neural applications. Sensors and Actuators A 2001;90:202-211.

[216] Jiang GQ, Mishler D, Davis R, Mobley JP, Schulman JH. Zirconia to Ti-6Al-4V braze joint for implantable biomedical device. J Biomed Mater Res Part B: Appl Biomater 2005;72B: 316–321.

[217] Dowling RD, Park SJ, Pagani FD, Mohr F-W. HeartMate VE LVAS design enhancements and its impact on device reliability. European Journal of Cardio-Thoracic Surgery 2004; 25(6):958–963.

[218] Takami Y, Yamane S, Makinouchi K, Niimi Y, Sueoka A, Nosé Y. Evaluation of platelet adhesion and activation on materials for an implantable centrifugal blood pump. Artif Organs 1998;22(9):753-758.

[219] Spiliopoulos K, Giamouzis G, Karayannis G, Karangelis D, Koutsias S, Kalogeropoulos A, Georgiopoulou V, Skoularigis J, Butler J, Triposkiadis F. Current Status of Mechanical Circulatory Support: A Systematic Review. Cardiology Research and Practice 2012, Article ID 574198, 12 pages, doi:10.1155/2012/574198.

[220] Myllymaa S. Novel micro- and nano-technological approaches for improving the performance of implantable biomedical devices. Publications of the University of Eastern Finland. Dissertations in Forestry and Natural Sciences. University of Eastern Finland. P122.

[221] Olga L; Péter B; George KS; Jósef B. Porous hydroxyapatite and aluminium-oxide ceramic orbital implant evaluation using CBCT scanning: a method for in vivo porous structure evaluation and monitoring. International Journal of Biomaterials 2012; 1-9: 1687-8787.

[222] Mitsuo A, Aizawa T. Thermal oxidation and characterization for surface layers of Al implanted TiN films. Ion Implantation Technology Proceedings, 1988 International Conference on IEEE. Date of Conference: Dec 1999;2:865–868.

[223] Sedrakyan A, Normand ST, Dabic S, Jacobs S, Graves S, Marinac-Dabic D. Comparative assessment of implantable hip devices with different bearing surfaces: systematic appraisal of evidence. BMJ 2011;343:d7434-7446.

[224] Defibrillator Risks eHow.com http://www.ehow.com/facts_7438880_defibrillator-risks.html#ixzz23258fVn4.

[225] Thamaraiselvi TV, Rajeswari S. Biological evaluation of bioceramic materials - a review. Trends Biomater Artif Organs 2004;18(1);9-17.

[226] Patel NR, Gohil PP. A Review on biomaterials: scope, applications & human anatomy significance. International Journal of Emerging Technology and Advanced Engineering 2012; 2(4), 2250-2259.

Chapter 6

Amelioration of Blood Compatibility and Endothelialization of Polycaprolactone Substrates by Surface-Initiated Atom Transfer Radical Polymerization

Shaojun Yuan, Gordon Xiong, Ariel Roguin, Swee Hin Teoh and Cleo Choong

Additional information is available at the end of the chapter

1. Introduction

Attempts to develop synthetic vascular grafts for the replacement of diseased vascular sections have been an area of active research over the past decades [1]. However, thrombosis formation as a result of platelet adhesion to the luminal surface of synthetic graft and restenosis caused by host inflammatory remain a challenge, especially for small-diameter (<6 mm) graft replacement [2,3]. Therefore, the haemocompatibility of the biomaterial used in the graft is a prerequisite for clinical success. As the result, various strategies have been developed to improve the blood compatibility of biomaterial surfaces, including the surface immobilization of anti-coagulants such as heparin [4] and sulfated silk fibroin [5], the incorporation of polyethylene oxide or negatively charged side chains [6,7], and surface passivation with protein layers, such as albumin [8]. Despite the efficacy of these approaches in preventing acute thrombogenesis, concerns remain on the drug elution lifespan, with possible consequence of late thrombosis [9]. To avoid undesirable blood-material interaction, the seeding of autologous endothelial cells (ECs) onto the luminal surface of the graft is considered to be an ideal approach to increase the patency of synthetic grafts [10]. Many studies have indicated that endothelial cells release factors that regulate thrombogenesis and platelet activation [11], while delayed or absent stent endothelialization has been implicated in late thrombosis and adverse clinical outcomes [13]. Thus, rapid endothelialization of vascular grafts is of great importance for blood-contacting vessels for long-term patency.

Due to its slow degradation rates in vivo (2-4 years) [14], good mechanical strength, and biocompatibility with vascular cell types [15,16], polycaprolactone (PCL) is currently being extensively investigated as scaffolds for vascular tissue engineering applications [17-21]. However, the intrinsic hydrophobicity and poor cytocompatibility of PCL substrates lead to poor affinity for cell adhesion, thereby restricting their applications as blood-contacting devices. Consequently, surface modification of PCL is necessary to improve cell adhesion and proliferation. Functional polymer brushes containing reactive hydroxyl (-OH), carboxyl (-COOH) or amine (-NH2) groups have been successfully grafted onto the PCL surfaces using γ-ray irradiated, ozone or photo-induced polymerization grafting to introduce hydrophilicity [9,16,22-24]. These flexible reactive groups on the polymer brushes are well-suited to conjugate bioactive macromolecules for improved cytocompatibility. However, γ-ray irradiated, ozone or photo-induced polymerization grafting of polymer brushes has several limitations, including low density of grafting due to steric hindrance, uncontrollable graft yield of polymer brushes, and undesired formation of a covalent bond between reactive groups on the polymer brushes and the surface [25]. Hence, an alternative grafting approach that allows control over brush density, polydispersity and composition is desired.

One such alternative is the use of surface-initiated atom transfer radical polymerization (ATRP) approach to covalently graft polymer brushes in a tunable and controllable manner [26]. This approach allows the preparation of well-defined dense polymer brushes containing reactive pendant groups (e.g. -OH, -COOH, or epoxide groups), and provides highly reactive binding sites for functional biomolecules.[27] As a result, surface-initiated ATRP provides a promising approach to fabricate PCL substrates with well-defined polymer brushes of controlled length and density, as well as tunable grafting density of biomacromolecules. However, to the best of our knowledge, only few studies have been devoted to modifying biodegradable polyester polymers using surface-initiated ATRP to improve their cytocompatibility or blood compatibility [27,28]. Also, the functionality of the attached cells was not thoroughly investigated in those studies.

As such, the aim of the current study is to utilize the surface-initiated ATRP method to tailor PCL substrates with dense functional P(GMA) brushes and high-density immobilized gelatin to improve their properties for cell attachment and proliferation. Each functionalization step was ascertained by XPS, AFM and water contact angle measurements. The cytocompatibility of the functionalized PCL substrates was evaluated using human umbilical vein endothelial cells (HUVECs) and the effect of different surface properties on the regulation of the thrombogenicity of the attached cells was also investigated.

2. Materials and methods

2.1. Materials

Polycaprolactone pellets (PCL, average M_n 45000), 1,6-hexanediamine (98%), glycidyl methacrylate (GMA, >97%), 2-bromoisobutyrl bromide (BIBB, 98%), 2,2'-bipyridine (bpy, 98%), dichloromethane (anhydrous, >99.8%), triethylamine (TEA, 98%), isopropyl alcohol, hexane (anhydrous, >95%), copper (I) bromide (CuBr, 99%), copper (II) bromide (CuBr$_2$, 98%), and gelatin (Porcine skin, Type A) were obtained from Sigma-Aldrich Chemical Co. (St. Louis,

MO, USA), and were used without further purification. GMA was passed through a silica gel column to remove the inhibitor, and stored under a nitrogen atmosphere at -4°C. All the other chemical reagents and solvents were used as received. Human Umbilical Vein Endothelial cells (HUVECs, ATCC CRL-1730™) were purchased from American Type Culture Collection (Manassas, VA, USA). Cell culture medium (MCDB131), heparin and paraformaldehyde (4%, v/v) were obtained from Sigma-Aldrich Chemical Co. Medium supplements, such as Foetal Bovine Serum (FBS), penicillin, amphotericin, bovine brain extract, streptomycin, and Trypsin-EDTA (0.25%), were purchased from Life Technologies (Carlsbad, CA, USA). LIVE/DEAD® cell viability assay reagent, AlamarBlue™ reagent, tissue thromboplastin (human brain extract), ellagic acid, and DAF-FM Diacetatewere obtained from Life Technologies. The P-selectin assay reagents were obtained from Serotec Co. (Kidlington, Oxford, UK).

2.2. Aminolysis of PCL film substrates and immobilization of ATRP initiator

Polycaprolactone (PCL) films were prepared by solution casting method using previously established methods [29]. Briefly, 5 g of the PCL pellets was dissolved in 40 ml of dichloromethane to form the PCL solution. The polymer solution was then cast onto the glass substrate with predetermined thickness using the automatic film applicator (PA-2105, BYK). The solvent was removed at room temperature by slow evaporation over a 24 h period, and was further dried in a vacuum oven for another 24 h at 35 °C to obtain the translucent PCL films with a thickness of about 150 μm. The resultant PCL films were cut into round-shaped specimens with a diameter of 2 cm. The activation of PCL substrates was performed by aminolysis treatment using a procedure previously described [30,31]. Briefly, the PCL films were immersed in a 10% (w/w) 1,6-hexanediamine and isopropanol mixture at 40 °C for a predetermined time. After aminolysis treatment, the resultant PCL-NH$_2$ surfaces were thoroughly rinsed with copious amounts of deionized water and isopropanol, respectively, to remove free 1,6-hexanediamine, and dried in a vacuum oven at 30 °C for 24 h.

The introduction of an alkyl halide ATRP initiator on the PCL-NH$_2$ surface was accomplished through the reaction of the amino groups with 2-bromoisobutyrate bromide (BIBB) [32]. The PCL-NH$_2$ films were immersed in 30 ml of anhydrous hexane solution containing 1.0 ml (7.2 mmol) of triethylamine (TEA). After 30 min of degassing with nitrogen, the reaction mixture was cooled in an ice bath, and 0.89 ml (1.65g, 7.2 mmol) of BIBB was added dropwise via a syringe. The reaction was allowed to proceed with gentle stirring at 0 °C for 2 h and then at room temperature for 12 h. The resulting surface (referred to as the PCL-Br surface) was washed thoroughly with copious amounts of hexane, ethanol, and finally deionized water, in that order, and was subsequently dried in a vacuum oven under reduced pressure at ambient temperature overnight.

2.3. Surface-initiated ATRP of GMA and immobilization of gelatin

For the grafting of P(GMA) brushes from the PCL-Br surfaces, surface-initiated ATRP of GMA was performed using a [GMA (3 ml)]:[CuBr]:[CuBr$_2$]:[Bpy] molar feed ratio of 100:1.0:0.2:2.0 in 5 ml of methanol/water mixture (5/1, v/v) at room temperature in a Pyrex® tube. The reaction was allowed to proceed for 0.5 to 3 h to produce the PCL-g-P(GMA) surfaces. After the prescribed reaction time, the films were removed and washed sequentially with copious amount of methanol and deionized water, followed by immersing in methanol for about 48 h to ensure the complete removal of the physically-adsorbed reactants or polymers. For the immobilization of gelatin onto the pendant epoxide groups of the P(GMA) brushes, the PCL-g-P(GMA) films were incubated in 10 ml of the phosphate buffered saline (PBS, pH 7.4) containing 3 mg/ml gelatin. The reaction was allowed to proceed at room temperature for 24 h under continuous stirring to produce the corresponding PCL-g-P(GMA)-c-gelatin surfaces. After the reaction, the gelatin-immobilized PCL films were washed thoroughly with PBS solution and deionized water to remove the physically adsorbed (reversibly-bound) gelatin, prior to being dried in a vacuum oven under reduced pressure overnight.

2.4. Grafting density of the P(GMA) brushes and immobilized gelatin

The grafting density of the P(GMA) brushes and the amount of immobilized gelatin on the PCL substrates was determined by the grafting yield (GY) using the following equation [27,33]:

$$GY = \frac{W_a - W_b}{A} \tag{1}$$

Where Wa and Wb are the weights of the dry film after and before graft polymerization (or immobilization of gelatin) respectively, and A is the film area (about 3.2 cm^2). For each GY measurement, a minimum of three pieces of PCL films was used and the resulting values were averaged.

2.5. Surface characterization

The composition of the functionalized PCL films was determined by X-ray photoelectron spectroscopy (XPS). All the XPS spectra were recorded on a Krato AXIS Hsi spectrometer with a monochromatic Al Kα X-ray source (1486.6 eV photons), using procedures similar to those described previously [32]. The N 1s core-level signal can be used as an indicator of the immobilized gelatin. The [N]/[C] ratio, as determined from the sensitivity-factor-corrected N 1s and C 1s core-level XPS spectral area, indicated the relative abundance of the immobilized gelatin on the PCL substrates. Static water contact angles of the functionalized PCL film surfaces were measured at 25 °C and 60% relative humidity using a sessile drop method with 3 μl water droplets on a FTÅ 200 contact angle goniometer (First Ten Angstroms Inc., Portsmouth, VA, USA). The contact angles reported were the mean values from four substrates, with the value of each substrate obtained by averaging the contact angles for at least three surface locations. The surface topography of the functionalized PCL substrates was investigated by atomic force microscope (AFM). A multimode scanning probe microscope equipped with a NanoscopeIIIa controller (Digital Instrument, Santa Barbara, USA) was used to capture the AFM images in air. 10 μm scans were recorded in tapping mode with a silicon cantilever. The drive amplitude was about 300 mV, and the scan rate was between 0.5 and 1.0 Hz. The arithmetic mean of the surface roughness (R_a) was determined by Nano-scope software.

2.6. Cytocompatibility of the functionalized PCL substrates

Human umbilical vein endothelial cells (HUVECs, ATCC CRL-1730™) were cultured in gel-atin-coated T25 flasks containing MCDB131 cell culture medium supplemented with Foetal Bovine Serum, 0.2% Bovine Brain Extract, 0.25 ug/ml amphotericin, 0.1 mg/ml heparin, 100 U/ml penicillin, and 100 ug/ml streptomycin, in a CO_2 environment at 37°C. The MCDB131 medium was changed every other day. Upon 90% culture confluency, cells were harvested by trypsinization using 0.25% Trypsin-EDTA. ECs between 4-6 passages were used for sub-sequent experiments.

2.6.1. Cell proliferation

The pristine and functionalized PCL films were sterilized by immersing into 75% (v/v) etha-nol solution for 60 min, and then rinsed thrice with sterile PBS, followed by MCDB131 medi-um incubation overnight. Gelatin-coated coverslips (0.1%) were used as positive controls. Cell viability and proliferation was determined using the AlamarBlue™(AB) assay. 0.5 ml of EC cell suspension (2×10^4 cells/ml) was seeded into each well of 24-well plate containing the pristine and functionalized PCL films, and incubated in a 5% CO_2 environment at 37 °C for 1, 3, 5 and 7 days. The cell culture medium was changed every other day. After the predeter-mined incubation period, culture media was removed from the wells, and 0.5 ml of the AB solution (10% AB solution in culture media without FBS) was added to the wells. The plates were incubated in a 5% CO_2 atmosphere at 37°C for 4 h and the fluorescence density was measured using a microplate reader (Model 680, Bio-Rad Laboratories, Inc. Hercules, CA, USA) at an excitation wavelength of 570 nm and an emission wavelength of 580 nm. Cell numbers were calculated using standards derived from seeding known quantities of cells and correlating with fluorescence emission.

2.6.2. Cell imaging

In vitro qualitative analysis of cell coverage and viability was performed using a LIVE/DEAD® viability/cytotoxicity assay to assess the extent of endothelialization on the function-alized PCL surfaces. For this procedure, calcein AM (4 mM in anhydrous dimethyl sulfox-ide, DMSO) and EthD-1 (2 mM in DMSO/H2O, 1:4 v:v) were added to PBS (1:1000 ratio) to produce a LIVE/DEAD® staining solution. The cell-seeded PCL samples, obtained after 7 days cell culture, were first washed thrice with PBS to eliminate the nonadherent cells, fol-lowed by staining using 0.1 ml of LIVE/DEAD staining solution. After incubation in a 5% CO_2 atmosphere at 37°C for 30 min, the samples were visualized by Nikon Image Ti fluores-cence microscope (emission at 515 nm and 635 nm (Nikon Instruments, Tokyo, Japan) to ac-quire fluorescent images using NIS-Elements Br software.

2.7. Blood compatibility of the bare and endothelialized PCL substrates

The hemolysis rate, coagulant activity, nitric oxide (NO) production, and platelet activation of the bare and endothelialized PCL films with various surface functionalizations were investigated to evaluate their blood compatibility. The endothelialized PCL substrates were obtained by culturing ECs (2×10^4 cells/ml) for 7 days on surface-functionalized PCL films using the procedures described above.

2.7.1. Hemolysis rate test

The pristine and functionalized PCL samples were immersed in diluted blood solution containing 2% fresh anticoagulated (ACD) human blood and 98% physiological salt solution and incubated at 37o for 1 h. After centrifugation at 3000 rpm for 5 min, the absorbance of solution was recorded as D_t. Under the same conditions, the solution containing 2% ACD blood and 98% physiological salt solution was used as a negative reference, and the solution containing 2% ACD blood and 98% distilled water was used as a positive reference. These absorbances were recorded as D_{nc} and D_{pc}, respectively. The hymolysis rate α of the samples was calculated using the following equation:

$$\alpha = \frac{D_t - D_{nc}}{D_{pc} - D_{nc}} \times 100\% \tag{2}$$

2.7.2. Coagulation assays

Whole blood of healthy human volunteers was mixed with 3.8% sodium citrate at a volume ratio of 1:9. The blood was centrifuged at 3000 rpm for 15 min at room temperature to obtain platelet-poor plasma (PPP). Aliquots of 500 µl of PPP were added to be in contact with the surfaces of each bare or endothelialized PCL substrate for 10 min at 37°C. The PPP was then collected and added with tissue thromboplastin (human brain extract) for prothrombin time (PT) tests, or added with a partial thromboplastin reagent (ellagic acid) for activated partial thromboplastin time (APTT) test. Subsequently, the fibrin clot formation time was determined by an automatic coagulation analyzer (Sysmex CA-7000). PPP that was not exposed to the PCL substrates was used as a blank sample.

2.7.3. Nitric Oxide (NO) secretion by HUVEC

ECs cultured for 7 days on the functionalized PCL substrates were washed twice with PBS and incubated at 37°C with trypsin-EDTA (0.25%) solution for cell detachment. The resultant ECs were serum-starved overnight in serum-free medium. After incubation with fresh serum-free medium for 6 h, the medium was removed and DAF-FM diacetate (Molecular Probes, D-23842) was added to the medium to effect a final concentration of 10 µM. The medium was subsequently incubated at 37 °C for 1 h, followed by detection of fluorescence using Glomax 20/20 luminometer equipped with a blue fluorescent module. The end product of DAF-FM diacetate and NO is a benzotriazole derivative with a fluorescence excitation and emission maxima of 495 and 515 nm, respectively. Fluorescence units were normalized to cell numbers.

2.7.4. Platelet activation determination by P-selectinassay

Platelet activation by the bare and endothelialized PCL substrates was investigated using the P-selectin (CD62P) assay. Briefly, 100 µl of fresh human platelet rich plasma (PRP) was incubated with the bare or 7-day endothelialized PCL substrates at 37°C for 2 h. At the end of incubation, the films were thoroughly with copious amounts of PBS solution thrice, followed by adding 40 µl of anti-CD62P (1:100, v:v) to each film, and then incubated at 37°C for 1 h. After being washed thrice with PBS solution, the films were each incubated with 40 µl of horseradish peroxidase-conjugated sheep anti-mouse polycolonal antibody at 1:100 (v:v) at 37°C for 1 h. Subsequently, the PCL films were reacted with 150 µl of 3,3',5, 5'-tetramethylbenzidine (TMB) chromogenic solution for 10 min. The color reaction was terminated by adding of 100 µL of 1 M H_2SO_4, and the optical densities (OD) were measured at 450 nm using a Varioskan Flash Microplate Reader (Thermo Fisher Scientific, Waltham, MA, USA).

2.7.5. Gene and protein expression of vWF and activity of MMP-2 in ECs cultured on functionalized PCL surfaces

For the real-time qPCR of von Willebrand factor (vWF) and matrix metalloproteinase-2 (MMP-2), the total RNA was extracted from the ECs after 7 days in culture, reverse-transcribed into cDNA and analyzed as described above. The expression of vWF and MMP-2 was normalized to the housekeeping ribosomal protein L27 (rpl27). Endothelial cells treated with 10 ng /ml TNF were used as positive controls.

For the immunoblot detection of vWF protein, cells were lyzed in protein lysis buffer (0.1% sodium dodecyl sulfate, 0.5% triton X-100, and 0.5% sodium deoxycholate dissolved in pH 7.4 PBS) and resolved using a denaturing 10% SDS-PAGE. The proteins were then blotted onto a nitrocellulose membrane and after blocking with 5% non-fat milk in tris-buffered saline with 0.1% Tween (TBS-T), the membrane stained using a rabbit anti-human vWF antibody at 1:5000 and subsequently with anti-rabbit HRP-conjugated antibody at 1:10,000 in TBS-T. The vWF was then visualized after developing using chemiluminescence on X-ray film. For determination of the MMP-2 activity, proteins were extracted from trypsinized cells using the protein lysis buffer before resolving by electrophoresis through a 10% SDS-PAGE copolymerized with 0.1% gelatin as substrate for enzymatic digestion. The molecular sizes of gelatinolytic activities were determined using protein standards (Fermentas, Pre-stained PAGE rulers). Upon completion of gel running, the gel was incubated with 100 mL renaturation buffer containing 2.5% triton X-100 for 1 h at room temperature with agitation. The gel was subsequently incubated in 100 ml of development buffer containing 50 mM Tris base, 200 mM NaCl, 5 mM CaCl2, and 0.02% Brij-35 overnight at 37 °C. Developed gel was then stained by the Coomassie Blue and gelatinolytic activities of MMP-2 were determined by the transparent bands appeared at the molecular weight of approximately 68 kDa and 98 kDa, respectively.

2.8. Statistical analysis

Each experiment was carried out with four replicates (n = 4), and the data are presented as mean ± standard deviation (SD) unless of otherwise stated. Statistical analysis was carried out by means of one-way analysis of variance (ANOVA) with Tukey's post hoc test. The confidence levels of 95% (p<0.05) and 99% (p<0.01) were used and no adjustments were made for multiple comparisons.

3. Results and discussion

Polycaprolactone (PCL) films with gelatin-coupled poly(glycidyl methacrylate) (P(GMA)) brushes were prepared via the following reaction sequence (Fig. 1): (a) active amine groups were introduced to the PCL film surfaces by the aminolysis reaction, (b) the immobilization of an alkyl bromide ATRP initiator was achieved via TEA-catalyzed condensation reaction between the amine groups on the aminolyzed PCL substrates and 2-bromoisobutyryl bromide (BIBB), (c) well-defined P(GMA) functional brushes were covalently grafted from the ATRP initiator-immobilized PCL surface via surface-initiated ATRP of GMA, (d) cell-adhesive gelatin was directly coupled to the pendant active epoxide groups of the grafted P(GMA). Details of each functionalization step are discussed below.

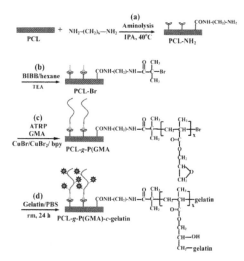

Figure 1. Schematic illustration of the process of (a) aminolysis of PCL substrates to introduce the free amino groups (the PCL-NH$_2$ surface), (b) immobilization of a alkyl bromine-containing initiator via condensation reaction to give the PCL-Br surface, (c) surface-initiated atom transfer radical polymerization (ATRP) of GMA from the PCL-Br surface to produce the PCL-g-P(GMA) surface, and (d) subsequently covalent conjugation of gelatin to obtain the PCL-g-P(GMA)-c-gelatin surface.

3.1. Aminolysis of PCL substrates and immobilization of ATRP initiator

Aminolysis represents an easy-to-perform chemical technique to engraft amino groups along the polyester chains, and hence has been widely used in the surface modification of scaffolds for tissue engineering applications [31,34]. In this study, PCL substrates were activated by the aminolysis reaction to introduce active amine groups. The relative amount of amine groups on the aminolyzed PCL (defined as the PCL-NH$_2$) surface was quantitatively determined by XPS measurements. The [N]/[C] ratio, as determined from sensitivity factor-corrected N 1s and C 1s core-level XPS spectral area, increases with the aminolysis time and reaches the maximal value after 1 h, which is estimated to be about 0.043 (Figs. 2). The result is consistent with the data reported previously [35,36]. As a degradation reaction, the aminolysis reaction is found to proceed preferentially at the amorphous regions of polymer in diamine solution during the initial period [37]. At longer aminolysis time, the decrease in bound amine groups may be caused by chain scission, formation of oligomers and other low mass fragments that are removed from the surface during reaction and the rinsing process [38]. Thus, the optimal aminolysis time for PCL film was found to be 1 h, and this reaction time was chosen for the subsequent surface modification and cell studies.

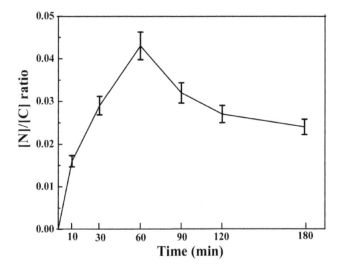

Figure 2. The [N]/[C] ratio of the aminolyzed PCL surface as a function of aminolysis time determined by XPS measurements. The analysis reaction of PCL films proceeded at 40°C in 10 wt% 1,6-hexanediamine/2-propanol solution. Error bars represent the standard deviation over separate measurement on three PCL films. The optimized aminolysis time was observed at 1 h with the [N]/[C] ratio of 0.043.

The chemical composition of the PCL film surfaces at various stages of surface modification was ascertained by XPS. Figs. 3a-3c show the respective wide scan, C 1s, and N 1s core-level spectra of the pristine PCL and PCL-NH$_2$ surfaces from 1 h of aminolysis. The C 1s core-level spectra of the pristine PCL can be curve-fitted into three peak components with binding energies (BEs) at about 284.6, 286.2 and 288.7 eV, attributable to the C-H, C-O, and O=C-O species, respectively (Fig. 3b) [39]. The area ratio of [C-H]:[C-O]:[O=C-O] is around 5.0:1.1:1.0 (Table 1), which is in good agreement with the theoretical value of 5:1:1 for the polycaprolactone structures. The appearance of N 1s signal in the wide scan spectrum (Fig. 3a) and an additional peak component at 285.5 eV, attributable to C-N species, in the curve-fitted C 1s core-level spectrum (Fig. 3c) indicate the successful introduction of amine groups onto the PCL substrates after 1 h of aminolysis. The only peak component found at the BE of 399.6 eV in the N 1s core-level spectrum is associated with the free amine group on the PCL-NH$_2$ film surface (Fig. 3c') [38]. The decrease in static water contact angles of the PCL substrates from 93 ± 2° to 66 ± 3° is consistent with the presence of amine groups on the PCL-NH$_2$ surface (Table 1). The amine groups on the aminolyzed PCL surface can not only improve surface hydrophilicity, but also offer the active sites for further functionalization.

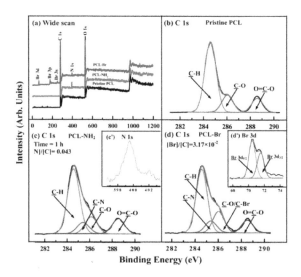

Figure 3. Wide scan and C 1s core-level curve-fitted XPS spectra of the (a,b) pristine PCL, (c,d) PCL-NH$_2$ from 1 h of aminolysis, and (e,f) PCL-Br surfaces. Insets of (d') and (f') correspond to the N 1s and Br 3d core-level XPS spectra of the PCL-NH$_2$ and PCL-Br surfaces, respectively.

The immobilization of a uniform monolayer of initiators on the solid surface is indispensible in the surface-initiated ATRP process [40]. An alkyl bromide ATRP initiator was introduced onto the PCL-NH$_2$ surface via TEA-catalyzed condensation reaction to produce the PCL-Br surface. Successful introduction of the alkyl bromide-containing ATRP initiator onto the PCL substrates can be deduced from the appearance of three additional signals with BEs at about 70, 189 and 256 eV, attributable to Br 3d, Br 3p, and Br 3s, respectively, in the wide scan spectrum of the PCL-Br surface (Fig. 3a) [41]. The [Br]/[C] ratio, as determined from the Br 3d and C 1s core-level spectral area ratio, was about 3.17×10^{-2} (Fig. 3d). The corresponding Br 3d core-level spectrum of the PCL-Br surface with a Br 3d$_{5/2}$ BE of 70.4 eV is consistent with the presence of the alkyl bromide species [41] (Fig. 3d'). The alkyl bromide-immobilized PCL surface became more hydrophobic, as static water contact angle increased noticeably to $85 \pm 3°$ (Table 1).

Sample	GY^g(µg/cm^2) (mean± SD^h)	[Br]/[C]^i	[N]/[C]^i	Surface composition^j (molar ratio)	WCA^k (degree)
Pristine PCL^a	–	–	–	[C-H]:[C-O]:[O=C-O] = 5:1.1:1.0 (5:1:1)	93±2
PCL-NH$_2$ ^{b}	–	–	0.043	[C-H]:[C-N]:[C-O]:[O=C-O] = 4.7:0.7:1.1:1.0	66±3
PCL-Br^c	–	3.17×10^{-2}	–	[C-H]:[C-N]:[C-O/C-Br]:[O=C-O] = 5.0:0.9:1.7:1.0	85±3
PCL-g-P(GMA)1^d	6.31±1.32	9.29×10^{-3}	–	[C-H]:[C-O]:[O=C-O] = 3.8:2.8:1.0 (3:3:1)	62±4
PCL-g-P(GMA)2^e	14.76±2.63	4.72×10^{-3}	–	[C-H]:[C-O]:[O=C-O] = 3.1:3.0:1.0 (3:3:1)	61±5
PCL-g-P(GMA)1-c-gelatin^f	2.63± 0.52	–	0.169	[C-H]:[C-N]:[C-O]:[O=CNH]: [O=C-O] = 3.5:1.5:1.7:1.0:0.7	37±3
PCL-g-P(GMA)2-c-gelatin^{pala}	3.79±0.73	–	0.203	[C-H]:[C-N]:[C-O]:[O=CNH]: [O=C-O] = 3.1:1.5:1.4:1.0:0.3	35±4

^{a} Pristine PCL refers to the cleaned PCL film after rigorous wasing with alcohol/water solution and deionized water, ^{b} PCL-NH$_2$ was obtained after 1 h of aminolysis in a 10% (w/w) 1,6-hexanediamine/isopropanol solution at 40 ºC, ^{c} PCL-Br was obtained after the PCL-NH$_2$ surface reacted with 2-bromoisobutyryl bromide (BIBB) in dried hexane containing 1:1 (molar ratio) BIBB and triethylamine (TEA), ^{d,e} Reaction conditions: [GMA]:[CuBr]:[CuBr$_2$]:[bpy]=100:1:0.2:2 in methanol-water solution (1:1, v:v) at room temperature for 1 and 3 h to produce the PCL-g-P(GMA)1 and PCL-g-P(GMA)2 surfaces, respectively, ^{f} Reaction conditions: the PCL-g-P(GMA)1 and PCL-g-P(GMA)2 surfaces incubated in PBS (pH 7.4) solution containing the gelatin at a concentration of 3 mg/mL at room temperature for 24 h, ^{g} GY denotes the grafting yield, and is defined as GY = (W$_a$ - W$_b$)/A, where W$_a$ and W$_b$ corresponds to the weight of the dry films before and after grafting of polymer brushes, respectively, and A is the film area (about 3.2 cm2), ^{h} SD denotes standard deviation, ^{i} Determined from the corresponding sensitivity factor-corrected element core-level spectral area ratios, ^{j} Determined from the curve-fitted C 1s core-level spectra. Theoretical values are shown in parentheses. ^{k} WCA denotes static water contact angles.

Table 1. Grafting yield, surface composition, and water contact angles of the pristine PCL and surface-functionalized PCL surfaces

3.2. Surface-initiated ATRP of GMA and immobilization of gelatin

P(GMA) is an effective surface linker to immobilize biomolecules, such as proteins, antibodies or enzymes, for tissue engineering applications [42]. Fig. 4 shows the respective wide scan, C 1s and Br 3d core-level spectra of the PCL-g-P(GMA) surface from 1 and 3 h of ATRP reaction. The C 1s core-level spectra of the PCL-g-P(GMA) surface can be curve-fitted into three peak components with BEs at 284.6, 286.2 and 288. 7 eV, attributable to C-H, C-O and O=C-O, respectively (Figs. 4b and 4d). For the PCL-g-P(GMA)1 surface from 1 h of ATRP, the area ratio of [C-H]:[C-O]:[O=C-O] is about 3.8:2.8:1.0 (Table 1), which is slightly different from the theoretical value of 3:3:1 for the GMA unit structure. The deviation in peak component area ratio of C 1s core-level spectrum of the PCL-g-P(GMA)1 surface suggests that the thickness of the P(GMA) brushes is less than the probing depth of XPS technique (about 8 nm in an organic matrix) [41]. Increasing the reaction time to 3 h leads to a [C-H]:[C-O]:[O=C-O] ratio of about 3.1:3.0:1.0, which is close to the theoretical value of the GMA repeat unit structure (Table 1). This is an indication that the P(GMA) brushes were thicker than the probing depth of XPS technique. It has been reported that the thickness of the P(GMA) brushes grafted on the silicon surface is around 30 nm after 3 h of ATRP of GMA under similar reaction conditions [41]. The presence of P(GMA) brushes leads to decrease in static water contact angles to $62 \pm 4°$ and $61 \pm 5°$, respectively, for the PCL-g-P(GMA)1 and PCL-g-P(GMA)2 surfaces, owing to the presence of hydrophilic epoxide groups [43].

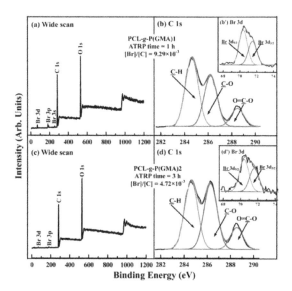

Figure 4. Wide scan, C 1s, and Br 3d core-level curve-fitted XPS spectra of the (a,b,b') PCL-g-P(GMA)1 from 1 h of ATRP reaction and (c,d,d') PCL-g-P(GMA)2 from 3 h of ATRP reaction. Successful grafting of P(GMA) polymer brushes can be deduced from the area ratios of [C-H]:[C-O]:[O=C-O] peak components comparable to the theoretical value of 3:3:1 of GMA molecular structure.

The grafting yield (GY) was measured to evaluate the kinetics of polymer chain growth in this study. As shown in Fig. 5, an approximate linear increase in GY of the grafted P(GMA) chains with polymerization time could be observed for the PCL-Br surface. The result suggests that the chain growth from the PCL-Br surface proceeds in a controlled and well-defined manner. The GY values of the PCL-g-P(GMA)1 and PCL-g-P(GMA)2 surfaces are about 6.31 ± 1.32 and 14.76 ± 2.63 $\mu g/cm^2$ (Table 1), respectively. The persistence of the Br 3d core-level signal (Figs. 4b' and 4d') is consistent with the fact that the living chain end from the ATRP process involves a dormant alkyl halide group, which can be readily reactivated to initiate the block copolymerization [25]. However, the molecular weight and molecular weight distribution of the surface-graft polymers cannot be determined with sufficient accuracy without precise cleavage of the grafted P(GMA) from the film surfaces [27].

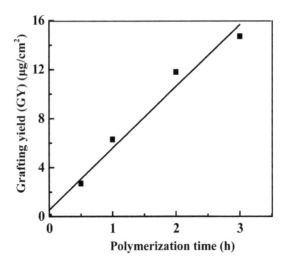

Figure 5. A linear relationship between the grafting yield (GY) of the P(GMA) brushes with the surface-initiated ATRP time. The polymer chain growth was tuneable by varying reaction time.

Nucleophilic reactions involving –NH$_2$ moieties of biomolecules and the pendant epoxide groups have been widely reported [44]. In this work, cell-adhesive gelatin was directly coupled to the pendant epoxide groups of the PCL-g-P(GMA)1 and PCL-g-P(GMA)2 surfaces to produce the corresponding PCL-g-P(GMA)1-c-gelatin and PCL-g-P(GMA)2-c-gelatin surfaces, respectively. Fig. 6 shows the respective wide scan, C 1s and N 1s core-level spectra of the gelatin-immobilized PCL surfaces. The corresponding curve-fitted C 1s core-level spectrum was composed of five peak components with BEs at about 284.6, 285.5, 286.2, 288.2 and 289.1 eV, attributable to the C-H, C-N, C-O, O=CNH, and O=C-O species [41], respectively (Figs. 6b and 6d). The C-N peak component is associated with the linkages in gelatin itself, as well as the linkage between P(GMA) and gelatin. The O=CNH peak component is ascribed to the peptide bonds in gelatin. The above results and the appearance of a strong N 1s signal with BE at 399.6 eV (Figs. 6b' and 6d'), characteristic of amine species, are consistent with the fact that gelatin has been covalently immobilized on the P(GMA) brushes. The surface wettability of the PCL substrates is significantly improved after the immobilization of gelatin, as water contact angles decrease to 37 ± 2° (for the PCL-g-P(GMA)1-c-gelatin) and 35 ± 3°(for the PCL-g-P(GMA)2-c-gelatin) (Table 1). It is reported that gelatin contains large amount of glycine (Gly) and proline (Pro) which are hydrophilic amino acids [45]. The hydroxyl groups (-OH) generated in the ring-opening reaction of epoxide groups by coupling of gelatin could have also contributed to the lower water contact angle of the PCL-*g*-P(GMA)-*c*-gelatin surfaces.

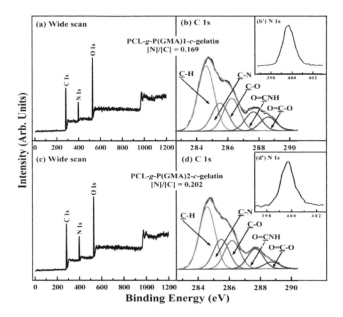

Figure 6. Wide scan, C 1s and N 1s core-level curve-fitted XPS spectra of the (a,b,b') PCL-*g*-P(GMA)1-c-gelatin and (c,d,d') PCL-*g*-P(GMA)2-c-gelatin surfaces. The appearance of two additional peak components of C-N and O=CNH as a result of immobilized gelatin.

3.3. Surface topography

The changes in topography of the PCL film surfaces after each functionalization step were investigated by AFM. Fig. 7 shows the representative AFM height images of the pristine PCL and functionalized PCL surfaces with scanned areas of 10 μm × 10 μm. The pristine PCL film surface is relatively uniform and smooth with a root-mean-square surface roughness values (R_a) of about 19 nm (Fig. 7a). After the aminolysis treatment, the R_a value increases to 31 nm (Fig. 7b). The observation that aminolysis caused a noticeable increase in surface roughness is in agreement with the findings by other groups [30,35]. The existence of shallow pits is probably the result of the penetration of hexanediamine molecules into the PCL films, since it has been previously reported that the aminolysis reaction can take place at a depth of around 50 μm [23,30]. After graft polymerization of GMA, obvious increases in R_a values are observed on the PCL-*g*-P(GMA)1 (56.9 nm, Fig. 7c) and PCL-*g*-P(GMA)2 surfaces (67.8 nm, Fig. 7e), and characteristic fiber-like features of polymer brushes are also visible on the P(GMA)-grafted film surfaces (Figs. 7c and 7e). The subsequent coupling of gelatin to P(GMA) brushes resulted in a further slight increase in surface roughness of PCL substrates, as R_a values increase to 59 nm and 71.5 nm for the PCL-g-P(GMA)1-c-gelatin and the PCL-g-P(GMA)2-c-gelatin surfaces, respectively.

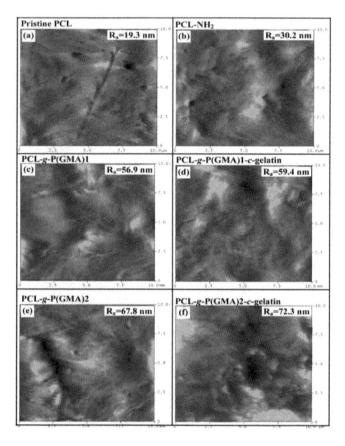

Figure 7. Representative two-dimensional (2D) AFM images of (a) pristine PCL, (b) PCL-NH₂, (c) PCL-g-P(GMA)1 from 1 h of ATRP, (d) PCL-g-P(GMA)2 from 3 h of ATRP, (e) PCL-g-P(GMA)1-c-gelatin, and (f) PCL-g-P(GMA)2-c-gelatin surfaces. The arithmetical mean roughness (R_a) of different PCL substrates was obtained from a scan size of 10 μm × 10 μm.

3.4. Endothelial cells proliferation and surface endothelialization

The adhesion and proliferation of endothelial cells (ECs) on the functionalized PCL surfaces was quantitatively determined by the AlamarBlueTM (AB) assay, and the results are shown in Fig. 8. The pristine PCL film surface is the least conducive for supporting cellular growth, since only a marginal increase in cells over 7 days of culture was observed. The cells attached to the PCL-NH₂ film surfaces showed a slight improvement in proliferation as compared to the pristine PCL surface. This result is consistent with previous findings that the presence of amine groups on the PCL surfaces leads to a positive effect on cell proliferation [23,30], albeit to a limited extent. Despite the improvement in surface hydrophilicity and roughness, the grafting of P(GMA) brushes onto the PCL film surfaces did not lead to an enhancement in EC proliferation behavior, which is probably associated with the cytotoxicity and mutagenicity of epoxides groups to ECs [46]. Besides the fact that polymer surfaces with moderate hydrophilicity of water contact angles in a range of 30-70° and rougher nano-topography are favorable for cell attachment and proliferation [47,48], other factors (e.g. biological cues) may also be required for positive cell interaction with material substrates. This hypothesis was confirmed by the observation that the gelatinized P(GMA)-grafted PCL substrates exhibited higher affinity and proliferation for ECs as compared to the surfaces that did not contain the bioactive gelatin motifs.

In fact, the proliferation rates of the PCL-g-P(GMA)1-c-gelatin and PCL-g-P(GMA)2-c-gelatin surfaces were comparable to that of the gelatin-coated coverslips (positive controls). Cell proliferation on the gelatin-immobilized PCL surfaces was not only significantly enhanced, but also found to be positively correlated to the amounts of immobilized gelatin. The PCL-g-P(GMA)2-c-gelatin surface exhibited more pronounced enhancement in cell adhesion and proliferation than that of the PCL-g-P(GMA)1-c-gelatin surface, as the longer ATRP reaction time allowed for more gelatin to be attached. This result suggests that an increase in surface density of the immobilized gelatin can lead to an increase in EC proliferation over time. This phenomenon is probably associated with the fact that immobilization of gelatin provides many epitopes or ligands for cell adhesion molecules, such as integrins, thus mimicking the natural extracellular environment that is favorable for EC adhesion, spreading and proliferation.

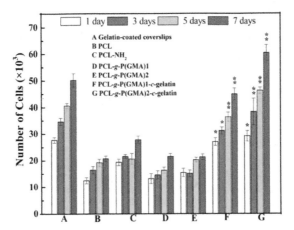

Figure 8. EC proliferation profile on the gelatin-coated coverslips, pristine PCL and functionalized PCL surfaces after 1, 3, 5 and 7 days of incubation at 37 °C in a 5% CO_2 atmosphere as determined by the AlamarBlue™(AB) assay. Data presented as means ± SD. *$p<0.05$ and **$p<0.01$ refers to statistically significant difference compared with the pristine PCL surface. The cell proliferation rate of ECs seeded on the gelatin-immobilized surfaces was significantly improved as compared to that the pristine PCL film.

The visualization of EC coverage on the functionalized PCL surfaces enabled a good assessment of the efficacy of endothelialization over the entire surface. Fig. 9 shows the representative fluorescence images of LIVE/DEAD-stained ECs on the pristine PCL and functionalized PCL film surfaces after 7 days of culture. The sparse coverage of ECs on the pristine PCL substrate further confirmed the unfavorable surface properties of pristine PCL for cell adhesion and proliferation (Fig. 9b). Poor endothelialization was also observed on the aminolyzed PCL (Fig. 9c) and P(GMA)-grafted PCL surfaces (Fig. 9d). The dense growth of ECs on the PCL-*g*-P(GMA)1-*c*-gelatin (Fig. 9e) and PCL-*g*-P(GMA)2-*c*-gelatin (Fig. 9f) surfaces indicated significant improvement in EC coverage for the gelatin-immobilized PCL surfaces. The observed denser coverage of ECs on the PCL-*g*-P(GMA)2-*c*-gelatin surfaces compared to the PCL-*g*-P(GMA)1-*c*-gelatin surfaces meant that the efficacy of endothelialization is positively correlated to the amount of immobilized gelatin. Taken together, the results suggest that the higher the surface concentration of immobilized gelatin, the better the endothelialization efficacy of the material within a given period of time.

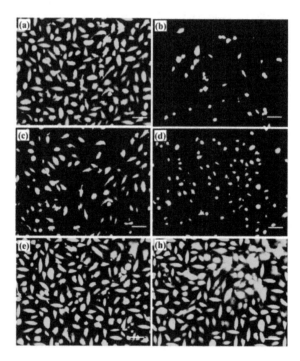

Figure 9. Fluorescence images of LIVE/DEAD-stained ECs on the (a) gelatin-coated coverslips (positive control), (b) pristine PCL, (c) PCL-NH$_2$, (d) PCL-*g*-P(GMA)2, (e) PCL-*g*-P(GMA)1-*c*-gelatin, and (f) PCL-*g*-P(GMA)2-*c*-gelatin after 7 days of incubation in cell suspension (2×10^4 cells/ml). Scale bar: 20 μm. Rapid endothelialization was observed for the gelatin-immobilized PCL surfaces.

3.5. Blood compatibility tests

3.5.1. Hemolysis rate test

Hemolysis rate is an important factor for characterization of the blood compatibility. The lower the hemolysis rate, the better the blood compatibility. Figure 10 shows the hemolysis rate of the pristine PCL and surface-functionalized PCL samples. It can be seen that the hemolysis rate of the functionalized samples has no substantial improvement. The gelatin-immobilized PCL substrates even show a relatively higher hemolysis rate than those of the pristine PCL and PCL-NH$_2$ surfaces. This result is consistent with the previous findings that gelatin exhibited somewhat hemostatic effect by nature. However, the hemolysis rate of the gelatin-immobilized PCL samples is approximately 3%, far below the accepted threshold value of 5% for biomaterial applications. Thus, the gelatin-immobilized samples can be used as a novel material with good hemocompatibility.

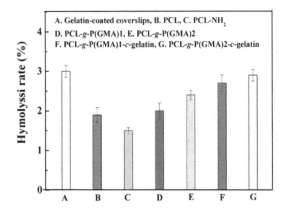

Figure 10. Hemolysis rate of the pristine PCL and surface-functionalized PCL samples. Data presented as means ± SD, n=3.

3.5.2. Coagulation activity on the bare and endothelialized PCL substrates

Blood coagulation, particularly under conditions of relatively low flow, has been recognized to be one of the main problems of vascular occlusion [49]. Activated coagulation factors influence the clotting time through extrinsic, intrinsic and common coagulation pathways. Prothrombin time (PT) is used to evaluate deficiencies in the extrinsic factor, and represents the time for blood plasma to clot after the addition of thromboplastin (activator of the extrinsic pathway) [50]. Activated partial thromboplastin time (APTT) is used to evaluate the intrinsic factors, such as VIII, IX, XI and XII, and common coagulation pathway factors V, X and II [50]. Both PT and APTT are commonly used to screen for adverse activation of the coagulation pathways on the vascular grafts and to evaluate their haemocompatibility in vi-

tro. Thus, the PT and APTT values of the bare and endothelialized PCL substrates with various surface modifications were measured.

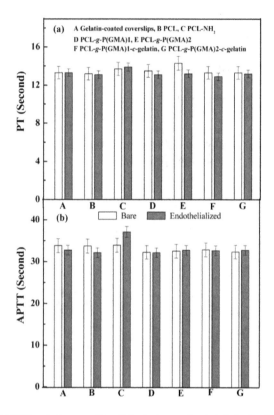

Figure 11. a) PT and (b) APTT results (means ± SD, n=3) for the bare and endothelialized surfaces of pristine PCL and surface-functionalized PCL, The coagulation activity of all surfaces was found to be in the normal range for healthy blood plasma.

The normal ranges of PT and APTT for healthy blood plasma are 12.0-14.5 s and 27.0-35.6 s, respectively [51]. Fig. 11 shows the PT and APTT results for the bare and endothelialized PCL substrates with various surface modifications. For the bare PCL and functionalized PCL surfaces, both PT and APTT are all within the normal ranges of coagulation time. None of the PCL substrates was found to affect the coagulation pathways significantly, and no discernible effect was observed in the presence of gelatin, indicating that surface functionalization activated neither the intrinsic nor the extrinsic coagulation pathways. This result is consistent with previous findings by other groups that cell-adhesive proteins and peptides do not affect or convert blood coagulation pathways [51,52]. Even after the PCL substrates were coated with a layer of ECs, the PT and APTT readings were still observed to be in the normal range of the clinical reference, and no significant differences in the coagulant activities were observed on the endothelialized PCL substrates as compared to the bare PCL substrates. The results also revealed that the ECs cultured on the pristine PCL and functionalized PCL surfaces remained unactivated and did not exhibit procoagulation phenotypes. Hence, it could be concluded that the presence of the monolayer of ECs had no effect on the intrinsic or the extrinsic coagulation pathways.

3.5.3. Nitric Oxide (NO) production

Nitric oxide (NO) is an important regulator of vascular tone and platelet adhesion and the continuous NO release by ECs prevents thrombogenesis [53]. In this study, the NO secretion of the ECs on the pristine PCL and functionalized PCL surfaces were measured. As shown in Fig. 12, the amount of NO secreted by ECs on the gelatin-immobilized PCL surfaces was significantly higher than those on the pristine PCL, aminolyzed and P(GMA)-grafted PCL surfaces. The amount of NO production of the ECs seeded on the PCL-g-P(GMA)2-c-gelatin surface was around 2-fold higher than that on the PCL-g-P(GMA)1-c-gelatin surfaces, indicating that the improved NO production observed for ECs grown on the gelatin-immobilized PCL surface may be positively correlated to the amount of covalently immobilized gelatin. The above results suggest that a high density of immobilized gelatin led to the enhancement in NO secretion.

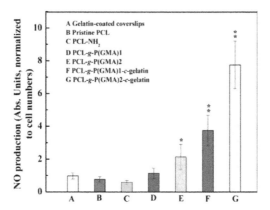

Figure 12. The amount of NO production for the ECs seeded on the pristine and functionalized PCL substrates. Data presented as means ± SD, n=3. *$p<0.05$ and **$p<0.01$ corresponds to statistically significant difference as compared to the pristine PCL.

3.5.4. Platelet activation on the bare and endothelialized PCL substrates

Apart from coagulation pathways, platelet activation is considered another important criterion in assessing blood compatibility of the biomaterial surface. The activation of attached platelet results in platelet aggregation and the formation of a thrombus [54]. The subendothelial collagens (i.e., types I - IV) have been found to interact directly with platelets to trigger their activation for thrombogenic initiation [55]. As gelatin is a derivative of collagen, one downside of using gelatin-immobilized surfaces could be the detrimental adhesion and activation of platelets, which could initiate clotting. Therefore, the extent of platelet activation by the different biomaterial surfaces was studied.

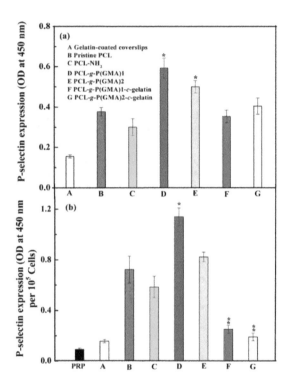

Figure 13. P-selectin expression for the (a) bare and (b) endothelialized surfaces of the pristine and functionalized PCL substrates. Plasma rich platelet (PRP) was used as positive control. *$p<0.05$ and **$p<0.01$ corresponds to statistically significant difference compared with the pristine PCL surface.

In this study, platelet activation on the bare and endothelialized PCL substrates was determined using the P-selectin assay, since P-selectin is one of intracellular granular molecules released upon platelet activation and stimulation [5], For the bare PCL substrates, the amount of activated platelets on the gelatin-immobilized PCL surfaces was comparable to those of the pristine PCL surfaces (Fig. 13a). In contrast, platelet activation was found to be significantly higher on the P(GMA)-grafted PCL surfaces, indicative of an increased risk for thrombogenesis. The results suggest that the immobilization of gelatin on the P(GMA)-grafted PCL surfaces not only rendered them with adhesion-promoting properties, but also decreased the risk of inducing the activation of platelets. It has been reported previously that the biological motifs immobilized on the polymers could not bind effectively with the platelet integrin unless their separation distances was between 1.48-2.2 nm [56], and that polymers with small spacer, such as lauric acid-conjugated GRGDS, exhibited no increase in activation [57]. Here, the gelatin was directly conjugated onto the grafted P(GMA) brushes (small spacer), and thus the gelatin motif could not gain access to the binding sites of the platelet integrin (such as $\alpha2\beta1$). In addition, it is probable that the other surface properties (e.g. enhanced hydrophilicity) were also responsible for reduced platelet activation activity.

In the case of the endothelialized PCL substrates, the amount of activated platelets on the gelatin-immobilized PCL surfaces was significantly reduced with respect to the other endothelialized PCL substrates (Fig. 13b), indicative of good anti-thrombogenic behavior of the EC confluent layer. This result is consistent with the high level of NO production by ECs on the gelatinized PCL surface. The P-selectin expression on the endothelialized pristine PCL and PCL-NH$_2$ surfaces was higher than those on the bare substrates (Fig. 13b), which is line with the well-established fact that subconfluent EC layers were more thrombogenic in nature [13]. The platelet activation was significantly enhanced on the endothelialized P(GMA)-grafted PCL surfaces, as observed by the high levels of P-selectin expression, which is an indication of an increased risk of thrombogenesis for those surfaces. Overall, the above results showed that the thrombogenicity of a biomaterial is influenced by both EC confluency and the surface properties of the biomaterial. Consequently, it can be concluded that the immobilization of gelatin on the P(GMA) brushes prevented platelet activation, but that the presence of the P(GMA) brushes alone led to a pro-thrombogenic surface.

3.5.5. Expression and activity of vWF and MMP-2 of EC on the surface-functionalized PCL samples

In order to further investigate the thrombogenicity of endothelialized surfaces, we performed real-time PCR tests and protein immunoblotting on factors that mediate platelet adhesion to ECs. The expression of von Willebrand factor (vWF) on endothelial cells promotes platelet adhesion and high or abnormal expression of vWF has been implicated in pathological conditions such as thrombosis [58]. Matrix metalloproteinase-2 (MMP-2) is another factor known to be involved in platelet aggregation, as well as to have important roles in the degradation and remodeling of the endothelial extracellular matrix [59, 60]. 7 days after the seeding of ECs, the relative expression of both vWF and MMP-2 mRNA in the EC on both PCL-g-P(GMA)1-c-gelatin and PCL-g-P(GMA)2-c-gelatin surfaces were downregulated when compared to the ECs on PCL-g-P(GMA) surfaces and gelatin-coated coverslips (Fig. 14a and 14c). Immunoblotting of the vWF protein produced in ECs, also, suggest that it is lower in ECs on PCL-g-P(GMA)-c-gelatin surfaces in comparison to PCL-g-P(GMA) surfaces but differed where the vWF expression of ECs on the pristine PCL surface and gelatin-coated coverslip could not be detected (Fig. 14b). Nevertheless, these results suggest that pro-thrombogenic factors could be increased on bare PCL-g-P(GMA) surfaces and the conjugation of gelatin could help to reduce thrombogenicity

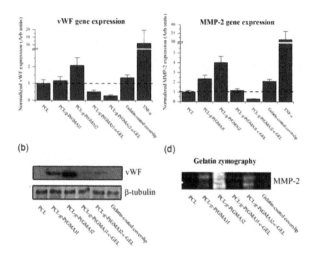

Figure 14. Real-time qPCR revealed that the expression of (a) vWF and (c) MMP-2 in ECs on PCL-g-P(GMA)-c-gelatin surfaces is lower when compared to PCL-g-P(GMA) surfaces and gelatin-coated coverslips. Expression levels are normalized using the housekeeping gene rpl27 and taken relative to ECs on pristine PCL (dotted line) (mean ± SD, n=3). Endothelial cells treated with TNF-αfor 6 h were used as a positive control for the expression of both genes. (c) Immunoblotting of vWF protein expressed in ECs on PCL-g-P(GMA)-c-gelatin is also reduced when compared to PCL-g-P(GMA) surfaces, thus corroborating the real-time PCR results.

4. Conclusion

This study described the successful biofunctionalization of PCL substrates with tunable surface densities of covalently-immobilized gelatin by surface-initiated ATRP of glycidyl methacrylate (GMA). Kinetics studies revealed that the grafting yield of the functional P(GMA) brushes increased linearly with polymerization time, and the amount of immobilized gelatin increased with the concentration of epoxide groups on the P(GMA) brushes. The significant improvement in the adhesion and proliferation of ECs on the gelatin-immobilized PCL substrates were found to be positively correlated to the amount of covalently immobilized gelatin. Blood compatibility tests demonstrated that the ECs cultured on the gelatin-immobilized-P(GMA) surfaces exhibited low platelet activation and significantly increased nitric oxide (NO) production, although the coagulation pathways were not affected both before and after EC coverage. Overall, the high surface-density of immobilized gelatin obtained by surface-initiated ATRP on the PCL surfaces is favorable for EC attachment and proliferation. The attached ECs maintained an unactivated and non-thrombogenic phenotype that mimics the EC lining of a healthy blood vessel. Hence, such a surface may have huge potential for vascular graft applications.

Acknowledgements

This research is supported by the Singapore National Research Foundation under CREATE programme: The Regenerative Medicine Initiative in Cardiac Restoration Therapy (NRF-Technion).

Author details

Shaojun Yuan[1,2*], Gordon Xiong[2], Ariel Roguin[3], Swee Hin Teoh[4] and Cleo Choong[2*]

*Address all correspondence to: yuanshaojun@gmail.com

*Address all correspondence to: cleochoong@ntu.edu.sg

1 Multi-phases Mass Transfer & Reaction Engineering Lab, College of Chemical Engineering, Sichuan University, Chengdu, China

2 School of Materials Science and Engineering, Nanyang Technological University, Singapore

3 Department of Cardiology, Rambam Medical Center, B. Rappaport Faculty of Medicine, Technion – Israel Institute of Technology, Israel

4 School of Chemical and Biomedical Engineering, Nanyang Technological University, Singapore

References

[1] Chlupac J, Filova E, Bacakova L. Blood vessel replacement: 50 years of development and tissue engineering paradigms in vascular surgery. *Physiol Res.* 2009;58:S119-S139.

[2] Mitchell SL, Niklason LE. Requirements for growing tissue-engineered vascular grafts. *Cardiovasc Pathol* 2003;12(2):59-64.

[3] Wang XW, Lin P, Yao QH, Chen CY. Development of small-diameter vascular grafts. *World J. Surg.* 2007;31(4):682-689.

[4] Sharkawi T, Darcos V, Vert M. Poly(DL-lactic acid) film surface modification with heparin for improving hemocompatibility of blood-contacting bioresorbable devices. *J. Biomed. Mater. Res. A* 2011;98A(1):80-87.

[5] Liu HF, Li XM, Niu XF, Zhou G, Li P, Fan YB. Improved hemocompatibility and endothelialization of vascular grafts by covalent immobilization of sulfated silk fibroin on poly(lactic-co-glycolic acid) scaffolds. *Biomacromolecules* 2011;12(8):2914-2924.

[6]   Lee JH, Oh SH. MMA/MPEOMA/VSA copolymer as a novel blood-compatible mate-rial: Effect of PEO and negatively charged side chains on protein adsorption and pla-telet adhesion. *J. Biomed. Mater. Res.* 2002;60(1):44-52.

[7]   Lee JH, Ju YM, Kim DM. Platelet adhesion onto segmented polyurethane film surfa-ces modified by addition and crosslinking of PEO-containing block copolymers. *Bio-materials* 2000;21(7):683-691.

[8]   Amiji M, Park K. Surface modification of polymeric biomaterials with poly(ethylene oxide), albumin and heparin for reduced thrombogenicity. *J Biomater Sci-Polym Ed* 1993;4(3):217-234.

[9]   Chong MSK, Teoh SH, Teo EY, Zhang ZY, Lee CN, Koh S, Choolani M, Chan J. Be-yond cell capture: antibody conjugation improves hemocompatibility for vascular tissue engineering applications. *Tissue Eng. Part A* 2010;16(8):2485-2495.

[10] Ku SH, Park CB. Human endothelial cell growth on mussel-inspired nanofiber scaf-fold for vascular tissue engineering. *Biomaterials* 2010;31(36):9431-9437.

[11] Wu KK, Thiagarajan P. Role of endothelium in thrombosis and hemostasis. *Annu Rev Med* 1996;47:315-331.

[12] Lijnen HR, Collen D. Endothelium in hemostasis and thrombosis. *Prog. Cardiovasc. Dis* 1997;39(4):343-350.

[13] McGuigan AP, Sefton MV. The influence of biomaterials on endothelial cell thrombo-genicity. *Biomaterials* 2007;28(16):2547-2571.

[14] Woodruff MA, Hutmacher DW. The return of a forgotten polymer - polycaprolac-tone in the 21st century. *Prog. Polym.Sci.* 2010;35(10):1217-1256.

[15] Sung HJ, Meredith C, Johnson C, Galis ZS. The effect of scaffold degradation rate on three-dimensional cell growth and angiogenesis. *Biomaterials* 2004;25(26):5735-5742.

[16] Chong MSK, Chan J, Choolani M, Lee CN, Teoh SH. Development of cell-selective films for layered co-culturing of vascular progenitor cells. *Biomaterials* 2009;30(12): 2241-2251.

[17] Serrano MC, Portoles MT, Vallet-Regi M, Izquierdo I, Galletti L, Comas JV, Pagani R. Vascular endothelial and smooth muscle cell culture on NaOH-treated poly (epsilon-caprolactone) films: A preliminary study for vascular graft development. *Macromol Biosci* 2005;5(5):415-423.

[18] de Valence S, Tille JC, Mugnai D, Mrowczynski W, Gurny R, Moller M, Walpoth BH. Long term performance of polycaprolactone vascular grafts in a rat abdominal aorta replacement model. *Biomaterials* 2012;33(1):38-47.

[19] Tillman BW, Yazdani SK, Lee SJ, Geary RL, Atala A, Yoo JJ. The in vivo stability of electrospun polycaprolactone-collagen scaffolds in vascular reconstruction. *Biomateri-als* 2009;30(4):583-588.

[20] Walpoth BH, Moller M. Tissue engineering of vascular prostheses. *Chirurg* 2011;82(4):303-310.

[21] Serrano MC, Pagani R, Pena J, Vallet-Regi M, Comas JV, Portoles MT. Progenitor-derived endothelial cell response, platelet reactivity and haemocompatibility parameters indicate the potential of NaOH-treated polycaprolactone for vascular tissue engineering. *J Tissue Eng Regen Med* 2011;5(3):238-247.

[22] Ma ZW, Gao CY, Gong YH, Shen JC. Chondrocyte behaviors on poly-L-lactic acid (PLLA) membranes containing hydroxyl, amide or carboxyl groups. *Biomaterials* 2003;24(21):3725-3730.

[23] Zhu YB, Gao CY, Liu YX, Shen JC. Endothelial cell functions in vitro cultured on poly(L-lactic acid) membranes modified with different methods. *J. Biomed. Mater. Res. A* 2004;69A(3):436-443.

[24] Shin YM, Kim KS, Lim YM, Nho YC, Shin H. Modulation of spreading, proliferation, and differentiation of human mesenchymal stem cells on gelatin- immobilized poly(L-lactide-co-epsilon-caprolactone) substrates. *Biomacromolecules* 2008;9(7): 1772-1781.

[25] Edmondson S, Osborne VL, Huck WTS. Polymer brushes via surface-initiated polymerizations. *Chem Soc Rev* 2004;33(1):14-22.

[26] Coessens V, Pintauer T, Matyjaszewski K. Functional polymers by atom transfer radical polymerization. *Prog. Polym.Sci.* 2001;26(3):337-377.

[27] Xu FJ, Yang XC, Li CY, Yang WT. Functionalized polylactide film surfaces via surface-initiated ATRP. *Macromolecules* 2011;44(7):2371-2377.

[28] Jiang H, Wang XB, Li CY, Li JS, Xu FJ, Mao C, Yang WT, Shen J. Improvement of hemocompatibility of polycaprolactone film surfaces with zwitterionic polymer brushes. *Langmuir* 2011;27(18):11575-11581.

[29] Tiaw KS, Teoh SH, Chen R, Hong MH. Processing methods of ultrathin poly(epsilon-caprolactone) films for tissue engineering applications. *Biomacromolecules* 2007;8(3): 807-816.

[30] Zhu YB, Gao CY, Liu XY, Shen JC. Surface modification of polycaprolactone membrane via aminolysis and biomacromolecule immobilization for promoting cytocompatibility of human endothelial cells. *Biomacromolecules* 2002;3(6):1312-1319.

[31] Causa F, Battista E, Della Moglie R, Guarnieri D, Iannone M, Netti PA. Surface investigation on biomimetic materials to control cell adhesion: the case of RGD conjugation on PCL. *Langmuir* 2010;26(12):9875-9884.

[32] Yuan SJ, Wan D, Liang B, Pehkonen SO, Ting YP, Neoh KG, Kang ET: Lysozyme-coupled poly(poly(ethylene glycol) methacrylate)-stainless steel hybrids and their antifouling and antibacterial surfaces. *Langmuir* 2011;27(6):2761-2774.

[33] Zhu YB, Gao CY, Shen JC. Surface modification of polycaprolactone with poly(meth-acrylic acid) and gelatin covalent immobilization for promoting its cytocompatibility. *Biomaterials* 2002;23(24):4889-4895.

[34] Chang KY, Hung LH, Chu IM, Ko CS, Lee YD. The application of type II collagen and chondroitin sulfate grafted PCL porous scaffold in cartilage tissue engineering. *J. Biomed. Mater. Res. A* 2010;92A(2):712-723.

[35] Zhang HN, Hollister S. Comparison of bone marrow stromal cell behaviors on poly(caprolactone) with or without surface modification: studies on cell adhesion, survival and proliferation. *J Biomater Sci-Polym Ed* 2009;20(14):1975-1993.

[36] Gabriel M, Amerongen GV, Van Hinsbergh VWM, Amerongen AVV, Zentner A. Direct grafting of RGD-motif-containing peptide on the surface of polycaprolactone films. *J Biomater Sci-Polym Ed* 2006;17(5):567-577.

[37] von Burkersroda F, Schedl L, Gopferich A. Why degradable polymers undergo surface erosion or bulk erosion. *Biomaterials* 2002;23(21):4221-4231.

[38] Bech L, Meylheuc T, Lepoittevin B, Roger P. Chemical surface modification of poly(ethylene terephthalate) fibers by aminolysis and grafting of carbohydrates. *J. Polym Sci Pol Chem* 2007;45(11):2172-2183.

[39] Moulder J F, Sobol FE, Bomben KD. Handbook of X-ray photoelectron spectroscopy. Eden Prairie, Minn: Perkin-Elmer Corp.; 1992.

[40] Siegwart DJ, Oh JK, Matyjaszewski K. ATRP in the design of functional materials for biomedical applications. *Prog. Polym.Sci.* 2012;37(1):18-37.

[41] Xu FJ, Cai QJ, Li YL, Kang ET, Neoh KG. Covalent immobilization of glucose oxidase on well-defined poly(glycidyl methacrylate)-Si(111) hybrids from surface-initiated atom-transfer radical polymerization. *Biomacromolecules* 2005;6(2):1012-1020.

[42] Chan K, Gleason KK. Photoinitiated chemical vapor deposition of polymeric thin films using a volatile photoinitiator. *Langmuir* 2005;21(25):11773-11779.

[43] Wang T, Kang ET, Neoh KG, Tan KL, Cui CQ, Lim TB. Surface structure and adhesion enhancement of poly(tetrafluooethylene) films after modification by graft co-polymerization with glycidyl methacrylate .*J. Adhes. Sci. Technol.* 1997;11(5):679-693.

[44] Eckert AW, Grobe D, Rothe U. Surface-modification of polystyrene-microtitre plates via grafting of glycidylmethacrylate and coating of poly-glycidylmethacrylate. *Biomaterials* 2000;21(5):441-447.

[45] Xia Y, Boey F, Venkatraman SS. Surface modification of poly(L-lactic acid) with biomolecules to promote endothelialization. *Biointerphases* 2010;5(3):FA32-FA40.

[46] Marquard H, Selkirk JK, Sims P, Kuroki T, Heidelbe C, Huberman E, Grover PL. Malignant transformation of cells derived from mouse prostate by epoxide and other derivatives of polycylic hydrocarbons. *Cancer Res* 1972;32(4):716-720.

[47] Cheng ZY, Teoh SH. Surface modification of ultra thin poly(ε-caprolactone) films using acrylic acid and collagen. *Biomaterials* 2004;25(11):1991-2001.

[48] Arima Y, Iwata H. Effect of wettability and surface functional groups on protein adsorption and cell adhesion using well-defined mixed self-assembled monolayers. *Biomaterials* 2007;28(20):3074-3082.

[49] van der Zijpp YJT, Poot AA, Feijen J. ICAM-1 and VCAM-1 expression by endothelial cells grown on fibronectin-coated TCPS and PS. *J. Biomed. Mater. Res. A* 2003; 65A(1):51-59.

[50] Kamal AH, Tefferi A, Pruthi RK. How to interpret and pursue an abnormal prothrombin time, activated partial thromboplastin time, and bleeding time in adults. *Mayo Clin Proc* 2007;82(7):864-873.

[51] Liu YA, Wang W, Wang J, Wang YL, Yuan Z, Tang SM, Liu M, Tang H. Blood compatibility evaluation of poly(D,L-lactide-co-beta-malic acid) modified with the GRGDS sequence. *Colloid Surf B-Biointerfaces* 2010;75(1):370-376.

[52] Hansson KM, Tosatti S, Isaksson J, Wettero J, Textor M, Lindahl TL, Tengvall P. Whole blood coagulation on protein adsorption-resistant PEG and peptide functionalised PEG-coated titanium surfaces. *Biomaterials* 2005;26(8):861-872.

[53] Graves JE, Greenwood IA, Large WA. Tonic regulation of vascular tone by nitric oxide and chloride ions in rat isolated small coronary arteries. *Am J Physiol-Heart Circul Physiol* 2000;279(6):H2604-H2611.

[54] Allen RD, Zacharski LR, Widirstky ST, Rosenstein R, Zaitlin LM, Burgess DR. Transformation and motility of human-platelets - details of the shape change and release reaction observed by optical and electron-microscopy. *J Cell Biol* 1979;83(1):126-142.

[55] Saelman EUM, Nieuwenhuis HK, Hese KM, Degroot PG, Heijnen HFG, Sage EH, Williams S, McKeown L, Gralnick HR, Sixma JJ. Platelet-adhesion to collagen type-I through type-VIII under condtions of stasis and flow is mediated by $\alpha 2\beta 1$-integrin. *Blood* 1994;83(5):1244-1250.

[56] Hu B, Finsinger D, Peter K, Guttenberg Z, Barmann M, Kessler I, Escherich A, Moroder L, Bohm J, Baumeister W, Sui SF. Intervesicle cross-linking with integrin alpha(IIb)beta(3) and cyclic-RGD-lipopeptide. A model of cell-adhesion processes. *Biochemistry* 2000;39(40):12284-12294.

[57] Kidane AG, Punshon G, Salacinski HJ, Ramesh B, Dooley A, Olbrich M, Heitz J, Hamilton G, Seifalian AM. Incorporation of a lauric acid-conjugated GRGDS peptide directly into the matrix of a poly(carbonate-urea)urethane polymer for use in cardiovascular bypass graft applications. *J. Biomed. Mater. Res. A* 2006;79A(3):606-617.

[58] Brill A, Fuchs TA, Chauhan AK, Yang JJ, De Meyer SF, Köllnberger M, et al. von Willebrand factor–mediated platelet adhesion is critical for deep vein thrombosis in mouse models. *Blood*. 2011; 117(4):1400-1407.

[59] Kazes I, Elalamy I, Sraer J-D, Hatmi M, Nguyen G. Platelet release of trimolecular complex components MT1-MMP/TIMP2/MMP2: involvement in MMP2 activation and platelet aggregation. Blood. 2000; 96(9):3064 –3069.

[60] Ben-Yosef Y, Lahat N, Shapiro S, Bitterman H, Miller A. Regulation of endothelial matrix metalloproteinase-2 by hypoxia/reoxygenation. Circulation Research. 2002; 90(7):784 –791.

Chapter 7

In Vitro Blood Compatibility of Novel Hydrophilic Chitosan Films for Vessel Regeneration and Repair

Antonello A. Romani, Luigi Ippolito,
Federica Riccardi, Silvia Pipitone, Marina Morganti,
Maria Cristina Baroni, Angelo F. Borghetti and
Ruggero Bettini

Additional information is available at the end of the chapter

1. Introduction

Tissue and organ failure treatments include drug therapy, surgical repair, medical devices but they do not always provide satisfactory restoration of organ function.

At present transplants represent an actual solution in treating organ failure once overcoming immunological rejection even though its application is largely affected by the paucity of available donors.

In the vascular field, currently, the best graft performance is given by saphenous vein autografts [1] whose main failures are related to thrombosis development, emboli production, and intimal hyperplasia. Synthetic non-bio-resorbable vascular prosthesis (such as Dacron® or extended-PTFE) exhibited very low incidences of thrombosis or hyperplasia and showed good clinical results in medium- and large-diameter graft sites.

Strategies based on polymeric materials (synthetic or natural) appear to be a valid alternative for the production of tissue graft materials. However, synthetic polymers are not able to induce any biological response leading to tissue regeneration, due to the lack of biomimetic activity. On the contrary, natural biodegradable polymeric supports, resembling extracellular matrix component, can provide a useful platform in tissue engineering and regenerative medicine applications [2-5].

Among them, chitosan (CS) a biodegradable [6], non-amphiphilic polymer of D-glucosamine obtained by partial de-acetylation of chitin [3], has shown interesting properties including bio-mimetism due to the similarity of is structure with that of glycosaminoglycanes [4].

Kind *et al.* [7] reported that it promotes plasma protein adsorption, platelet adhesion and activation, and thrombus development [8]. The positive charged CS surface induces a great degree of platelet adhesion. In fact, the Food and Drug Administration approved its use as haemostatic dressing for reducing haemorrhage [9-11]. Furthermore, it has been reported that the negatively charged-modified surface of CS prolongs clot formation after re-calcification of plasma [12].

Up to now, few data, often conflicting, on the haemocompatibility of negative charged-modified surfaces of CS films are available[11,12].

In a previous work [13] we developed novel CS hydrogel prepared in the presence of phosphate salts and relatively high amount of disaccharides such as D-(+)raffinose or D-(+)saccharose and investigated the physico-chemical characteristics as well as the cytocompatibility of films obtained with this hydrogel. These sugars were not retained in the final structure of the film but were able to act as viscosity modifiers during the solidification/gelation process. The interference of salts and disaccharides resulted in smooth, amorphous film with improved hydrophilicity and cytocompatibility compared to CS films produced with the same procedure but in low viscosity milieu. Differentiated human cells showed a great affinity for these sugar-modified chitosan (smCS) films, thus suggesting their candidature as promising biomaterial for tissue regeneration and repair.

The aim of the present study was to investigate qualities and aspects of the haemocompatibility (platelet activation, haemolysis and activation of coagulation cascade) of smCS films produced according to Bettini*et al.* [13]. Moreover, the cytotoxicity of fragmented smCS was investigated in view of its bio-resorbability.

These films were compared to materials able to activate platelets and induce thrombus formation such as plastic (standard polystyrene for cell culture) and glass (cover slips) as well as a material able to trigger cell death such as latex.

2. Methods

2.1. Production of sugar-modified chitosan films

Chitosan solution was prepared as described in [13]. Briefly, four grams of chitosan powder (Chitosan 95/50 HMC⁺· Germany) were dissolved in a 1% (w/v) acetic acid aqueous solution until complete dissolution. Dibasic sodium phosphate (7.5 mM), sodium dihydrogen phosphate (22 mM), potassium dihydrogen phosphate (1.5 mM), sodium chloride (125 mM) and potassium chloride (2mM) were then sequentially added. The solution was filtered under vacuum using a 0.8 μM filter. Finally, D-(+) raffinose pentahydrate (290 mM) or D-(+) sucrose (290 mM) were added to the solution and allowed to dissolve for 2 hours under gentle stirring. About one mL of this solution was poured into a circular mould (1 cm diameter) and dried at 45 °C for 45 minutes in a ventilated oven. The obtained dry film was placed in a 5% (w/v) KOH aqueous solution for 12 hours then, washed in distilled water until neutrality of the wash water.

2.2. Wettability

Contact angle measurements were performed at room temperature with a goniometer (AB Lorentzen & Wettre, Germany) on the surface of smC film in comparison to glass cover slip and plastic (standard polystyrene culture plates) to evaluate the wettability of the surface. Briefly, a drop (4 µL) of human serum was placed on the surface of the specimen. Images of the serum drop were recorded within 10 seconds of deposition by means of a digital camera (FinPix S602 Zoom, Fuji film, Japan). Digital pictures were analysed by ImageJ 1.43v software (NIH, USA) for angle determination. At least five measurements, taken at different positions on each specimen, were carried out on both left and right side of the drop and averaged.

2.3. Atomic force microscopy

Atomic force microscopy (AFM) images of the films were analysed by AFM Nanoscope IIIA (Digital Instruments Inc., USA). Point probe silicon cantilever tip was used in contacting mode by the accompanying software to determine the surface roughness of investigated surfaces. The roughness parameters of each sample was evaluated on three scanned areas of 10µm x 10µm each.

2.4. Procurement and processing of blood perfusates

This procedure was conducted in accordance with the tenets of the Declaration of Helsinki. Following the indication of Italian DLgs no.196/03 (Codex on Privacy) in order to guarantee the respect of the privacy of the patients and the confidentiality of the donors' information. Blood (3.5-4 mL/test) was drawn by venipuncture from four healthy volunteers and added with tri-sodium citrate (0.109 M, 3.2% final concentration) in a 9:1 volumetric ratio to prevent coagulation. Whole blood was used for the haemolysis and thrombus formation tests.

Platelet-rich plasma (PRP) was obtained by centrifugation (400xg for 10 minutes, at room temperature) while platelet-poor plasma (PPP, platelets less than 10.000/µL) by centrifugation at 2000xg for 20 minutes at room temperature.

Coagulation- and factor XII-assays were performed with platelet-poor plasma isolated from whole blood. For platelet function studies, PRP was volume adjusted with PPP to obtain a final physiologic stock platelet count of $3 \cdot 10^5$ platelets µL^{-1}.

2.5. Cell proliferation

Human endothelial cells derived from foetal umbilical vessels (HUVEC) were provided by the American Type Culture Collection (Rockville, MD, USA). Cell monolayer were cultured in complete medium (D-MEM containing antibiotics and 10% foetal calf serum) supplemented with 50 µg mL^{-1} of endothelial cell growth factor (Sigma-Aldrich, USA) and kept in a incubator at 37 °C in a water-saturated atmosphere with 5% CO_2. Endothelial cells were seeded onto smCS films as well as on tissue culture plates (TCPS, Corning, USA) or glasses (20x20 mm, ForLab, Carlo Erba, Italy,) at a density of 1–2.5 10^4 cells cm^{-2} in 24-well plates. After 1, 3 and 7 days, the monolayer was rinsed twice with phosphate buffer solution, PBS, and cells detached from the substrate by 0.02% trypsin in PBS. The number of adherent cells was then, counted with a Burkerhaemocytometer.

2.6. Cell morphology

For morphological characterization, endothelial cells cultured on smCS films were examined by contrast-phase microscopy. After 7 days, the cell monolayer adherent to the film was gently washed with PBS three times. Then, the film was fixed with 2.5% glutaraldehyde in PBS for 1 h at 4 °C. After thorough washing with PBS, the cells were dehydrated through graded alcohol series and positioned under the microscope (Zeiss AxioPhot, Germany) for observation and image recording (Zeiss AxioCam, Germany).

2.7. Cytotoxicity test

Endothelial cells were grown until confluence. The smCS films was cut in small pieces (0.5x0.5 mm) and placed in direct contact with the cell layer for 72 hours. Cells were detached and the resulting suspension was counted in a Burkerhaemocytometer after proper dilution.

Duplicate cell counts on each suspension from 3 culture wells were performed for each substrate investigated. Not less than 50 cells were scored for each counting. Counts from triplicate seeding differed by not more than 10% among replications throughout the experiments.

2.8. Haemolysis assay

Two positive controls, copper and deionised water, and a negative control, glass cover slip, were used in this study, SmCS films were dried and washed three times with PBS and then sterilized by soaking in 75% (v/v) ethanol for 15 minutes. Then, washed 5 times in sterile PBS and kept in the same buffer until use. Thereafter, the samples were put in vacutainers containing sodium citrate (0.109 M, 3.2% w/v final concentration) (Greiner Bio-One International AG, Austria) in which 3.5 mL of healthy volunteers blood was finally collected. The substrates were incubated with blood at 37 °C, with gentle shaking twice every 30 minutes. After 3 hours, 1.5 mL of each vacutainer was centrifuged at 740xg for 10 minutes at room temperature. The obtained pellet was re-centrifuged at 3000g for 15 minutes at room temperature. The haemolyses was quantified on a ADVIA 2120 system (Siemens-Bayer, Germany) using a colorimetric assay.

2.9. Coagulation assays

Human whole blood (3.5 mL) from a healthy volunteer was collected and mixed with an aqueous solution containing sodium citrate, then the human whole blood was centrifuged at 1500g for 15 min at room temperature to separate the blood corpuscles, and the resulting

PPP was used to study the coagulating ability of the CS film. All tests were performed on *IL Coagulation and ELECTRA™* system (Instrumentation Laboratories, USA). The level of Prothrombin Time (PT), activated Partial Thromboplastin Time (aPTT) and Thrombin Time (TT) were determined by using three different kits (Instrumention Laboratory USA): HemosIL ™ RecombiPlasTin 2G is a high sensitivity thromboplastin reagent based on recombinant human tissue factor (RTF) for the quantitative determination in human citrate plasma of Prothrombin Time (PT); HemosIL ™ SynthASil is a high synthetic phospholipids reagent for the *in vitro* determination of APTT (Activated Partial Thromboplastin Time). After incubation at 37 °C for an optimized period of time, calcium is added to trigger the coagulation process and the time required for clot formation is determined; HemosIL ™ Thrombin Time was used for the determination of TT in human citrated plasma.

2.10. Erythrocytes adhesion assay

SmCS films (10x10 mm) were equilibrated in PBS for 1 hour at 37°C. A washed-erythrocytes stock suspension containing $3 \cdot 10^5$ mL^{-1} was poured on plastic and smCS film surfaces and incubated for 30 minutes. The incubation volume was kept low (100 µL) to (a) minimize the floating population of erythrocytes and (b) maintain the total erythrocytes count at a level such as to prevent saturation-levels of adhesion and (c) to prevent other still suspended erythrocytes from contacting the surface. After that, the specimens were rinsed with PBS, fixed with glutaraldheyde and detached from surface with 1% sodium dodecyl sulphate, SDS. Ten microliters of recovered erythrocytes suspension were counted with a Burkerhaemocytometer.

2.11. Platelet adhesion assay

SmCS films, plastic and cover slips glass were sterilized with 75% (v/v) ethanol solution. Then air dried under a laminar-flow hood and rehydrated with 1 mL of sterile PBS for 1 hour. The surfaces were overlaid with 300 µL PRP at 37 °C for 2 hours. Then, the films were washed three times in PBS with mild shaking to remove non- or poorly-adherent platelets. After that, the specimens were rinsed with PBS, fixed with glutaraldheyde and cells detached with 1% SDS. Ten microliters of recovered platelets suspension were counted with a Burkerhaemocytometer.

3. Platelet immunofluorescence

The platelet count in the PRP was adjusted to 300.000 µL-1 by dilution with homologous PPP. After 1 hour contact of PRP with the different specimens at 37 °C, samples were washed with PBS, followed by fixation with 3% (w/v) paraformaldehyde and incubated with 1% (w/v) BSA in PBS. Labelling of the platelets was performed with a mouse monoclonal antibody CD62P (anti-P-Selectin, Santa Cruz Biotechnology, USA) at dilution 1:100, followed by 1:200 diluted monoclonal goat anti-mouse IgG antibody, FITC conjugated (Sigma-Aldrich, USA).

4. Platelet morphology

The platelets-coated testing surfaces were fixed with freshly prepared 2.5% glutaraldehyde for 20 minutes. After washing with PBS, the samples were dehydrated in a graded-ethanol series (50, 70, 90, and 100% v/v) for 15 minutes each and allowed to dry at room temperature. The platelet-attached surfaces were carbon sputter coated under vacuum to a thickness of 100–200 Å and examined at 10 kV using a Cambridge StereoScan 200 microscope (Cambridge Scientific Instruments, UK).

4.1. Platelet aggregation

The blood samples were collected in tubes containing PPACK (D-phenylalanyl-L-prolyl-L-arginine chloromethyl ketone) as anticoagulant. Platelet aggregation was measured by means of light transmission aggregometry using Born's turbidimetric procedure and the PPACK-4 Platelet Aggregation Chromogenic Kinetic System (Helena Laboratories, USA). Briefly, 250 μL of PRP were incubated with specimen surfaces for 10 (baseline) and 60 minutes. Thereafter,the PRP were placed in a cuvette containing a metal stir bar in the absence or in the presence (positive control) of the pro-aggregation agent, adenosine diphosphate (ADP) 20 μM. Upon the addition of ADP the platelets started to aggregate thus increasing light transmission through the sample. The degree of platelet aggregation was expressed as the maximum percentage change in light transmission from PPP used as baseline. The obtained values were expressed as mean of two measurements.

4.2. Complement activation assay

The test, based on Complement Reagents Kit (Siemens Healthcare Diagnostic, Germany) was performed on BCT Siemens coagulometer (Siemens, Germany). The test focused on the ability of the complement system to lyse a standard suspension of sheep erythrocytes, sensitized with a rabbit anti-serum against sheep erythrocytes. Briefly, 1 mL of fresh blood samples previously incubated for 1 hour with different substrates were incubated with sensitized erythrocytes to investigate the complement activation. Diminished levels of individual components (e.g. due to prior activation by a foreign surface) result in a prolongation of the time taken for lyses. The time necessary for the lyses of a defined amount of erythrocytes is used as basis for determining the complement activity [14,15]. The results were evaluated using a reference curve prepared by a serial dilution of standard plasma with isotonic saline to give 100% of complement activity, 75% (75% of plasma + 25% saline) down to 10% of complement activity (10% of plasma + 90% saline).

4.3. Statistical analysis

Data were expressed as means ± standard deviation (SD). Where not differently stated, measurements were conducted at least in triplicate. Chi-square test or Student's t-test on unpaired data was used to assess the statistical significance of the difference between the results obtained from the tested specimens (Kaleida-Graph, Synergy Software, USA). Statistical significance was assumed at a confidence level of 95% ($p < 0.05$).

5. Results

5.1. Physico-chemical characterisation

As already stated, the sugar added to the chitosan solution during the preparation of the smCS film was not retained in the final structure of the film.This assumption was mainly based on FT-IR spectra analysis for the identification of the absorption bands relevant to vibration of functional groups of chitosan [13]. The addition of phosphate salts and D-(+) raffinose to the chitosan solution used for film preparation led to non dramatic modifications in the IR spectrum of chitosan. The observation of the 1700-1500 cm^{-1} region evidenced that the amide I band (C=O in amide group) wavenumber was lower than the value for chitosan powder (1664 cm^{-1}) for all the prepared films and particularly for those prepared from a solution that did not contain the sugar [13]. This was interpreted as the result of a lower mobility of the C=O group in the film due to its involvement in the week bound formation in the solid structure. The incorporation of phosphate salts and significant amount of sugar in the chitosan solution used for film preparation reduced this effect. On the other hand, the amino group band of films prepared from a solution that did not contain the sugar was at a lower wavenumber (1588 cm^{-1}) than from chitosan powder (1592 cm^{-1}), while it was practically unchanged in film prepared from the sugar containing solution (1590 cm^{-1}).

D-(+)raffinose FT-IR spectrum evidenced characteristics bands at 2936 and 1649 cm^{-1}. Interestingly, no trace of this bands was found in the FT-IR spectra of the chitosan film prepared from solutions containing D-(+)raffinose. Similarly, no trace of the characteristic series of peaks between 2994 and 2914 cm^{-1} of the sucrose powder was found in the spectrum of the film prepared from a solution containing a high amount of sucrose [13].

These observations allowed to conclude that the excipients added to chitosan in the film forming solutions though not retained in the solid film, interact or interfere with chitosan chains during the film formation likely acting as viscosity modifiers during the solidification/gelation process.

5.2. Wettability

Contact angle measurements were performed by using serum droplets on plastic surface and on smCS film. As expected, plastic showed the least wettable surfaces with significantly higher contact angle (50° ± 6.3) compared to smCS film (15° ± 0.1) (Chi Square P< 0.001), thus confirming the high hydrophilicity of smCS [13].

The hydrophilicity of the sm CS film was also investigated by measuring the swelling index in water at the equilibrium according to the following equation:

$$S_w = \frac{W_s - W_d}{W_s} x100 \tag{1}$$

where W_s and W_d represent the weight of the fully hydrated and the dry film respectively. The smCS film afforded a degree of swelling at the equilibrium more than 3 order of magnitude (1285%) higher than that of the dry film. These data confirmed the very high hydrophilicity of the films obtained by adding a sugar to the solution used for the film preparation.

5.3. Roughness (AFM measurements)

The AFM analysis (Figure 1) revealed that the plastic specimen exhibited rather low surface roughness (average= 28 nm) in contrast to smCS film that showed a roughness approximately 1.7-fold higher, around 50 nm. It is interesting to note the almost regular appearance of groove and pits in smCS compared with plastic surface.

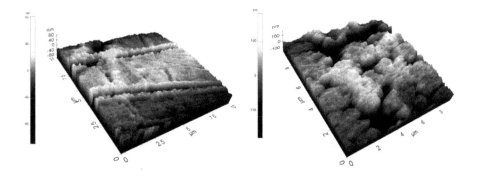

Figure 1. AFM 3D image of (A) standard colture plastic dish (plastic) and (B) smCS film surfaces.

5.4. Adhesion and proliferation assay of endothelial cells

As shown in Figures 2 endothelial cells attached (A), extended and proliferated (B) very well on all surfaces tested. Cell attachment (panel A, C) and proliferation (panel B) on smCS films were comparable to control cells grown on standard tissue culture surface (plastic). Contrast-phase microscopy showed that cells were well attached to the different surfaces and closely packed maintaining their original shapes. Moreover, endothelial cells did not evidence any morphological indication of cell death 72 hours after seeding (panel D). The counts of cells showed little variation for the three surfaces used. In the case of plastic surface (control) the growth of HUVEC reached the values of 21284 ± 650 cm^{-2}, while in the case of smCS reached a lower value of 19805 ± 305 cm^{-2} similarly to that obtained on glass surface (19543 ± 1050 cm^{-2}).

5.5. In vitro cytotoxicity

Data relevant to cell growth in the presence of small pieces of smCS film or latex (positive control) are reported in Table 1.

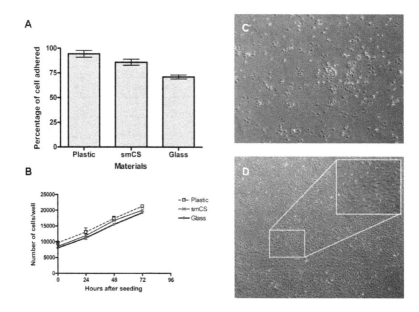

Figure 2. A) Percentage of cells adhered after 24 hoursand (B) proliferation assay of endothelial cells on the different surfaces tested. Pictures taken at the optical microscope, in phase contrast (40x), showing the morphology of endothelial cells 8 hours (C) and 72 hours (D) after seeding on smCS film.

	Hours after seeding			
	0	24	48	72
Latex (positive control)	10000 (± 239)	924 (± 25)	714 (±16)	50 (±30)
smCS	10000 (± 360)	11420 (±100)	16070 (±290)	18570 (± 200)

Table 1. Number of endothelial cells attached to the different substrates in the presence of latex or smCS film fragments.

The initial plating corresponds to the number of cells attached to the substrate 6 hours after their inoculation into the well. The measured plating efficiency was around 95%. When smCS fragments were present in the colture medium, a progressive increase of cell numbers was observed, while in the presence of latex a progressive detachment was noticed with almost all plated cells detached from the substratum after 72 hours.

These results indicate that smCS film were not cytotoxic while latex, as expected, was found to markedly affect endothelial cell survival.

5.6. Haemolysis assay

Haemolysis of red blood cells was used to evaluate the membrane damaging potential of the surface of the smCS film. Two positive controls, distilled water and Copper, and one nega-tive control, glass, were used.

Substrate	Haemolysis (%)
Distilled Water	97 (± 5)
Copper	7 (± 2)
Plastic	5 (± 1)
Glass	2 (± 1)
smCS	1 (±3)

Table 2. Percentage of haemolysis measured on different substrates. The tested surfaces were incubated with whole blood for 1 hour. Distilled water was used as positive control.

As shown in Table 2, distilled water resulted in about 100% haemolysis, while Copper led to 7% haemolysis. Glass and smCS film caused negligible haemolysis (within the experimental error) indicating very low membrane damaging properties of smCS material.

5.7. Blood coagulation assay

The effects of the biomaterial on coagulation process were tested by means of the (aPTT), the (PT) and the (TT) selected as reliable measurements of the capacity of blood to coagulate through the intrinsic, extrinsic and common coagulation mechanisms, respectively. As shown in Figure 3 the values obtained for PT, TT and aPTT were similar to those observed for human plasma, thus indicating that all materials tested, including smCS, did not affect coagulation pathways.

Substrates	Erythrocyte lyses time (seconds)
Plasma (control)	35.4
Glass	38.2
Plastic	35.7
SmCS film	36.3

Table 3. Erythrocyte lyses time determined by plastic and glass surfaces in comparison with smCS film.

5.8. Complement activation assay

The erythrocyte lyses time observed and reported in Table 3 shows no significant difference among the material studied and the control. The data presented demonstrate that smCS is a nonreactive biomaterial that does not directly activate complement.

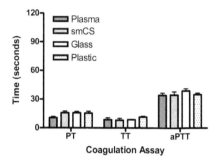

Figure 3. Effect of the different surfaces on coagulation time tested by means of the (aPTT), the (PT) and the (TT).

5.9. Erythrocytes and platelets adhesion assay

In Table 4 the number of cells detached with SDS from the different surfaces after adhesion test is reported. The smCS film presented a lower overall erythrocyte and platelet adhesion in comparison to plastic surface.

Materials	Surface Adhesion	
	Erythrocytes μL^{-1}	Platelets μL^{-1}
Plastic	40 (± 13)	11(± 8)
Glass	-	17 (± 6)
smCS	8 (±3)	5 (± 2)

Table 4. Numbers of erythrocytes and platelets adhered to the studied surfaces

The test showed a high significant difference in the number of adhered erythrocytes on materials studied ($p<0.0001$): the erythrocyte adhesion on smCS film was about 5 fold less than the adhesion on plastic surface. A similar behaviour was observed for platelets. In fact, the platelets recovered from plastic and glass surfaces ranged from 2 to 3 fold more than platelets recovered from smCS film surface.

5.10. Platelet aggregation

This test was performed in order to investigate the ability of plastic, smCS film and glass surfaces to induce platelet aggregation. The presence of ADP (adenosine-diphosphate, a pro-aggregation agent) determined a normal profile of platelets aggregation (range 90-95% after 5 minutes of incubation). Subsequently, the influence of materials on platelets aggregation in the absence of ADP was studied. There were no differences between materials observed at baseline (10 min) and after 1 hour of incubation with the substrates. smCS induced slightly higher aggregation of platelets (5-6%) compared to plastic (2.5%) or glass (less than 2%). However, these differences have to be considered with caution, as the coefficient of variation estimated with human plasma in the absence of ADP was around 10%.

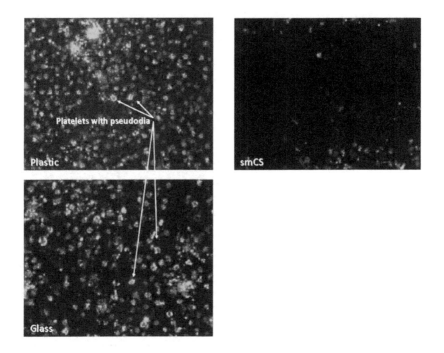

Figure 4. Fluorescence microscopy (100X)images of human platelets immunodecorated with CD62P (p-Selectin). Arrows indicate the presence of pseudopodia.

5.11. Platelet activation assay

Platelet activation was studied by the membrane expression of P-Selectin using the CD62P antibody. The expression of P-Selectin was evident on platelets adherent to plastic and glass surfaces and was negligible on platelets settled on smCS films (Figure 4).

On glass and plastic (see arrows) the analysis of morphology showed several fully spread platelets expressing pseudopodia with the occurrence of focal clumps. This was also evident when platelets were examined by Scanning Electron Microscopy, SEM (Figure 5B and 5C).

SmCS film (Figure 5A) induced very limited morphological changes over the 90 minutes of contact: platelets remained mostly discoid without the occurrence of pseudopodia.

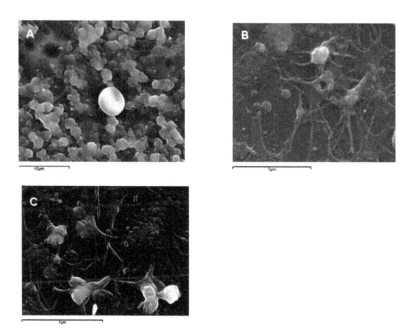

Figure 5. Scanning Electron Microscope images of platelets incubated onto different surfaces. (A) smCS film, (B) plastic, (C) glass.

6. Discussion

For blood-contact applications, haemocompatibility is largely determined by specific interactions with blood and its components [16]. Many, if not all, blood-contacting biomaterials are able to cause different undesired host responses like thrombosis, inflammatory reactions and infections.

The coagulation system and platelets are the main factors for thrombus formation on biomaterials and represent a major unmet problem in the design of vascular implants and blood-handling systems [17].

It is known that the endothelium is an active organ that maintains vessels integrity and prevent thrombosis and intimal hyperplasia [18,19]. Hence, biomaterials able to promote *in situ* endothelialisation of implants would be highly desirable.

Studies involving in vitro endothelialisation of grafts with cultured endothelial cells prior to implantation have shown that a confluent endothelium is able to prevent trombogenic complications and improves long-term patency [20,21]. Thus, taking into account that the endothelialisation of the blood-contacting polymeric materials is an important pre-requisite for the success of the synthetic vascular grafts [22] we firstly investigated the ability of endothelial cells to adhere and proliferate on smCS film. The results obtained, in agreement with those shown in our previous paper [13], showed only little variation among the surfaces tested (glass, plastic and smCS). However, from the cell proliferation and morphology it was very difficult to discriminate difference in cytophilicity among the surfaces tested. Furthermore, the presence of fragmented smCS did not induce any decrement in the total number of endothelial cells compared to latex that, on the contrary, strongly affected cell survival.

The high hydrophilicity of smCS, indicated by the low contact angle, could ease the interaction with the bipolar extra-cellular matrix proteins such as fibronectin and vitronectin. Furthermore, the reduced cationic nature, due to a water shell does not allow anionic proteins such as collagen and fibronectin to dissociate from CS surface in a physiological environment. This aspect is in agreement with the conclusion of [23] who reported that a hydrophilic surface is good for anti-non-specific protein adsorption. It was recently reported that the affinity for water of the cell-material interface seems to be a chief parameter in controlling cell adhesion, migration and differentiation [24].

Stevens and George [25] recognized that cells are sensitive to microscale patterns of chemistry and topography, and Dalby [26] noted that cell behaviour is directly influenced by the surface structures such as grooves, pits, or ridges.

In this paper AFM images of smCS films evidenced a topographically patterned surface. In the light of the above reported literature, this observation can be used to speculate about the enhanced adhesion and proliferation of vascular cells compared to conventional, CS films previously observed in [13].

Surface properties such as wettability, surface topography and charge are known to affect endothelial cells attachment and growth [8]likely by altering the rate of the amount of adsorbed proteins and their conformational changes [27,28]. The effect of surface materials on erythrocyte aggregation and platelet adhesion/activation becomes a chief parameter in haemocompatibility studies.

Several years ago Malette and co-workers [29] ascribed the pro-coagulation properties of chitosan to the negative charged surface of erythrocytes, while [30]showed that chitosan may induce the adhesion of erythrocytes.

In the present study, the surface of smCS films induced only a limited erythrocytes agglomeration, thus indicating that smCS surface neither captures erythrocytes nor forms a three-dimensional network structure with these cells.

The lack of erythrocyte aggregation may be likely due to a polymer chains rearrangement that masks the cationic nature of chitosan surface. Such a rearrangement can be ascribed to the larger amount of water in smCS films as described in [13].

One of the most important findings of this work is the observed difference in platelets morphology seeded on smCS in comparison with glass or plastic. On the latter surfaces platelets appeared flat with interconnecting pseudopodia coupled to strong P-Selectin membrane expression.On the contrary, the platelets on smCS films were discoidal, and neither pseudopodia formation nor a P-Selectin membrane translocation was observed.

This finding could be attributed to a new conformation of the adsorbed plasma proteins on glass or plastic that could have facilitated platelet aggregation. Indeed, it is well known that the surface topography can induce a spatial reorganization of adsorbed proteins as well as how this phenomenon occurs [31]. In contrast, when the adsorbed proteins maintain their native state, they do not support platelet adhesion and aggregation [32].

The absence of platelet activation on smCS surfaces suggests this outcome.

As far as the surface morphology is concerned, it has been reported that platelets adhere in similar manner on smooth and rough surfaces when tested under static conditions [33]. Similarly Ward et al. [34] concluded that it is not the roughness *per se* which affects the platelet adhesion.

One decade ago, Suzuki and Minami [35,36] showed that Chitosan depleted complement proteins from plasma, suggesting that chitosan activates complement. A greater depletion of complement activity was seen for a highly de-acetylated form of chitosan [36]. It is however, important to note that the results obtained about the complement activation were based on binding and depletion assays. This complement depletion can equally be explained by assuming a tight binding to the chitosan surface without activation [37].

The results presented here indicate that although large amounts of serum were deposited on smCS surface no activation of the complement system occurred, suggesting that the complement is not directly activated by the smCS surface in the process of blood coagulation.

Haemolysis testing of biomaterials has been advocated for, and used in, standard biological safety testing of materials for more than 30 years. The results of test for haemolysis should be considered with care even if they represent the only recommended test for some medical devices as stated in Part 4 of ISO 10993 guideline.

Different papers have reported that chitosan promotes surface-induced haemolysis likely through an electrostatic interactions [38]. In the present work, in the presence of whole blood smCS triggered less than 5% of haemolysis that, along with the low erythrocyte adhesion, indicates a wide safety margin in blood contacting applications and suitability for vascular implants.

In the process of haemostasis, the activation of platelet adhesion and aggregation could represent an initial and critical step. Here we showed that the surface of smCS films does not interfere with coagulation mechanism and supportswell endothelial cell adhesion and proliferation even if [39] reported that the haemostatic mechanism of chitosan may be independent of the classical coagulation cascade.

7. Conclusion

In this paper we demonstrated that the simple introduction of a viscosity modifier, such as a polysaccharide, during the process of production of chitosan films affords chitosan structures (smCS film) with improved capability to induce surface endothelialisation.

This structure is moreover, characterized by a high degree of haemocompatibility and does not induce clots formation.

These findings are of particular interest as they add new information with respect to the presently available literature and they put new light on the use of chitosan for producing surfaces that has to get in contact with blood.

As a matter of fact, the haemostatic properties of chitosan have to be considered more carefully as we have demonstrated that they could be dramatically reduced by an improvement of the hydrophilicity of the chitosan film surface.

Finally, from the results presented in this work, we can conclude that the sugar modified chitosan film could be envisaged as a new material for the design the luminal portion of vessel prosthesis based on a natural and bio-resorbable polymer.

Acknowledgements

This work was partially supported by a grant from Emilia Romagna Region, Italy, through its *"Programma di Ricerca Regione Università 2007-2009 Area Tematica 1B Medicina Rigenerativa"*.

Author details

Antonello A. Romani[1], Luigi Ippolito[2], Federica Riccardi[3], Silvia Pipitone[4],
Marina Morganti[5], Maria Cristina Baroni[5], Angelo F. Borghetti[4] and Ruggero Bettini[6]

*Address all correspondence to: bettini@unipr.it

1 Department of Surgery, O.U. of General Surgery, University Hospital of Parma, Italy

2 Department of Pathology and Medicine of Laboratory University Hospital Parma, Italy

3 Department of Medicine poly-specialist 2, University Hospital Parma, Italy

4 Department of Experimental Medicine, University of Parma, Italy

5 Department of Internal Medicine and Biomedical Sciences, University of Parma, Italy

6 Department of Pharmacy, University of Parma, Italy

References

[1] Baig K, Fields RC, Gaca J, Hanish S, Milton LG, Koch WJ, Lawson JH. A porcine model of intimal-medial hyperplasia in polytetrafluoroethylene arteriovenous grafts. J Vasc Access 2003;4:111–7.

[2] Hardy JG, Scheibel TR. Silk-inspired polymers and proteins. Biochem. Soc. Trans. 2009;37:677–81.

[3] Chandy T, Sharma CP. Chitosan--as a biomaterial. Biomater Artif Cells Artif Organs 1990;18:1–24.

[4] Shi C, Zhu Y, Ran X, Wang M, Su Y, Cheng T. Therapeutic Potential of Chitosan and Its Derivatives in Regenerative Medicine. Journal of Surgical Research 2006;133:185–92.

[5] Ramshaw JAM, Peng YY, Glattauer V, Werkmeister JA. Collagens as biomaterials. J Mater Sci Mater Med 2009;20 Suppl 1:S3–8.

[6] Hirano S, Tsuchida H, Nagao N. N-acetylation in chitosan and the rate of its enzymic hydrolysis. Biomaterials 1989;10:574–6.

[7] Kind GM, Bines SD, Staren ED, Templeton AJ, Economou SG. Chitosan: evaluation of a new hemostatic agent. Curr Surg 1990;47:37–9.

[8] van Wachem PB, Hogt AH, Beugeling T, Feijen J, Bantjes A, Detmers JP, van Aken WG. Adhesion of cultured human endothelial cells onto methacrylate polymers with varying surface wettability and charge. Biomaterials 1987;8:323–8.

[9] Wedmore I, McManus JG, Pusateri AE, Holcomb JB. A special report on the chitosan-based hemostatic dressing: experience in current combat operations. J Trauma 2006;60:655–8.

[10] Ong S-Y, Wu J, Moochhala SM, Tan M-H, Lu J. Development of a chitosan-based wound dressing with improved hemostatic and antimicrobial properties. Biomaterials 2008;29:4323–32.

[11] Rao SB, Sharma CP. Use of chitosan as a biomaterial: studies on its safety and hemostatic potential. J. Biomed. Mater. Res. 1997;34:21–8.

[12] Sagnella S, Mai-Ngam K. Chitosan based surfactant polymers designed to improve blood compatibility on biomaterials. Colloids Surf B Biointerfaces 2005;42:147–55.

[13] Bettini R, Romani AA, Morganti MM, Borghetti AF. Physicochemical and cell adhesion properties of chitosan films prepared from sugar and phosphate-containing solutions. Eur J Pharm Biopharm 2008;68:74–81.

[14] Kolde HJ, Deubel R. Development of a rapid kinetic assay for the function of the classical pathway of the complement system and for C2 and C4. J Clin Lab Immunol 1986;21:201–7.

[15] Siedentopf HG, Lauenstein K, Fischer H. [On the automatic registration of hemolysis by serum complement and lysolecithin]. Z. Naturforsch. B 1965;20:569–74.

[16] Angelova N, Hunkeler D. Rationalizing the design of polymeric biomaterials. Trends Biotechnol. 1999;17:409–21.

[17] Brash JL. The fate of fibrinogen following adsorption at the blood-biomaterial interface. Ann. N. Y. Acad. Sci. 1987;516:206–22.

[18] Risler NR, Cruzado MC, Miatello RM. Vascular remodeling in experimental hypertension. ScientificWorldJournal 2005;5:959–71.

[19] Myhre HO, Halvorsen T. Intimal hyperplasia and secondary changes in vein grafts. Acta Chir Scand Suppl 1985;529:63–7.

[20] Pollara P, Alessandri G, Bonardelli S, Simonini A, Cabibbo E, Portolani N, Tiberio GA, Giulini SM, Turano A. Complete in vitro prosthesis endothelialization induced by artificial extracellular matrix. J Invest Surg 1999;12:81–8.

[21] Crombez M, Chevallier P, Gaudreault RC, Petitclerc E, Mantovani D, Laroche G. Improving arterial prosthesis neo-endothelialization: application of a proactive VEGF construct onto PTFE surfaces. Biomaterials 2005;26:7402–9.

[22] Bengtsson L, Rådegran K, Haegerstrand A. A new and simple technique to achieve a confluent and flow resistant endothelium on vascular ePTFE-grafts using human serum. Eur J Vasc Surg 1994;8:182–7.

[23] Lu D, Lee S, Park K. Calculation of Solvation Interaction Energies for Protein Adsorption on Polymer Surfaces. J Biomat Sci-Polym E 1991;3:127–47.

[24] Ayala R, Zhang C, Yang D, Hwang Y, Aung A, Shroff SS, Arce FT, Lal R, Arya G, Varghese S. Engineering the cell-material interface for controlling stem cell adhesion, migration, and differentiation. Biomaterials 2011;32:3700–11.

[25] Stevens MM, George JH. Exploring and engineering the cell surface interface. Science 2005;310:1135–8.

[26] Dalby M, McCloy D, Robertson M, Wilkinson C, Oreffo R. Osteoprogenitor response to defined topographies with nanoscale depths. Biomaterials 2006;27:1306–15.

[27] Steele JG, Dalton BA, Johnson G, Underwood PA. Adsorption of fibronectin and vitronectin onto Primaria and tissue culture polystyrene and relationship to the mechanism of initial attachment of human vein endothelial cells and BHK-21 fibroblasts. Biomaterials 1995;16:1057–67.

[28] Burmeister J, Vrany J, Reichert W, Truskey G. Effect of fibronectin amount and conformation on the strength of endothelial cell adhesion to HEMA/EMA copolymers. J. Biomed. Mater. Res. 1996;30:13–22.

[29] Malette WG, Quigley HJ, Gaines RD, Johnson ND, Rainer WG. Chitosan: a new hemostatic. Ann. Thorac. Surg. 1983;36:55–8.

[30] Klokkevold PR, Lew DS, Ellis DG, Bertolami CN. Effect of chitosan on lingual hemostasis in rabbits. J. Oral Maxillofac. Surg. 1991;49:858–63.

[31] Curtis A, Wilkinson C. New depths in cell behaviour: reactions of cells to nanotopography. Biochem Soc Symp, vol. 65, 1999, pp. 15–26.

[32] Tanaka M, Motomura T, Kawada M, Anzai T. Blood compatible aspects of poly (2-methoxyethylacrylate)(PMEA)--relationship between protein adsorption and platelet adhesion on PMEA surface. Biomaterials 2000; 21:1471-1481.

[33] Zingg W, Neumann AW, Strong AB, Hum OS, Absolom DR. Effect of surface roughness on platelet adhesion under static and under flow conditions. Can J Surg 1982;25:16–9.

[34] Ward CA, Forest TW. On the relation between platelet adhesion and the roughness of a synthetic biomaterial. Ann Biomed Eng 1976;4:184–207.

[35] Minami S, Suzuki H, Okamoto Y, Fujinaga T, Shigemasa Y. Chitin and chitosan activate complement via the alternative pathway. Carbohyd Polym 1998;36:151–5.

[36] Suzuki Y, Okamoto Y, Morimoto M, Sashiwa H, Saimoto H, Tanioka S, Shigemasa Y, Minami S. Influence of physico-chemical properties of chitin and chitosan on complement activation. Carbohyd Polym 2000;42:307–10.

[37] Marchand C, Bachand J, Perinet J, Baraghis E, Lamarre M, Rivard GE, De Crescenzo G, Hoemann CD. C3, C5, and factor B bind to chitosan without complement activation. J Biomed Mater Res A 2010;93A:1429–41.

[38] Yao K, Li J, Yao F. Chitosan-Based Hydrogels: Functions and Applications. 1st ed. CRC Press; 2011.

[39] Khan T, Peh K, Ch'ng H. Mechanical, bioadhesive strength and biological evaluations of Chitosan films for wound dressing. J Pharm Pharm Sci 2000;3:303–11.

Chapter 8

Cell Adhesion to Biomaterials: Concept of Biocompatibility

M. Lotfi, M. Nejib and M. Naceur

Additional information is available at the end of the chapter

1. Introduction

Cell adhesion is a dynamic process that results from specific interactions between cell surface molecules and their appropriate ligands. Adhesion can be found between adjacent cells (cell-cell adhesion) as well as between cells and the extracellular matrix (ECM) (cell-matrix adhesion). Adhesion is an extremely important concept in both practical and theoretical terms. Unfortunately, there is no completely satisfactory definition of the term that fulfils the needs of both the theoretical surface chemist and the practicing technologist. It is assumed as a state in which two bodies (usually, but not necessarily dissimilar) are held together by intimate interfacial contact in such a way that mechanical force or work can be applied across the interface without causing the two bodies to separate.

Cell membrane are crucial to the adhesion of the cell and therefore to its life. Indeed, plasma membrane encloses the cell, defines its boundaries, and maintains the essential differences between the cytosol and the extracellular environment. In all cells the plasma membrane also contains proteins that act as sensors of external signals, allowing the cell to change its behavior in response to environmental cues; these receptors transfer information rather than ions or molecules across the membrane. Plasma membrane has the structure of a thin film of lipid and protein molecules linked together mostly through non covalent interactions. These lipid molecules are arranged as a continuous bilayer and are responsible for the basic structure of the membrane and the protein molecules embedded into it control most of the functions of the membrane. In the plasma membrane some proteins serve as structural links that connect the membrane to the cytoskeleton and/or to either the extracellular matrix (ECM) or an adjacent cell, while others serve as receptors to detect and transducer chemical signals in the cell's environment [1].

Besides keeping a multicellular organism together, cell adhesion is also a source of specific signals to adherent cells; their phenotype can thus be regulated by their adhesive interactions. In fact, most of the cell adhesion receptors were found to be involved in signal transduction. By interacting with growth factor receptors they are able to modulate their signaling efficiency. Therefore, gene expression, cytoskeletal dynamics and growth regulation all depend, at least partially, on cell adhesive interactions [2].

In this chapter, I tried to find a possible correlation between polyelectrolyte multilayer films and human gingival fibroblasts to test these biomaterials biocompatibility. This represents a fundamental step needed to know about a possible use in a biological field (i.e. as implant). For that purpose, I characterized each solid surface used as a surface on which fibroblasts were cultured; by calculating their surface free energy and evaluating their chemical heterogeneity, roughness and wettability using contact angle measurement. Thereafter, I followed the adhesion of fibroblasts, their proliferation and their morphology.

2. Polyelectrolyte multilayer film

2.1. Biomaterials: Generality and interest

During a consensus conference in 1986, a definition was given for biomaterials. Indeed, a biomaterial is «a non-living material used and designed to be integrated with biological systems». Biomaterials are defined according to their domain of use and regroup metals and alloys, ceramics, polymers (i.e. collagen)[3].

Biomaterials were used since the pharaoh's time to replace injured and affected organs. Pharaoh had used pure natural materials but presenting integration's problems. Since that, researches had grown up rapidly in this field in order to design the "ideal" material which will be more accepted by the human body. The designed material was referred to as "biomaterial" afterwards and will recover a lot of biomedical applications for implants and tissues injuries covering.

Biomaterials' design must take into account the purpose and the place of its use. This biomaterial must have a well defined shape depending on his position within the body. Indeed, for orthopedic usage, a biomaterial must conform to some criteria and regulations such as: a good mechanical structure, a good resistance to corrosion and metal fatigue. For vascular surgery, a biomaterial must not induce thrombosis, in odontology a biomaterial must withstand changes that can occur to temperature (coffee, cool drinks), to pH (alcohol, lemon…) and to the buccal cavity [4].

Making reliable and cheap biomaterials is being a new challenge for researchers and industries. In fact, the infallibility of every biomaterial depends on the materials from which it's made of. Consequently, there's a great demand in developing new suitable biomaterials (or making the existing ones better) used in multidisciplinary fields and involving physics, chemistry and biology.

In this study, the biomaterials used for fibroblasts adhesion are made of polyelectrolytes using the layer-by-layer technique based on alternating oppositely charged polyelectrolytes on glass probes (more details are shown in paragraph III.2).

2.2. Polyelectrolytes

Polyelectrolytes are highly charged nanoscopic objects or macromolecules. Their electric charge density appears as more or less continuous, when it is seen from distances to the macromolecule equal to several times to the intercharge distance, giving them the polyelectrolytic character. Obviously, their properties will be extremely different according to their geometry. Massive spherical objects will behave like colloids, whereas linear flexible objects will keep some of the macromolecular polymeric character [5]. They are defined as materials for which the solution's properties in dissolvent presenting a high permittivity are governed by electrostatic interactions for distances superior to the molecular dimensions [6]. Polyelectrolytes are by no way a mere superposition of electrolytes and polymers properties. New and rather unexpected behaviours are observed:

• Whereas polymers exhibit only excluded volume effects, the long ranged coulomb interactions, which are present in polyelectrolytes, give rise to new critical exponents.

• The main difference with electrolytes is that one kind of ions, the counterions are stuck together along a chain, and the collective contribution of the charged monomers causes a strong field in the vicinity of the chain, even at very low dilution.

These materials are widely used in industries as dispersive substances in aqueous medium, flocculants to aggregate sludge and industrial waste. Recently, they were used to make films by alternating thin layers of polymers of medical use such as dental prosthesis, fabrication of transplantable organs etc...

Polymers differ by their structure, their surface composition and their biological properties:

2.2.1. Biological properties

The biological properties reflect the origin of polymers. Indeed, one can distinguish three different origins for polymers [7]:

• Natural polymers coming from animal, vegetal and mineral origins

• Artificial polymers with natural basic components and chemically transformed functions in their units (monomers)

• Synthetic polymers presenting synthetic basic components which are often very similar to those of natural polymers

2.2.2. Physico-chemical properties

According to Oudet [7], polymers have different physical properties. The most important are their thermal conductivity reflecting polymers' behaviour under temperature changes.

The second interesting physical property is their optical reactions towards light (refraction, reflection angle, polarization, absorption…). Moreover, polymers are characterized by their ability as electrical conductors or insulators.

From the chemical point of view, Fowkes [8] presumed the existence of different polymers surface structure: polymers with polar surfaces (polyethylene), polymers with acid (polyimide) or basic (polystyrene) sites dominance and others are regrouping both acid and basic characters (polyamide). These surfaces are governed by specific (dispersive forces attraction) and non-specific interactions (acid-base interaction).

Polymers properties are strongly influenced by molecular interactions such as Van der Waals interactions (low energy bonds), hydrogen interactions (low energy bonds having an electrostatic origin) and ionic interactions due to electrostatic attractions and repulsions between ions or ionized groups.

2.3. Polyelectrolyte multilayer film

2.3.1. Generality

In recent years, polyelectrolyte multilayer film has been widely developed in different fields and for a variety of purposes. This kind of ultrathin film can be fabricated from oppositely charged polyelectrolytes using a method called self-assembly discovered by Decher and co-workers in 1992 and allows surface modification and therefore controlling their properties at the molecular (or even the atomic) level.

These films are of a great interest for covering biomaterials used as implants [9, 10] and therefore they will be in contact with cells [11]. Layer-by-layer assembly of polyelectrolytes is a simple and suitable method for coating different substrates such as glass, silicon, thermoplastic and even curved surfaces [12, 13].

It's known that biomaterials must present two main conditions to be admitted for integration in the biological system: to be biocompatible with this system and to have definite mechanical and electrical properties depending on their use [14]. The next implants generation has a tendency to be bioactive, besides its biocompatibility, thanks to substrate coating with bioactive substances.

2.3.2. Fabrication method and application fields

Multilayer polyelectrolyte films are made by alternating oppositely charged polyelectrolytes (polyanions and polycations) on glass slides (Figure 1).

Film's formation is based on charge overcompensation of the newly adsorbed polyions. Indeed, a polyanion (negative charge) added to a polycation (positive charge), previously deposited on the substrate, will neutralise the excess of positive charges and therefore create a new negatively charged polyelectrolyte layer. This step can be repeated as many times as the needed number of layers is reached [15].

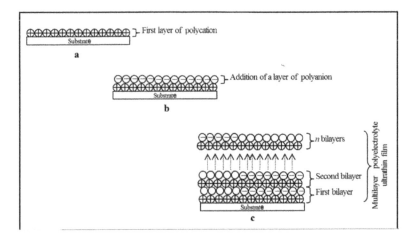

Figure 1. Layer-by-layer polyelectrolyte film's fabrication. This assembly method is based on alternating oppositely charge polyanion (positive charge) and polycations (negative charge) on a solid substrate. One bilayer consists in one polycation associated with one polyanion and the film is a set of n bilayers.

This adsorption mechanism is governed by electrostatic interactions which represent, besides other secondary interactions (hydrogen bond or dispersive force), a paramount parameter for the final structure of the formed film [16].

Polyelectrolyte multilayer films are used in different fields: orthopedic surgery (hip prosthesis...), cardiovascular (artificial heart, vascular prosthesis...), odontology (dental restoration...), ophthalmology (contact lenses...), urology (catheters, artificial kidney...), endocrinology (artificial pancreas, biosensors...), aesthetic surgery and other domains [17].

2.4. Polyelectrolyte film surface characterization

This study is possible by investigating surface wettability and calculating surface free energy. Indeed, wettability is the aptitude of a substrate to be coated by a thin liquid film while dipped in a liquid solution. This method is used to follow the substrate behaviour in relation to its environment and can be done thanks to the contact angle measurement. In this paper we are interested in the dynamic contact angle method using Wilhelmy plate method, treated later. This method, besides giving information about substrate surface hydrophilicity and hydrophobicity, allows us to evaluate the surface roughness and chemical heterogeneity. Moreover, with the results found, we measured the polyelectrolyte film's surface free energy according to Van Oss theory.

2.4.1. Contact angle measurement

There are a variety of simple and inexpensive techniques for measuring contact angles, most of which are described in detail in various texts and publications and will be mentioned only briefly here. The most common direct methods (Figure 2) include the sessile drop (a), the captive bubble (b) and the tilting plate (c). Indirect methods include tensiometry and geometric analysis of the shape of a meniscus. For solids for which the above methods are not applicable, such as powders and porous materials, methods based on capillary pressures, sedimentation rates, wetting times, imbibition rates, and other properties, have been developed [18].

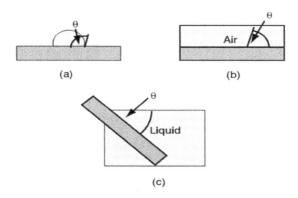

Figure 2. The more common systems of contact angle measurement showing the sessile drop (a), the captive bubble (b) and the tilting plate (c). θ is the contact angle to be measured.

2.4.1.1. The sessile drop method

It's a static contact angle measurement method which consists in putting down a liquid drop on the solid plate we want to characterize its surface by measuring the contact angle made by the drop on this surface. Indeed, when a drop of a liquid is putted down on a solid surface; three phases system occurs: solid, liquid and gas (Figure 3).

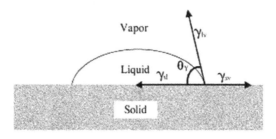

Figure 3. Static contact angle measurement with the sessile drop method

The drop's profile is being changed depending on the physico-chemical characters of the solid surface, on the adhesion forces newly created at the interface solid/liquid and on the cohesion forces of the liquid. This change will affect the contact angle value revealing the surface state (hydrophobic or hydrophilic, rough or smooth, homogeneous or heterogeneous…) and the different forces occurred are linked together according to Young's equation [19]:

$$\gamma_{sv} = \gamma_{sl} + \gamma_{lv} cos\theta,$$

Where $\gamma_{sv,}$ γ_{sl} and γ_{lv} represent the "surface tensions" of the interface solid/gas, solid/liquid and liquid/gas, respectively, and θ represents the contact angle.

2.4.1.2. The captive bubble method

It's a derivative of the sessile drop method and consists in making an air bubble (or a bubble from a less dense and non miscible liquid such as dodecane, octane and octadecane) on a solid surface immersed in pure water or in other liquid with a well known physico-chemical characters. So, it's possible to measure the contact angle made by this bubble with the immersed solid surface (see Figure 2).

2.4.1.3. The tilting plate method

The tilting plate method is to slowly tilt a contact angle sample until the sessile drop on it begins to move in the downhill direction. At that time, the downhill contact angle is the advancing angle and the uphill angle the receding contact angle [20].

The principal alternative to the tilting plate method is having the dispense needle remain immersed in the sessile drop and pumping in until the drop expands in base area and pumping out until the drop contracts in base area. Often the tilting plate measurement is carried out on an instrument with a mechanical platform that tilts the stage and the camera together.

It has been shown that these methods are a subject of controversy. However, the dynamic contact angle measurement using the Wilhelmy plate method has been shown to be easier for use and gives more information about the surface characterized.

2.4.1.4. The dynamic contact angle method: The tensiometer

In our study, we used the Wilhelmy plate method (Tensiometer 3S, GBX, France) which allows a dynamic measurement of the contact angle hysteresis. Indeed, the tensiometer used for the measurement will measure the force applied to the substrate while immerged in a liquid thanks to a balance where the substrate was hanged (Figure 4)

In each case, the polyelectrolyte film coated glass slide was immersed into and then drawn out of the measurement liquid. Therefore, the tensiometer will evaluate the advancing angle (θ_a) when the liquid moves forward the substrate surface and thereafter the receding angle (θ_r) when the liquid resorbs from the substrate. The difference between θ_a and θ_r is called contact angle hysteresis H ($H = \theta_a - \theta_r$) and is useful for understanding the wettability of the film. It gives us information about the surface film mobility, its reorganization and roughness [21].

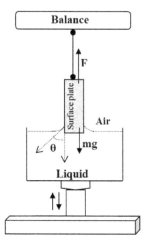

Figure 4. The Wilhelmy plate method for dynamic contact angle measurement. The surface plate is partially immerged in the up down moving liquid container. Curves (Loops) are automatically drawn by a software associated to the Tensiometer according to F = f (Immersion depth)

When a substrate is immersed in a liquid, three forces occur (see Figure 4): the gravity force, the upthrust buoyancy and the capillary forces. Therefore, by measuring the applied force according to the immersion depth and as we previously know the dimension of the substrate; one can calculate the wetting forces according to the equation [22]:

$$F = mg + p * \gamma_{LV} * \cos\theta - F_b \qquad (1)$$

Where F represents the force measured (mN/m), m is the substratum mass, g is the acceleration constant induced by the gravity, p is the substratum perimeter (cm²), γ_{LV} is the surface free energy (mN/m) of the liquid used for measurement (constant), θ: the contact angle between the liquid and the substratum (°) and F_b is the force related to the upthrust buoyancy.

Usually, we make several immersion/emersion cycles for the substratum we are investigating and the different loops (one loop corresponds to one immersion/emersion cycle) are drawn by a software associated to the Tensiometer according to Force = f (immersion depth). Moreover, the substratum weight is assumed to be nil by a direct correction fixing the pre-immersion force to the value of zero. Therefore, the previous equation ([Eq. 1]) becomes:

$$F_{(zero\ immersion)} = p * \gamma_{LV} * \cos\theta$$

As the surface energy of the liquid of measurement is previously known, therefore the contact angle could be deduced.

It has been shown that the contact angle changes depending on the nature of the film and on its charges and thickness. The nature of liquid of measurement, the speed and temperature of measurement are also involved in this change [23]. Indeed, the thickness of the film can affect its elasticity which will induce a difference in the liquid diffusion into this film and therefore the film's swelling level changes affecting the contact angle. A previous study made by Elbert et al.[24] has shown a clear effect of the film layers' number on the wettability of the film.

The liquid used for measurement can affect the surface wettability by the mean of its pH which varies from a liquid to another and controls the acid or base character as well as the liquid polarity. These parameters are responsible for the rearrangement of the biomaterial's groups at its contact. This reorganization is also depending on the liquid diffusion into the polymer and on the effect of solubilization induced by the liquid to this polymer. This phenomenon represents an interesting mechanism for explaining contact angle hysteresis especially when the liquid concerned is water. Indeed, water has small molecules which allow it to diffuse easily. Therefore, after diffusion into a polymer, water will confer its hydrophilic character to this polymer which is being to have some kind of elasticity responsible for the reorganization of its polar groups as a reaction to the high surface energy level of water which is responsible for the high energy level at the interface [25]. Concerning the dynamic contact angle measurement speed, it affects the contact period between the biomaterial and the liquid and therefore it will change the period of time needed for the rearrangement of the surface polar groups during contact with the liquid. As each film has its own defined reorganization time, therefore different contact angles were found for the same surface at different measurement speeds. Moreover, every polymer has a defined glass transition temperature (T_g) able to induce a change on the surface wettability depending on the temperature of measurement [26].

2.4.2. Surface free energy calculation

It's interesting to know the value of surface free energy of a biomaterial because it has an effect on wettability as shown by Van Oss [27]. While the contact between the biomaterial and the liquid generates an interface solid/liquid which will consume, during its formation, a defined energy called the interface energy. The reversible adhesion force represents, therefore, the difference in the energy level between the initial state characterized by two surfaces [28, 29]: solid surface with the energy (γ_s) and liquid surface with the energy (γ_l); and the final state (γ_{sl}).

The surface free energy is a kind of an attraction force of the surface which cannot be measure directly but calculated after contact angle measurement in different measurement liquids (with different surface free energies) according to Owends et Wendt or Van Oss' approaches. Their theories are complementary but Van Oss' approach has been shown to give more information. It consists in the following equation [27]:

$$\gamma_S = \gamma_S{}^{LW} + 2 \, (\gamma_S{}^+ . \gamma_S{}^-)^{\frac{1}{2}}$$

where γ_S represents the surface free energy of the biomaterial surface, $\gamma_S{}^{WL}$: the dispersive component and $\gamma_S{}^+$, $\gamma_S{}^-$ represent the polar components (acid- base).

The different components of the solid and the liquid surface free energies as well as the contact angle are related by this equation:

$$\gamma_L \, (1 + cos\theta) = 2 \, ((\gamma_S{}^{LW} . \gamma_L{}^{LW})^{\frac{1}{2}} + (\gamma_S{}^+ . \gamma_L{}^-)^{\frac{1}{2}} + (\gamma_L{}^+ . \gamma_S{}^-)^{\frac{1}{2}}),$$

This equation contains three unknown parameters: γ^{LW}, γ^+ and γ^-; the contact angle measurement must be done with three different measurement liquids in order to solve this equation and calculate the surface free energy of our polyelectrolyte film. For this purpose, we used three different liquids: water, diiodomethane and formamide.

2.4.3. Evaluation of the surface roughness and heterogeneity

Theses parameters are deduced from the shapes of the curves drawn (loops). Indeed, the more the surface is rough; the more the curve is deformed (non linear curve). However, the more the surface is smooth; the more the curve presents a linear shape (no deformations observed). Otherwise, a roughness of about 100 nm has been shown to induce contact angle hysteresis. As for surface heterogeneity, it can be concluded from the different contact angle hysteresis values measured in the case of a negligible roughness.

Concerning the different polyelectrolyte films used in this study, a previous investigation was made by Picart and coworkers [30]. They measured the roughness by the AFM technique, refractive index and thickness are estimated by optical waveguide light mode spectroscopy, and zeta potential is measured by streaming potential measurements. Indeed, these parameters give us information about the chemical heterogeneity of the polyelectrolyte used.

Many studies had observed an important dependence of the contact angle hysteresis on the surface composition and topography (roughness) [31, 32]. Therefore, the more the surface is rough; the more it's hydrophilic and vise versa and the more this surface is composed of small molecules, the less the liquid diffusion in the biomaterial surface is disturbed leading to a low contact angle value. According to Morra et al.[33], this is may be due to existence of two different effects while studying the wettability of rough and homogeneous biomaterials: the barrier effect, where hysteresis increases with increasing the surface roughness due to an important rigidity of the substrate, and the capillary attraction at the surface which can affect Young's concept. Indeed, the capillary effect induces an increase of both the advancing and receding contact angles in the case of a surface presenting a contact angle superior to 90° at the equilibrium state. In the opposite case (contact angle inferior to 90° at the equilibrium state), the inverse situation will happen and the contact angle variations will be less important than those corresponding to the barrier effect. Only in the case of a contact angle equals to 90°, the capillary effect is negligible.

2.5. Conclusion

When a drop of liquid is placed on a solid surface, the liquid will either spread across the surface to form a thin, approximately uniform film or spread to a limited extent but remain as a discrete drop on the surface. The final condition of the applied liquid to the surface is taken as an indication of the wettability of the surface by the liquid or the wetting ability of the liquid on the surface. The quantitative measure of the wetting process is taken to be the contact angle, which the drop makes with the solid as measured through the liquid in question.

The wetting of a surface by a liquid and the ultimate extent of spreading of that liquid are very important aspects of practical surface chemistry. Many of the phenomenological aspects of the wetting processes have been recognized and quantified since early in the history of observation of such processes. However, the microscopic details of what is occurring at the various interfaces and lines of contact among phases has been more a subject of conjecture and theory than of known facts until the latter part of this century when quantum electrodynamics and elegant analytical procedures began to provide a great deal of new insight into events at the molecular level. Even with all the new information of the last 20 years, however, there still remains a great deal to learn about the mechanisms of movement of a liquid across a surface.

3. Fibroblast cells

3.1. Human gingival fibroblasts

3.1.1. Generality

Fibroblasts are spindle-shaped connective-tissue cells of mesenchymal origin that secretes proteins and especially molecular collagen from which the extracellular fibrillar matrix of connective tissue forms. They have oval or circular nucleus and a little developed cytoplasm giving rise to long prolongation forms [34]. These cells do not have a basal lamina and their surfaces are often in contact with the fibers of the collagen. Their cytoplasm contains a rough endoplasmic reticulum, an important Golgi apparatus, few mitochondria and a little bit quantity of cytoplasmic filaments. Fibroblasts synthesize enormous quantities of the extracellular matrix constituents. Indeed, the majority part of the extracellular matrix components consists of collagen made in the intracellular space where fibroblasts sustain structural modifications.

3.1.2. Gingival tissue

It's the tissue that surrounds the necks of teeth and covers the alveolar parts of the jaws; broadly: the alveolar portion of a jaw with its enveloping soft tissues [35]. It consists in a pink connective tissue with fibrous collagen surrounded by an epithelial tissue. Its pink color changes from one person to another, depending on pigmentation, epithelium thickness, its keratinization level and on the underlying vascularization [36]. Fibroblasts are the basic component of the gingival chorion whose intercellular matrix is essentially formed by collagen and elastin.

3.2. Cell-Biomaterial: Interface and interactions

3.2.1. Biocompatibility concept

While a cell is in contact with a biomaterial, many reactions can occur and a sensing phenomenon will launch between this cell and the biomaterial [37]. Indeed, the cell has a signal network reached as a result of the surface exploration and sensing made in order to verify whether the new environment (biomaterial) is in accordance with its expected physiological conditions necessary for a normal biological activity [38]. Thus, before putting a new material in contact with a cell it's of a great importance to choose the corresponding material in such a way that this material obey the cell's norm by not being toxic or injurious and not causing immunological rejection. In one word, this material must be biocompatible.

The biological tolerance of a biomaterial led scientists to regroup the different parameters and mechanisms controlling the interface biomaterial/cell (or tissue) so that they can deduce a concrete and a common definition for biocompatibility concept. Indeed, biocompatibility includes the understanding of the interactive mechanisms relating the biomaterial with its biological environment. Generally, biocompatibility represents the ability of a material to be accepted by a living organism.

In 1987, Williams D.F suggested the following definition «biocompatibility is the ability of a material to be used with an appropriate and suitable reaction of the host for a specific application».

According to Exbrayat [39] « biocompatibility is a set of the different interrelations between a biomaterial and its environment, and their biological local or general consequences, immediate or delayed, reversible or definitive».

Indeed, biocompatibility is a group of networks that liaises between the biomaterial and its environment and takes into account the possible effect of this biomaterial on its environment and vice versa. Interactions existing in the interface biomaterial/biological environment differ by their intensity and their duration period depending both on the biomaterial and on the tissue in contact.

Characterizing the surface properties of a biomaterial before putting it in contact with a cell seems to be an obligation. This step allows us to know about different parameters and characters of this biomaterial (topography, roughness, surface energy etc.) in order to find a correlation with the cell behavior and therefore we can adjust these physico-chemical properties, when making the biomaterial, so that we have a normal and physiological cell behavior in contact with that biomaterial.

3.2.2. Cell adhesion

It is well known that during the contact between a cell and a material, information will be transferred from the material surface to the cell and this contact will induce, in return, an alteration to the material. This situation may cause material remodelling [40,22].

Cells adhere to surfaces through adhesion proteins (i.e. fibronectin, collagen, laminin, vitronectin) using specific cell receptors, called integrins, attached to the cell membrane. Indeed, when fibroblasts grow on a substrate, most of their cell surface is separated from the substratum by a gap of more than 50 nm; but at focal contacts, this gap is reduced to 10 to 15 nm. The main transmembrane linker proteins of focal contacts belong to the integrin family and the cytoplasmic domain of the integrin binds to the protein talin, which in turn binds to vinculin, a protein found also in other actin-containing cell junction. Vinculin associates with α-actinin and is thereby linked to an actin filament [1].

Besides their role as anchors, focal contacts can also relay signals from the extracellular matrix (ECM) to the cytoskeleton. Several protein kinases are localized to focal contacts and seems to change their activity with the type of the substratum on which the rest. These kinases can regulate the survival, growth, morphology, movement, and differentiation of cells in response to new environment. Figure 5 shows a possible arrangement of these different proteins during a focal contact.

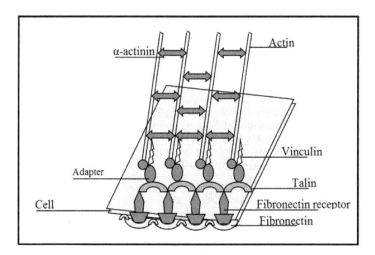

Figure 5. Adhesion proteins involved in focal contacts

The formation of focal contacts occurs when the binding of matrix glycoprotein, such as fibronectin, on the outside of the cell causes the integrin molecules to cluster at the contact site. Fibronectins are associated together by proteoglycans and constitute thins fibers of the extracellular matrix (ECM).

3.2.2.1. Extracellular matrix

The extracellular matrix (ECM) represents an important element in the processes of cell adhesion. Indeed, at this level, cell adhesion is under the control of a well defined zone in the cytoplasmic membrane called focal contact. At this zone, filaments of actin are linked to fibronectin through an intracellular complex of proteins, the adherence complex. The extracellular matrix (ECM) is made of different proteins such as fibronectins, collagen, laminin, vitronectin [41] and represents the mediator of cell adhesion thanks to its integrins.

Although the extracellular matrix generally provides mechanical support to tissues, it serves several other functions as well. Different combinations of ECM components tailor the extracellular matrix for specific purposes: strength in a tendon, tooth, or bone; cushioning in cartilage; and adhesion in most tissues. In addition, the composition of the matrix, which can vary, depending on the anatomical site and physiological status of a tissue, can let a cell know where it is and what it should do (environmental cues). Changes in ECM components, which are constantly being remodeled, degraded, and resynthesized locally, can modulate the interactions of a cell with its environment. The matrix also serves as a reservoir for many extracellular signalling molecules that control cell growth and differentiation. In addition, the matrix provides a lattice through or on which cells can move, particularly in the early stages of tissue assembly [42].

Many functions of the matrix require transmembrane adhesion receptors that bind directly to ECM components and that also interact, through adapter proteins, with the cytoskeleton. The principal class of adhesion receptors that mediate cell–matrix adhesion are integrins, a large family of $\alpha\beta$ heterodimeric cell surface proteins that mediate both cell–cell and cell–matrix adhesions and inside-out and outside-in signalling in numerous tissues.

3.2.2.2. Adhesion proteins and receptors in fibroblast cells

Different proteins and their receptors are involved in fibroblast cells adhesion process. The most important and known are fibronectins and their receptors; integrins:

• Fibronectins

  Fibronectins are dimers of two similar polypeptides linked at their C-termini by two disulfide bonds; each chain is about 60–70 nm long and 2–3 nm thick. The combination of different repeats composing the regions, another example of combinatorial diversity, confers on fibronectin its ability to bind multiple ligands [40].

  Fibronectins help attach cells to the extracellular matrix by binding to other ECM components, particularly fibrous collagens and heparan sulfate proteoglycans, and to cell surface adhesion receptors such as integrins. Through their interactions with adhesion receptors (e.g., $\alpha5\beta1$ integrin), fibronectins influence the shape and movement of cells and the organization of the cytoskeleton. Conversely, by regulating their receptor-mediated attachments to fibronectin and other ECM components, cells can sculpt the immediate ECM environment to suit their needs.

• Integrins

Integrins are the principle adhesion receptors; a large family of αβ heterodimeric cell surface proteins that mediate both cell–cell and cell–matrix. They are transmembrane proteins that mediate interactions between adhesion molecules on adjacent cells and/or the extracellular matrix (ECM). They have diverse roles in several biological processes including cell migration during development and wound healing, cell differentiation, and apoptosis. Their activities can also regulate the metastatic and invasive potential of tumor cells. They exist as heterodimers consisting of alpha and beta subunits. Some alpha and beta subunits exhibit specificity for one another, and heterodimers often preferentially bind certain cell adhesion molecules, or constituents of the ECM.

Although they themselves have no catalytic activity, integrins can be part of multimolecular signalling complexes known focal adhesions. The two subunits, designated as alpha and beta, both participate in binding.

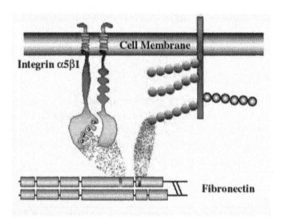

Figure 6. Fibronectin binding to its Integrin receptor (adapted from internet)

Integrins participate in cell-cell adhesion and are of great importance in binding and interactions of cells with components of the extracellular matrix such as fibronectin. Importantly, integrins facilitate "communication" between the cytoskeleton and extracellular matrix; allow each to influence the orientation and structure of the other. It is clear that interactions of integrins with the extracellular matrix can have profound effects on cell function, and events such as clustering of integrins activates a number of intracellular signally pathways.

3.2.3. Cell adhesion: The physical process

Biological systems exhibit electromagnetic activity in a wide frequency range from the static or quasistatic electric field to optical bands. Fröhlich [43] presumed that biological matter has anomalous polarization properties (e.g. induction of great electric dipole after electric field application). Static charge distribution of dipole and/or multipole nature exists (e.g. in protein molecules). Vibrations in biological molecules, therefore, generate an electromagnetic field [44]. Pokorny et al.[45], assume that the Fröhlich electromagnetic field can be a fundamental factor of cell adherence.

Surface topography is of an important interest in cell adhesion as well as its chemical composition. Indeed, it has been shown that cells adhere and proliferate depending on the surface roughness and the more the surface is rough the more cell adhesion and proliferation is better [46]. This effect depends on the cell type. For fibroblasts, they line up along the biomaterial surface microstructures and may adapt their shape with uneven surfaces.

Moreover, recent studies had shown that a weak change in the surface roughness may induce different cell reactions such as change in their shape and their way of adhesion [47, 48].

3.2.3.1. Forces involved in cell adhesion

According to Richards [49], cell adhesion to biomaterials is done thanks to focal adhesion sites which represent strict contact sites with the substrate in a so limited space. For fibroblasts, it has been shown the existence of a force called cohesion force responsible for keeping contact between cells themselves. However, this force is weaker than the adhesion force involved while a cell adheres to a biomaterial. This difference in force level depends on the cell type and on the nature of the biomaterial used for adhesion, and may explain the different ways of cell adhesion and spreading on different surface structures.

3.2.3.2. Surface free energy

Surface free energy is a thermodynamic measurement which contributes to the interpretation of the phenomena occurring in interfaces. It has an important effect on cell adhesion in the way that every change in its value induces the modification of the surface wettability, and therefore cell behaviour will be affected too [50, 51, 52].

Cell-biomaterial interface depends on the physico-chemical properties of the biomaterial and every change in the chemical composition or in the electric charge of the surface will affect its surface free energy.

3.2.4. Parameters involved in cell adhesion

3.2.4.1. Surface roughness

Surface roughness has been the subject of many studies as a deciding factor in the process of cell adhesion to biomaterials. Ponsonnet et al.[53] had studied the behaviour of fibroblast cells while adhering to titanium surface with different roughness; they found that cells had adhered to the surface using thin cytoplasmic structures. Indeed, these cells presented a flattened shape spreading practically over the substrate surface after adhesion to smooth surfaces. However, on rough surfaces, cell morphology was affected by the surface grooves and they were reoriented by the surface structure.

According to Richards [48], smooth titanium surfaces always increase fibroblasts adhesion and proliferation better than rough surfaces. They suggested that this kind of surfaces should be a better candidate for biological implant thanks to their ability to resist to bacterial infections. Indeed, their weak roughness is unfavourable to the adhesion of bacteria.

3.2.4.2. The electric charge effect

In the majority of the studies carried out about biomaterials made from polyelectrolyte film, as in our case, the electric charge effect is in proportion with the thickness of the film built and depends on the charged functional group of the polyelectrolyte used [54].

For Andrade [25], the notion of the nature of an electric charge is important to be mentioned but its effect is not significant and doesn't induce an efficient change on surface wettability. However, it has been shown that a better adhesion of cells was observed on negatively charged polyelectrolyte [55]. In reality, most of the existed cells and their corresponding adhesion proteins are negatively charged. Nevertheless, this charge can be without any effect in the case when functional groups become able to control cell adhesion mechanism by their hydrophilic or hydrophobic character as it will be shown later in this text. Dubois [56] presumed that an electric charge trapped within an insulating biomaterial, none associated to a particular chemical group, is able to affect its biological environment. Moreover, Maroudas [57] revealed the dependence of cell adhesion and spreading on a solid surface on the surface charge of the substrate.

3.2.4.3. Chemical composition

The different chemical components of a biomaterial must be studied and known before to start investigating cell adhesion to that biomaterial. Therefore, this step is fundamental for concluding about the biocompatibility of a given biomaterial and its effect on cell adhesion [58].

The wettability of a surface depends on the chemical composition of the material and each change than can occur at this level will disturb cell adhesion process [59]. Besides the effect of the biomaterial, the adhered cell type plays an important role in adhesion. Indeed, for the same biomaterial surface, different cell reactions were observed for two types of cells [60]; this kind of biomaterial seems to be biocompatible with one cell type but not tolerated by the other cell type.

According to Marmur [61], most of the materials in the nature are rough and heterogeneous and contact angle may change along the contact line with a value depending on the roughness and heterogeneity level.

3.2.4.4. Surface hydrophilicity and hydrophobicity

Contact angle measurement allows us to calculate surface free energy [62]. It also allows knowing about the polar or non polar nature of the interactions at the interface liquid/ solid. Moreover, one can deduce from it the hydrophilic or the hydrophobic character of a surface [63].

A study about polyelectrolyte films found that hydrophobic interactions on a surface induce the adsorption of proteins and stabilise the complex formed [64]. Indeed, it has been proved that myoglobin or lysozymes are able to adhere to polystyrene sulfonate (PSS) and form many layers. However, this adhesion was not possible when using another surface having the same electric charge as PSS but with a hydrophilic character. The electrostatic interactions between the protein complex and this hydrophilic surface were easily destructed after water rinsing. Thus, surface hydrophilicity and hydrophobicity are a determinant parameter for substrate wettability on account of the rearrangement of the functional groups at the surface of a biomaterial in contact with a cell [65, 66, 67]. Indeed, it has been shown that fibroblast cells adhere and proliferate better on biomaterials with a moderate hydrophilicity [68, 69].

Andrade [66] presumed that, in the case of deformable materials, an elasticity model of 3.5 10^5 dyn/cm^2 is necessary for avoiding contact angle change. A roughness below 0.1 μm has a negligible effect on contact angle. Most of the materials holding over than 20 to 30 % of water present a receding contact angle (θ_r), in water, near zero because of the hydrophilic character which dominates the interface in these conditions. The same author estimated that the majority of polymers have a changeable volume which can be the reason for contact angle change: this change is depending on the duration of the contact with water, on the nature of the liquid and on the temperature of measurement. Non existent contact angle hysteresis may be due to the duration of contact between the material and the liquid which is shorter or longer than the measurement time needed for recording contact angle change. Therefore, surface hydrophilicity and hydrophobicity depends on the volume blowing of the material, on the diffusion phenomenon and on the mobility and reorientation of the molecules on the material surface.

Some materials are able to go out of shape in contact with a liquid depending on their mechanical properties and on their relaxation time and temperature. So, what characterizes a polymer is its chemical composition, roughness, mobility, wettability, surface free energy and its electric charge [70].

3.2.4.5. Surface wettability: Contact angle hysteresis

Contact angle hysteresis is the result of contact angle change between the surface we are characterizing and another ideal surface physico-chemically homogeneous. It's the direct result of a different sensitivity to the wettability process of heterogeneous surfaces. According to Rupp et al.[71], the receding contact angle value (θ_r) is under the control of the small hydrophilic particles of the surface which are able to disturb or to delay the non wettability process. Indeed, when the hysteresis remains constant after many immersion and emersion cycles it's called thermodynamic (or true) hysteresis. However, in the opposite case, it's called kinetic hysteresis (see Figure 7).

Thermodynamic hysteresis is due to the surface roughness and heterogeneity. Nevertheless, kinetic hysteresis is caused by the adsorption mechanisms (due to the liquid phase), surface polar group's reorientation and surface deformation [24].

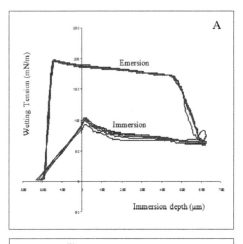

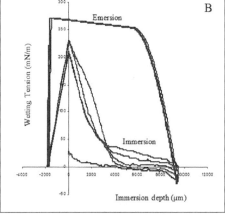

Figure 7. Immersion and emersion loops showing the two types of hysteresis: (A): thermodynamic hysteresis and (B): kinetic hysteresis. The sample is repeatedly immersed in the liquid leading to typical hysteresis loops. From each loop, wettability parameters (advancing and receding contact angle or wetting tension) can be calculated

Contact angle hysteresis is often assigned to the surface roughness and heterogeneity. Actually, a study made by Lam et al. [26], have shown that hysteresis is related to the molecules' mobility, the liquid diffusion and the surface swelling. These authors had observed a close dependence between the liquid molecules size and the liquid/material contact duration. Liquid resorption and retention are the direct causes of hysteresis. However, as the liquid surface free energy is higher that that of the material; therefore the liquid retention into the material will increase the material surface free energy and thus reduces the receding contact angle (θ_r). Indeed, liquids having smaller molecular chains (or smaller molecular weight) diffuse faster into the polymer surface leading to an important decrease in contact angle.

According to Shananan et al.[72], contact angle hysteresis is related to the polymer polarity. Indeed, when a polymer gets in touch with a polar liquid (water), it orients its mobile polar groups on the surface in order to increase the interfacial water/polymer energy and therefore decreasing the system surface free energy. In the other hand, when the polymer is contact with a non polar liquid, its functional groups conserve their state and will not reorient. These authors assumed the existence of two parameters behind hysteresis: the intrinsic polarity of the material and the mobility of its polar groups on the surface. Nishioka et al.[73], had observed that the advancing contact angle hysteresis is under the control of surface sites more hydrophobic than those controlling the receding contact angle hysteresis.

The contact angle hysteresis observed on hydrophilic and hydrated polymers is due to the polar groups' orientation on the interfaces polymer/liquid and polymer/air. This reorientation represents the polymer reaction to every environmental change (air, liquid). The receding contact angle (θ_r) depends on the contact duration with water, the environment temperature and on the glass transition temperature (T_g) of the material itself. Each material has its own glass transition temperature (T_g) allowing a defined molecular mobility sufficient for an important rearrangement [74].

3.3. Conclusion

The concepts of solid surfaces assumed that the surfaces in question were effectively rigid and immobile. Such assumptions allow one to develop certain models and mathematical relationships useful for estimating and understanding surface energies, surface stresses, and specific interactions, such as adsorption, wetting, and contact angles. It is assumed that the surfaces themselves do not change or respond in any specific way to the presence of a contacting liquid phase, thereby altering their specific surface energy [75]. Although such assumptions are (or may be) valid for truly rigid crystalline or amorphous solids, they more often than not do not apply strictly to polymeric surfaces.

In contact with condensed phases, especially liquids, surface relaxations and transitions can become quite important leading to a possible dramatically change in the interfacial characteristics of a polymer with possibly important consequences in a particular application. And since the processes are time-dependent, the changes may not be evident over the short span of a normal experiment. For critical applications in which a polymer surface will be in contact with a liquid phase, such as implant device for biomedical application, it is not only important to know the surface characteristics (e.g., coefficient of friction, adhesion, adsorption)under normal experimental conditions but also to determine the effects of prolonged (equilibrium) exposure to the liquid medium of interest. It is therefore important for biomedical as well as many other applications that the surface characteristics of a material of interest be determined under conditions that mimic as closely as possible the conditions of use and over extended periods of exposure to those conditions, in addition to the usual characterizations.

4. Experimental and results

4.1. Polyelectrolyte multilayer film preparation

Before use, glass slides were cleaned in 0.01 M SDS and then in 0.1 N HCl, both for 10 min in a boiling water bath, followed by a pure water rinse. Polyelectrolyte solutions were prepared by dissolution of the polyelectrolyte powders in 0.15 M NaCl (using ultrapure water filtered with a MilliQ system, Millipore) at a concentration of 1mg/l for PLL, PGA and HA and 5 mg/l for PEI, PSS and PAH. For all the films, the precursor layer was always PEI (polycation), followed by the alternate adsorption of polyanions/polycations for 12 min adsorption times and two rinses in the 0.15 M NaCl solution [76]. The glass slides held in a slide holder were dipped into the different polyelectrolyte baths for the preparation of three different types of film, ending either by the polycation or polyanion: $(PSS/PAH)_{10}$, $(PSS/PAH)_{10}$–PSS; $(PGA/PLL)_5$, $(PGA/PLL)_5$–PGA; and $(HA/PLL)_5$, $(HA/PLL)_5$–HA. Cleaning was made before film characterization. The films were all prepared at the same pH before being in contact with culture medium. Poly(styrene-4-sulfonate) (PSS,MW=70 kDa), Poly(allylamine hydrochloride) (PAH,MW=70 kDa) and Poly(ethyleneimine) (PEI,MW=70 kDa) are purchased from Aldrich. Poly(l-lysine) (PLL, MW=32 KDa) Poly(l-glutamic acid) (PGA, MW=72 KDa) were obtained from Sigma and Hyaluronan (HA,MW=400 kDa) from Bioiberica. Sodium dodecyl sulfate (SDS) was purchased from Sigma and sodium chloride (NaCl, purity ~ 99%) from Aldrich, glass slides (18x18 cm^2 square and 14x14 cm^2 disk), respectively, were obtained from CML, France.

4.2. Contact angle measurement and Surface Free Energy (SFE) calculation

The measurements were performed with a Wilhelmy balance for the characterization of solids using the 3S tensiometer and the corresponding software (GBX, France). For these experiments, the glass slides were coated with polyelectrolyte multilayer films on both sides. Before beginning the measurements, the films were washed in 18.2 MΩ Millipore water for 30–45 min in order to eliminate the NaCl traces that could modify the results. Samples were then dried at 30 °C for 2 h. The dynamic contact angle hysteresis was determined at 20°C for each film and five wetting/dewetting cycles were carried out at a 50 μm/s speed.

Three liquids were used as a probe for surface free energy calculations: diiodomethane, formamide (Sigma Chemical CO, St Louis, MO, USA) and distilled water. The final contact angle used for this calculation was the average of the 2nd to 5th cycle advancing contact angle (θ_a) and the surface free energies of the different films were calculated using the Van Oss (VO) approach, as usual with sessile drop method contact angles:

$$\gamma_S = \gamma_S^d + 2\,(\gamma_S^+ \cdot \gamma_S^-)^{\frac{1}{2}}$$

This method produces the dispersive (γ_S^d) and the polar acid–base (γ_S^+, γ_S^-) components. Solid and liquid SFE components and contact angle are related according to the equation below:

$$\gamma_L\,(1 + cos\theta) = 2\,((\gamma_S^d \cdot \gamma_L^{\ d})^{\frac{1}{2}} + (\gamma_S^+ \cdot \gamma_L^{\ -})^{\frac{1}{2}} + (\gamma_L^{\ +} \cdot \gamma_S^-)^{\frac{1}{2}})$$

Were γ_L is the SFE of the liquid and γ_s the SFE of the surface.

4.3. Cell adhesion, viability and morphology study

For adhered cell counting, image analysis was performed on a Quantimet 570 (Leica, UK) fitted to an epifluorescence microscope (Axioplan, Zeiss, DE) and a black-and-white charge-coupled device (CCD) camera (LH51XX-SPU, Lhesa Electronique, FR). The scanning was carried out using a ten times lens (NA=0.3) and a filter set adapted for propidium iodide fluorescence observation (BP 546/12 nm, DM 580 nm, LP 590 nm). Microscope focus and stage were motorized and software controlled.

The cell viability was determined with the MTT colorimetric assay. It was measured at 570 nm with a 96-well microplate reader (Becton Dinkinson, Lincoln Park, USA) on a spectrophotometer (Bio-Tek Instruments, Winooski, USA). The blank reference was taken for wells containing only the MTT solution.

The morphology of the cells was analyzed after 120 min (day 0), 2 and 7 days of culture using a scanning electron microscopy (Philips, EDAX XL-20) and phase contrast microscopy.

4.4. Results

4.4.1. Contact angle measurement

The different contact angle values found are shown in Table 1. Experiments were performed at 20 °C at a speed of 50 μm/s. One can observe that contact angle depends on the film's nature (physico-chemical composition) which differs from a polymer to another.

	Water	Formamide	Diiodomethane
Glass	43 ± 2	23 ± 3	43 ± 3.1
(HA/PLL)$_{10}$	12 ± 2	00	00
(HA/PLL)$_5$	81.9 ± 1.8	49.6 ± 2	43.5 ± 3
(HA/PLL)$_5$-HA	87.8 ± 1.2	00	45 ± 2.9
(PGA/PLL)$_5$	55.2 ± 3	14.7 ± 2.5	39.1 ± 1.2
(PGA/PLL)$_5$-PGA	44.1 ± 3.1	00	40.7 ± 1.6
(PSS/PAH)$_{10}$	49.2 ± 1.8	23.6 ± 3	00
(PSS/PAH)$_{10}$-PSS	53 ± 1.9	12.1 ± 3.3	00

Table 1. Dynamic contact angle

4.4.2. SFE values

SFE and its component's values are summarized in Table 2. (HA/PLL) films have the lowest SFE value and (PSS/PAH) films have the highest value. The outermost layer of the film does not have a great influence.

	(HA/PLL)$_5$	(HA/PLL)$_5$- HA	(PGA/PLL)$_5$	(PGA/PLL)$_5$- PGA	(PSS/PAH)$_{10}$	(PSS/PAH)$_{10}$- PSS	Glass	Thermanox
Surface Free Energy (mN/m)	42.4	44.95	53.3	48.26	57.1	58.9	50	35
Dispersive component (mN/m)	38.8	37.1	40.23	39.5	50.8	50.8	35	36
Acid component (mN/m)	1.2	11.85	3.56	9.46	0.46	1.7	3	3
Basic component (mN/m)	2.86	1.3	14.6	2.4	23.76	7	25	0
Acid-basic component (mN/m)	3.56	7.8	13.9	8.86	6.3	8.1	17	1

Table 2. Surface Free Energy (SFE) and its components for the different films used. The SFE of PSS/PAH is higher compared to the other films.

4.4.3. Cell adhesion

Figure 8 shows the percentage of fibroblasts that have adhered after 2 h in culture. The highest adhesion is found with (PGA/PLL)$_5$ film (95%) and the lowest on (HA/PLL)$_5$ film (49%).

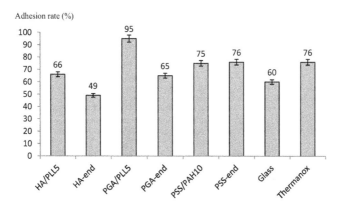

Figure 8. Fibroblast adhesion rate after 2 h in culture onto different films. The percentage represents the number of the adhered cells compared to the initial number of seeded cells.

4.4.4. Cell viability and proliferation rate

Cell viability was evaluated on the different types of film at different time intervals (0, 2 and 7 days) with the MTT assay (Figure 9A). The (PGA/PLL)$_5$–PGA films exhibited a good proliferation rate (Figure 9B) and the (PSS/PAH)$_{10}$ films were the most favorable to cell proliferation.

4.4.5. Cell morphology

Good adhesion is observed on (PGA/PLL)$_5$ film (Figure 10A) whereas bad adhesion was found on (HA/PLL)$_5$-HA film (Figure 10B). Typical morphology at day 2 on a (PGA/PLL)$_5$–PGA film is presented in Figure 10C. After seven days in culture, the difference in morphology for the cells that had adhered to the different films was even more striking. Cells in contact with (HA/PLL)$_5$–HA exhibit necroses (Figure 11A) whereas the cells exhibit elongated and spread morphologies on the highly proliferative (PSS/PAH)$_{10}$ films (Figure 11B).

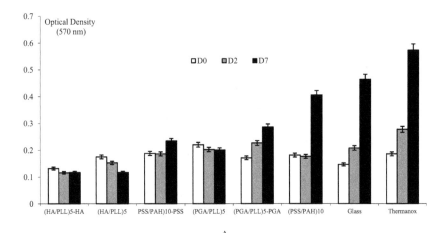

A

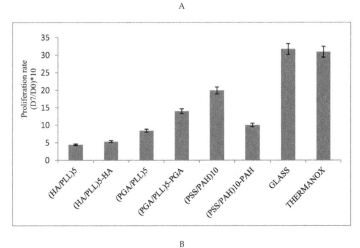

B

Figure 9. A. Cell viability (MTT test) on each film type followed over a seven day period at: day 0 (D0), day 2 (D2), and day 7 (D7), B. Proliferation rate on the different films as estimated by the ratio (D7/D0)

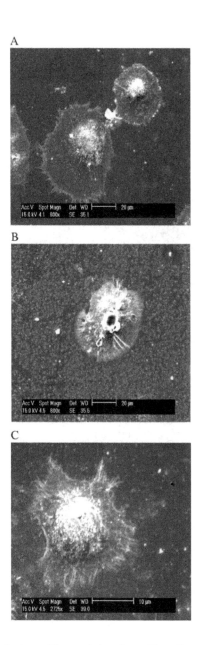

Figure 10. SEM images of cells adhering to different polyelectrolyte multilayer films. (A) (PGA/PLL)5(x800) on the first day, (B) HA/PLL)$_5$–HA (x800) on the first day, (C) (PGA/PLL)$_5$–PGA film observed on the second day (x2725).

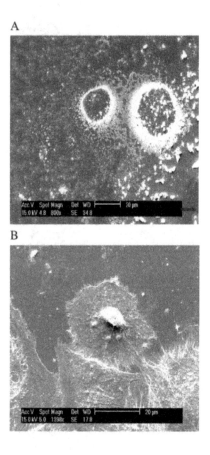

Figure 11. SEM images of cell morphology after seven days of culture. (A) (HA/PLL)$_5$–HA (x800) film, a (PSS/PAH)$_{10}$ film observed at different magnifications (B) (x1398): some areas are at confluency.

4.4.6. Correlation between cell adhesion and films SFE

No correlation was found between the wettability parameters or the SFE parameters and the fibroblast proliferation ratio. However, the adhesion rate at 2 h was correlated to both SFE basic component and the SFE acid component (Figure 12). For the adhesion rate, the SFE basic component is optimum at 15 mN/m (Figure 12A) whereas the acid one is optimum at about 5 mN/m (Figure 12B).

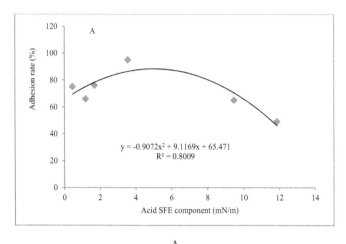

A

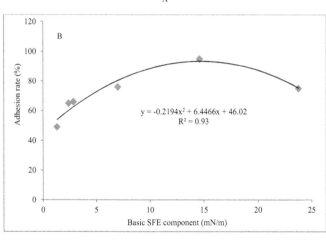

B

Figure 12. SEM images of cell morphology after seven days of culture. (A) (HA/PLL)₅–HA (x800) film, a (PSS/PAH)₁₀ film observed at different magnifications (B) (x1398): some areas are at confluency. Figure 12B. Correlation between cell adhesion rate and Basic SFE component. An optimum is found for 15 mN/m with good polynomial correlation (R^2=0.93)

4.5. General conclusion

Cell adhesion is a paramount parameter for the biomaterial tissue. These biomaterials, by their surface properties (chemical composition, topography, roughness, surface energy) hold the key of the control of the cell adhesion, proliferation and orientation. Thus, the concept of biocompatibility is seen imposed, it is primarily focused on the interface, sites of the interactions between cells and biomaterials.

The influence of different polyelectrolyte multilayer films (PEM) on gingival fibroblast cell response was studied. Roughness and hydrophobicity/hydrophilicity of the PEM were characterized by contact angle measurement. Polar (acid-basic) components of the surface free energy (SFE) were determined. Surface advancing and receding angles were measured and hysteresis was determined. Cell adhesion, viability and morphology were analyzed.

This work pointed out that cell adherence is a complex process modulated by numerous parameters. Usually, in cell adherence studies and particularly in biomaterial approaches, surface physico-chemical properties are analysed (chemistry, roughness, motility, wettability…).

In our work we tackled the subject of the cellular behavior in contact with a biomaterial by the characterization of the surface of this material. We were interested in physical (topography) and chemical (composition) properties of various polyelectrolyte multilayer films deposited on glass slides, with different charge densities scale and thickness. We have evaluated the wettability of theses biomaterials by measuring the contact angle hysteresis using the Wilhelmy balance tensiometry to study their physico-chemical characteristics in order to understand the effects of surface roughness and chemistry on the fibroblasts behavior. Epifluorescence microscopy, SEM, phase contrast microscopy and MTT test were used to study cell adhesion, proliferation and morphology in order to correlate the film's properties and the cultivated cells response.

Surface hydrophobicity and roughness were found to be unfavourable for both adhesion and proliferation. Adhesion and proliferation were found not to be correlated.

Author details

M. Lotfi[1], M. Nejib[2] and M. Naceur[3]

*Address all correspondence to: lotfi.mhamdi@gmail.com

1 Faculty of Medicine of Monastir, Tunisia, Laboratory of biophysics, Avicenne Avenue, Tunisia

2 Higher Institute of Agronomy of Chott Meriem, Laboratory of animal sciences, Sousse, Tunisia

3 Ecole Polytechnique of Montreal, Canada

References

[1] Aberts B, Bray D, Lewis J, Raff M, Roberts K, D. Watson J. Membrane structure, Molecular biology of the cell, 3rd edition, chapter 10, Garland publishing, Inc., 1994, 477.

[2] Rusciano D. Encyclopedic reference of cancer, p. 24, Manfred Schwab Ed. 2001

[3] Passuti N, Baqey C, Guillot F, Reach G. 2000. In www.frm.org

[4] Shabalovskaya S.A. Biocompatibility aspects of Nitinol as an implant material, Biomedical Materialsand Engeneering, 2002

[5] Durand-Vidal S, Simonin J.-P, Turq P. Polyelectrolytes, Electrolytes at interface, Vol. 1,chapter 6, Kluwer Academic Publishers, 2002, 331

[6] Mini-Encyclopedia of paper making. Wet-End Chemistry, Part Two: Definitions and Concepts

[7] Oudet Ch. Polymères, Structure et propriétés, Introduction, Masson, Paris, Milan, barcelone. 1994

[8] Fowkes F.M. Interface Acid-base/charge-transfer properties, Polymer surface dynamics, Vol.1, Joseph D. Andrade, Plenum Press, New York and London, 1983, 336-371

[9] De Groot C. J, Van Luyn M J. A, Van Dijk-Wolthuis W. N. E, Cadée J. A, Plantinga J. A, Den Otter W,Hennink W. E. In vitro biocompatibility of biodegradable dextran-based hydrogels tested with humanfibroblasts, Biomaterials, Vol. 22, Issue 11, 2001, 1197-1203

[10] Bell J.P, Schmidt R.G, Malofsky A, Mancini D. Controlling factors in chemical coupling of polymers to metals. J. adhesion Sci. Technol, Vol.5, N°10, 1991, 927-944

[11] Serizawa T, Kamimura S, Kawanishi N, Akashi M. Layer -by-layer assembly of Poly(vinyl alcohol) and hydrophobic polymers based on their physical adsorption on surfaces. Langmuir 2002

[12] Caruso F, furlong D N, Ariga K, Ichinose I, Kunitak T. Characterization of polyelectrolyte-protein multilayer films by atomic force microscopy, scanning electron microscopy and Fourrier transform infrared reflection adsorption spectroscopy. Langmuir 1998

[13] Kasemo B.N.L. J, Mattsson H. Surface spectroscopic characterization of titanium implant materials. Appl. Surf. Sci., 1990

[14] Rodil S.E, Olivares R, Arzate H, Muhl S. Properties of carbon films and their biocompatibility using in vitro tests, Diamond and Related Materials, Vol.12, Issues 3-7, 2003, 931-937

[15] Schaaf P, Voegel J. C. Films bioactifs destinés au recouvrement de biomatériaux et ciblant une régénération tissulaire : de nouvelles voies originales? Pathologie Biologie, Vol. 50, 2002, 189-193

[16] Hammond P.T. Recent explorations in electrostatic multilayer thin film assembly. Current Opinion in Colloid & Interface Science, Vol.4, 1999, 430-442

[17] Sedel L, Janot C, Biomatériaux, document found in internet, 1996

[18] Meyers D. Wetting and spreading, Surfaces, Interfaces, and Colloids: Principles and Applications, chapter 17, Second Edition. John Wiley & Sons, Inc., 1999, 419

[19] Young T. Philos. Trans. R. Soc. 95 (1805)65.

[20] www.firsttenangstroms.com. Tilting plate example, 3 February 2004

[21] Chen J, Luo G, Cao W. The study of layer-by-layer ultrathin films by the dynamic contact angle method. Journal of Colloid and Interface Science, Vol.238, 2001, 62-69

[22] Defay P, Peter G. Dynamic surface tension, Surface Colloid Sci., 1969; 3: 27-82

[23] Okano T, Yamada N, Okuhara M, Sakai H, Sakurai Y. Mechanism of cell detachment from temperature- modulated, hydrophilic-hydrophobic polymer surfaces. Biomaterials 16, 1995, 297-303

[24] Elbert D.L, Hubbel J.A. Self-assembly and steric stabilization at heterogeneous biological surfaces using adsorbing block copolymers, Chem. Biol, 5, 83-177

[25] Andrade J. The contact angle and interface energetics, surface and interfacial aspects of biomedical polymers, Vol.1, Joseph D .Andrade, Plenum Press, New York and London, 1983, 249-289

[26] Lam C. N. C, Wu R, Li D, Hair M.L, Neumann A.W. Study of the advancing and receding contact angles: liquid sorption as a cause of contact angle hysteresis. Advances in Colloid and Interface Science, Vol.96, 2002, 169-191

[27] Van Oss C.J. Hydrophobicity and hydrophilicity of biosurfaces. Current opinion in colloid and interface science, 1997, 503-512

[28] Takahara A. Block copolymers and hydrophilic city, Modern approaches to wettability: theory and applications, Malcolm E. Schrader and George Loeb. Plenum Press, New York, 1992, 206-210

[29] Kamusewitz H, Possart W, Paul D. The relation between Young's equilibrium contact angle and the hysteresis on rough paraffin wax surfaces. Colloids and Surfaces A: Physicochemical and Engineering Aspects, Vol.156, Issues 1-3, 15, 1999, 271-279

[30] Picart C, Ph. Lavalle Ph, Hubert P, Cuisinier F.J.G, Decher g, Schaaf p, Voegel J.C. Build-up mechanism for poly-L-lysine/Hyaluronine acid films onto a solid surface. Langmuir 2002

[31] Otsuka H, Nagasaki Y, Kataoka K. Dynamic wettability study on the functionalized PEGylated layer on a polylactide surface constructed by the coating of aldehyde-ended poly(ethylene glycol) (PEG)/ polylactide (PLA) block copolymer. Science and technology of advanced materials, 2000, 9-21

[32] Estarlich F.F, Lewey S.A, Nevell T.G, Torpe A.A, Tsibouklis J, Upton A.C. The surface properties of silicone and fluorosilicone coating materials immersed in seawater. Biofluing, Vol. 16, 263-275

[33] Morra M, Occhiello E, Garbassi F. Knowledges about polymer surfaces from contact angle measurements. Adv. Colloid Interfaces Sci.32, 1990, 79-116

[34] Vogler E.A. Wettability, Interfacial chemistry in biomaterials science, Ed. John C. Berg, Marcel Dekker, Inc, New York, Basel, Hong Kong, 1993

[35] Merriam-Webster's Collegiate® Dictionary. 10th edition with Merriam-Webster's Collegiate® Thesaurus. Version 3.0.327

[36] Comte V. PhD thesis, Faculty of Medicine of Lyon, March 18th 2003

[37] Castner D.G, Ratner B.D. Biomedical surface science: Foundations to frontiers. Surface Science, Vol.500, Issues 1-3, 2002, 28-60

[38] Jones F. H. Teeth and bones: applications of surface science to dental materials and related biomaterials. Surface Science Reports, Vol.42, Issues 3-5, 2001, 75-205

[39] Exbrayat P. Question C.E.S: La biocompatibilité des matériaux dentaires. Journal de Biomatériaux Dentaires, Vol.13. 1998

[40] Hubbel J.A. In situ material transformations in tissue engineering, Mat.Res.Soc.Bull, 21, 1996, 5-33

[41] El-Amin S.F, Lu H, Khan Y, Burems J, Mitchell J, S.Tuan R, Laurencin C.T. Extracellular matrix production by human osteoblasts cultured on biodegradable polymers applicable for tissue engineering. Biomaterials, 24, 2003

[42] Berk L, Kaiser M, Scott K, Darnell Z. Integrating cells into tissues, Molecular cell biology, 5th edition, Chapter 6, p.201

[43] Frölch H. Coherent electric vibrations in biological systems and cancer problem, IEEE Trans, 1978; MTT-26:613-617, 1978

[44] Pokorny J, Jandova. A, Sorfova J, Kobilkova J, Trojan S, Costato M, Milani M. Leukocytes of cancer patients give evidence of fundamental physical forces: a pathway for a new view. Laser & Technology, Vol.6, N° 1-2, 15-23, 1996.

[45] Pokorny J, Fiala J, Jandova A, Kobilkova J. Fröhlich electromagnetic field and adherence of leukocytes. 2nd Int. Meeting Microwaves in Med, 11-14 Oct. 1993, Rome

[46] Eisenbarth E, Meyle J, Nachtigall W, Breme J. Influence of the surface structure of titanium materials on the adhesion of fibroblasts, Biomaterials, 17. 1996

[47] Eisenbarth E, Linez P, Biehl V, Velten D, Breme J, Hildebrand H. F. Cell orientation and cytoskeleton organisation on ground titanium surfaces, Biomolecular Engineering, Vol.19, 2002, 233-237

[48] Schwartz J, Avaltroni M.J, Danahy M.P, Silverman B.M, Hanson E.L, Schwarzbauer J.E, Midwood K.S, Gawalt E.S. Cell attachment and spreading on metal implant materials, Materials science and engineering C, Vol.23, Issue 3, 2003, 395-400

[49] Richards R.G. The effect of surface roughness on fibroblast adhesion in vitro, Injury, Volume 27. Supplement 3, 1996, S

[50] Shelton R.M, Rasmussen A.C, Davies J.E. Protein adsorption at the interface between charged polymer substrata and migration osteoblasts. Biomaterials, 9, 1988, 24-29.

[51] Drummond C, Israelachvili J. Surface forces and wettability. Petroleum science and engineering, 2002, 123-133

[52] Satriano C, Carnazza S, Guglielmino S, Marletta G. Surface free energy and cell attachment onto ion- beam irradiated polymer surfaces. Article in press. Beam interactions with materials and atoms. 2003

[53] Ponsonnet L, Comte V, Othmane A, Lagneau C, Charbonnier M, Lissac M, Jaffrezic N. Effect of surface topography and chemistry on adhesion, orientation and growth of fibroblasts on nickel-titanium substrates. Materials Science & Engineering. 2002

[54] Elbert D, Herbert C.B, Hubbel J.A. Thin polymer layers formed by polyelectrolyte multilayer technique on biological surfaces. Langmuir, 1999

[55] Forest P, Master Diploma report, 2002

[56] Dubois J.C , PhD thesis, Faculty of Medicine of Lyon, 2002

[57] Maroudas N.G. Adhesion and spreading of cells on charged surfaces. J theor Biol, 49, 417-424, 1975

[58] Fischer D, Li Y, Ahlemeyer B, Krieglstein J, Kissel T. In vitro cytotoxicity testing of polycations: influence of polymer structure on cell viability and haemolysis. Biomaterials, 2003, 1121-1131

[59] Good R.J. Contact angle, wetting, and adhesion: a critical review. In: K.L. Mittal Editor, Contact Angle, Wetting and Adhesion VSP, Utrecht, the Netherlands (1993), 3–36.

[60] Troyen-Toth P, Vantier D, Haikel Y,Voegel J.C, Schaaf P, Chluba J, Ogier J. Viability, adhesion and bone phenotype of osteoblast-like cells on polyelectrolyte multilayer films, Wiley Periodical, Inc. 2001

[61] Marmur A. Equilibrium contact angles: theory and measurement. Colloids and Surfaces, Vol.116, 1996, 55-61

[62] Kwok D. Y, Neumann A. W. Contact angle interpretation in terms of solid surface tension. Colloids and Surfaces A: Physicochemical and Engineering Aspects, Vol.61, Issue 1, 2000, 31-48

[63] Lam C.N.C, Kim N, Hui D, Kwok D.Y, Hair M.L, Neumann A.W. The effect of liquid properties to contact angle hysteresis. Colloids and Surfaces A: Physicochemical and Engineering Aspects, Vol. 189, Issues 1-3, 2001, 265-278

[64] Kotov N.A. Layer-by-layer self-assembly: the contribution of hydrophobic interactions, Nanostructured Materials, Acta Metallurgica Inc., Vol.12, 1999, 789-796

[65] Warocquier-Cleront M.R, Legris C, Degrange M, Sigot-Luizard M.F. Correlation between substratum roughness and wettability, cell adhesion and cell migration. J. Biomed. Mater. Res., 36 (1), 1997, 99-108

[66] Andrade J, Gregonis D.E, Smith L.M. Polymer surface dynamics; surface and interfacial aspects of biomedical polymers, Vol.1, Joseph D. Andrade, Plenum Press, New York and London, 1983, 14-39

[67] Voegler .E. Structure and reactivity of water biomaterial surfaces, Advances in colloid and interface science. 1998

[68] Shelton R.M, Rasmussen A.C, Davies J.E. Protein adsorption at the interface between charged polymer substrata and migration osteoblasts, Biomaterials, 9, 1988, 24-29

[69] Janssen M.I,. Van Leeuwen M.B.M, Scholtmeijer K, van Kooten T.G, Dijkhuizen L, Wösten H.A.B. Coating with genetic engineered hydrophobin promotes growth of fibroblasts on a hydrophobic solid. Biomaterials, Vol.23, 2002, 4847-4854

[70] Hunter A, Archer C.W, Walker P.S, Blunn G.W. Attachment and proliferation of osteoblasts and fibroblasts on biomaterials for orthopedic use. Biomaterials, Vol.16, 4, 1995

[71] Rupp F, Scheideler L, G-Gerstorfer J. Effect of heterogenic surfaces on contact angle hysteresis: Dynamic contact angle analysis in material sciences, Chem. Eng. Technol. 25. 2002

[72] Shanahan M.E.R, Carre A, Moll S, Schultz J. Une nouvelle interprétation de l'hystérèse de mouillage des polymères. J. Chim. Phys. Chim. Biol.1996

[73] Nishioka G.M, Wesson S.P. A computer model for wetting hysteresis. 3. Wetting behavior of spatially encoded heterogeneous surfaces, Colloids and Surfaces, Vol.118, 1996, 247-256

[74] Orkoula M.G, Koutsoukos P.G, Robin M, Vizika O, Cuiec L. Wettability of CaCo3 surfaces, Colloids and surfaces. 1999

[75] Vold M.J, Vold R.D. Colloid and Interface Chemistry, Addison-Wesley, Reading, MA, Chapter 3, 198

[76] L. Mhamdi, C. Picart, C. Lagneau, A. Othmane, B. Grosgogeat, N. Jaffrezic-Renault and L. Ponsonnet. Study of the polyelectrolyte multilayer thin films properties and correlation with the behavior of the human gingival fibroblasts. Material sciences and engineering C 26, 2006, 273-281

Drug and Gene Delivery

Chapter 9

Nanoparticles Based on Chitosan Derivatives

Ylenia Zambito

Additional information is available at the end of the chapter

1. Introduction

A tremendous effort has been and is currently being devoted to the research in the field of pharmaceutical nanotechnology. Several peculiar properties of gelled polymeric nanosize (<1μm) particulate systems have been reported, among which the ability to encapsulate either small molecular weight or macromolecular active principles in mild conditions and protect them from degradation by the harsh pH conditions or enzymes they may encounter in the organism, promote transport of actives across mucosal barriers, undergo internalization by cells thereby carrying actives into them. Chitosan, a copolymer of glucosamine and N-acetylglucosamine, obtained by deacetylation of the naturally-occurring chitin, has been studied as a basic biomaterial for preparing pharmaceutical nanoparticles, because it is biodegradable and has a very low toxicity [1-5] besides an ability to promote transport of drugs, peptides and proteins across mucosal barriers [6-10]. The preparation procedures of chitosan nanoparticles, their characterization for drug encapsulation efficiency, physical and biopharmaceutical properties, and toxicity have been covered by recent reviews (11,12). Chitosan has been subjected to derivatization, taking advantage of the reactivity of the primary amino group in position 2, or the hydroxyl group in position 6 of its repeating unit, glucosamine. The derivatization changed the physicochemical, biopharmaceutical and biological properties of the parent chitosan and each derivative type lent itself to preparing nanoparticles with their own physical properties (size, shape, surface charge), drug encapsulation and release capability, biopharmaceutical and biological properties (mucoadhesivity, ability to promote drug transport across biological barriers, aptitude for internalization within cells, citotoxicity).

In the following sections the nanoparticles obtained from chitosan derivatives will be surveyed in respect to preparation procedures, interactions with cells and tissues, factors influencing biological properties, pharmaceutical applications.

2. Preparation procedures

2.1. Ionotropic gelation

Ionotropic gelation, that is by far the most used technique for preparation of nanoparticles from chitosan derivatives, was first reported in 1997 by Calvo et al. [13]. The basic concept is that a polycationic polymer in aqueous solution passes, in appropriate conditions, from sol to dispersed gel following electrostatic crosslinking with an adequate anionic substance. This technique has been used with several quaternized chitosans carrying fixed, pH-independent positive charges, the most known of which is N-trimethyl chitosan (TMC). Sodium tripoly-phosphate (TPP) has widely been employed as the ionotropic crosslinker [14-19].

The nanoparticles prepared by ionotropic gelation of quaternized chitosans with TPP were generally 200-300 nm in size, i.e., smaller than those obtained by the same method starting from plain chitosan which, by the way, showed lesser stability and tended to re-dissolve after some time from formation. The zeta potential was always positive, in the 10-20 mV range. The solution of the chitosan derivative into which the TPP solution was dripped would often contain a surfactant, usually Tween 80, to hinder nanoparticle aggregation and facilitate their re-dispersion after centrifugation. In fact, centrifugation was necessary to clear the particles of non-encapsulated drug.

The technique under discussion has also been used to prepare nanoparticles from thiolated derivatives of chitosan [20-23].

These polymers have shown mucoadhesive properties due to the ability of their thiol groups to form covalent disulfide bridges by reacting with the thiol residues present on the glyco-proteins of mucus. For this reason the nanoparticles derived from these chitosan derivatives were themselves endowed with mucoadhesivity. The thiolated nanoparticles formed by ionotropic gelation with TPP were stabilized via oxidation of thiols with H_2O_2 which formed interchain disulfide bonds. These would bestow gastroresistance on the particles, which would be particularly appropriate in case of oral administration of the nanoparticle formulation. However the presence of some non-oxidized thiols on the nanoparticle surface was needed to confer enhanced mucoadhesivity on such a surface. This goal was actually achieved by Bernkop-Schnurch et al. [21]. These authors also studied the crosslinker effect on nanoparticle size. Under similar preparation conditions, sizes in the 200-300 nm range were obtained with TPP as the crosslinker, whereas sizes beyond the micron resulted using Na_2SO_4.

2.2. Gelation from polyelectrolyte complex (PEC) formation

This method involved ionotropic gelation, just as described in the preceding section, only in the present case the crosslinker was a polyanionic polymer with charges opposite to those of the chitosan derivative, with which it formed a PEC. To this purpose N-carboxymethyl chitosan, poly(γ-glutamic acid), poly(aspartic acid) and hyaluronic acid were used as polyan-ions, while TMC and glycidyl trimethyl ammonium chitosan were the polycations [24-27]. In a case both the polyanion (hyaluronic acid) and the polycation (TMC) were thiolated and the nanoparticles were stabilized by the formation of interchain disulfide bonds [28].

2.3. Polymer-drug complexes

Some negatively charged active principles, such as insulin or gene drugs, when mixed with cationic chitosan derivatives in adequate proportions spontaneously formed nanoparticulate dispersions of insoluble complexes [29-34]. TMC nanoparticles obtained by ionotropic gelation with TPP in the presence of insulin were compared with nanoparticles obtained by PEC formation between TMC and insulin. In the latter instance higher encapsulation efficiency and zeta potential (positive), and smaller particle size were observed, which is particularly appropriate for particle internalization into cells. In addition, a higher stability in simulated intestinal fluid (pH 6.8) of the nanocomplex compared to the nanoparticles prepared with TPP resulted [31,32].

2.4. Self-assembly

Amphiphilic derivatives of chitosan in aqueous solution were found, at a critical aggregation concentration (CAC), to spontaneously arrange into nanoparticles of sizes in between 100-400 nm. Such derivatives were prepared by connecting hydrophobic structures to the chitosan or glycol chitosan backbone via the amino group of the chitosan repeating unit. Examples of the above amphiphilic derivatives are the following: glycol chitosan-5β-cholanic acid conjugate [35-40]; palmitoyl chitosan [41]; palmitoyl glycol chitosan [42]; oleoyl chitosan [43]. Other amphiphiles were prepared from chitosans bearing fixed positive charges, in the case of quaternary ammonium palmitoyl glycol chitosan [42], or negative fixed charges, as in the case of linoleic acid-modified O-carboxymethyl chitosan [44], or deoxycholic acid-modified N,O-carboxymethyl chitosan [45]. Usually, after suspending the polymer in an aqueous medium, probe sonication was applied to limit particle size. The formation of nanoparticles was monitored and the CAC determined fluorometrically, or through UV absorption spectra, or measuring the enthalpy change by a microcalorimeter [42,44,45].

The CAC for the hydrophobically modified chitosan derivatives is usually in the μM range, whereas the CMC of small-molecular weight surfactants is in the mM range. This is one of the most important characteristics of amphiphilic polymers, pointing to stability of the self-aggregates in dilute conditions, such as those the nanoparticles are supposed to encounter after administration to the organism. The CAC values of these polymers have been found to decrease with increasing hydrophobic content of derivatives [44]. In fact, the nanoparticles formed from these chitosan derivatives are characterized by a core-shell structure, i.e., a hydrophobic core in a hydrophilic shell. The drug incapsulation method was chosen on the basis of the hydrophilic or hydrophobic nature of the drug. With hydrophobic drugs the solution of polymer and drug in a water-miscible organic solvent was mixed with an aqueous medium and the organic solvent was cleared away by dialysis or evaporation [36,39,40]. Hydrophobic drugs having a fair water solubility and polar drugs have been loaded into nanoparticles via direct addition to the aqueous polymer dispersion [41,42,44,45]. The non-encapsulated drug has been separated by ultracentrifugation, filtration or dialysis.

3. Interactions with cells and tissues

3.1. Quaternized derivatives

Chitosan has been found to open the tight junctions connecting epithelial cells, through an interaction of its positively charged amino groups with negatively charged sites in the tight junctions, thereby promoting paracellular transepithelial absorption of drugs, peptides and proteins [10,46-57]. The major drawback of unmodified chitosan as an absorption promoter is its insolubility at physiological neutral pH. Therefore the primary amino groups of its repeating units have been quaternized to bestow fixed, pH-independent positive charges on the polymer, thus making it soluble and active as an absorption promoter at physiological pH. In fact, TMC was found to act as an enhancer of drug, peptide and protein permeability across intestinal, nasal, buccal, ocular epithelium [47, 58-66]. TMC was shown to promote not only paracellular but also transcellular drug absorption [66]. Other quaternized chitosan derivatives, namely, N-triethylchitosan (TEC) [68], N,N-dimethyl N-ethylchitosan (DMEC) [69] and N,N-diethyl N-methylchitosan (DEMC) [70] have been synthesized. Positively charged chitosan and its quaternized derivatives have also exhibited mucoadhesive properties, determined by ionic interactions with the negatively charged sialic acid residues of mucins at neutral or slightly alkaline pH [71].

Particles in the nanosize range have resulted from the interaction of quaternized chitosans with polyanions. Proteins or macromolecular drug models have been encapsulated in these nanoparticles. Ovalbumin (OVA) was encapsulated in nanoparticles, obtained by ionotropic gelation of TMC with TPP, and studied as a nasal delivery system for proteins [19]. No cytotoxicity of nanoparticles on Calu-3 cells, a model of human respiratory function, was evidenced, whereas a partially reversible cilio-inhibiting effect on the ciliary beat frequency of chiken trachea was observed. Confocal laser scanning microscopy (CLSM) of nasal epithelia and nasal associated lymphoid tissue (NALT), incubated with nanoparticles loaded with fluorescein-labelled albumin, showed the presence of fluorescent nanoparticles throughout the cytoplasm of these cells, indicating the transport of albumin-associated TMC/TPP nanoparticles across the nasal mucosa. These findings led the authors to point to these nanoparticles as a potential delivery system for transport of proteins through the nasal mucosa

Other authors studied similar TMC/TPP nanoparticles, loaded with fluorescein isothiocyanate dextran, molecular weight 4400 Da (FD4), as a model of macromolecular drugs [17]. In analogy with the free TMC, the TMC/TPP nanoparticles exhibited the property of opening the tight junctions between cells in the Caco-2 monolayer in vitro and the rat intestinal epithelium ex vivo, thus promoting the permeation of FD4 across the two epithelium models. The nanoparticles also shared, with the free TMC, the property of adhering to the intestinal mucosa. Using CLSM, Sandri et al. [17] showed internalization of their nanoparticles into Caco-2 cells and excised rat jejunum tissue.

Nanoparticles encapsulating fluorescein-labelled bovine serum albumin (BSA) were obtained by ionotropic gelation of alginate-modified TMC with TPP [16]. According to the authors the transport of alginate-modified TMC nanoparticles across the Caco-2 cell in vitro model of gastrointestinal (GI) epithelium was more efficient than that produced by non-modified TMC nanoparticles. However, alginate modification barely had any effect on the trans-epithelial electrical resistance or on paracellular protein transport. Then the hypothesis was made that alginate modification facilitated nanoparticle transport across the Caco-2 monolayer by the transcellular route (transcytosis) by virtue of a reduction of particle size to 100-200 nm (16). The supposedly permeated nanoparticles were assayed by measuring the fluorescence of fluorescein-labelled BSA, which was assumed to be completely associated with the particles. Similar nanoparticles as the above were loaded with urease, a vaccine protein against *Helicobacter pylori* infection. Immunization studies in mice showed that oral administration of urease-loaded TMC nanoparticles generated high titers of both IgG and S-IgA antibodies. The immunostimulating effect was caused by nanoparticle mucoadhesivity and transcytosis by M cells in gut associated lymphoid tissue [16].

OVA-loaded nanoparticles have been prepared from TMC using unmethylated CpG DNA as adjuvant and crosslinker, in place of TPP, for nasal vaccination in mice [15]. TMC/CpG/OVA showed similar physical properties as TMC/TPP/OVA in terms of particle size, zeta-potential and antigen release characteristics, but TMC/CpG/OVA induced a 10-fold higher IgG2a response than TMC/TPP/OVA, and a strong humoral and Th1 type cellular immune responses after nasal vaccination [15].

Nanoparticles derived from the polyelectrolytic complexation of TMC by the polyanionic mono-N-carboxymethyl chitosan (MCC), and loaded with fluorescein-labelled BSA were taken up into mouse Balb/c monocyte macrophages. Mice were nasally immunized with tetanus toxoid-loaded TMC/MCC complex nanoparticles. These were shown to induce both mucosal and systemic immune response [24].

Insulin was formulated into nanoparticles formed from quaternized chitosans such as TMC or DEMC via either ionotropic gelation with TPP, or polyelectrolyte complexation by the polyanionic insulin. The PEC method resulted in higher insulin loading efficiency and nanoparticle zeta-potential [31].

Similar nanoparticulate systems loaded with insulin were prepared from other quaternized chitosans, namely, N-triethyl chitosan (TEC) and N-dimethylethyl chitosan (DMEC), by the PEC method [30]. Insulin was transported ex vivo across the colon membrane of rats when it was formulated into nanoparticles made of quaternized derivatives, better than into those made of plain chitosan. In vivo colon absorption of insulin was enhanced by using insulin-loaded nanoparticles compared to free insulin. Insulin absorption from rat colon was evaluated by its hypoglycemic effect [30].

Poly(γ-glutamic acid) was used by Mi et al. [25] as the anionic polyelectrolyte complexing agent to prepare nanoparticles from TMC by the PEC method, for the oral delivery of insulin. According to the authors insulin was transported across the Caco-2 cell in vitro model of GI epithelium via the paracellular route. In fact, CLSM confirmed the opening of the tight junctions between cells caused by the nanoparticles. The authors propose a mechanism whereby the orally administered nanoparticles with mucoadhesive TMC on their surfaces may adhere and infiltrate into the intestinal mucus, mediate the opening of tight junctions between enterocytes, undergo disintegration, and release insulin, which would permeate through the paracellular pathway to the bloodstream. This hypothesis is contrasting with that, proposed by Chen et al. [16], of protein being carried by TMC/alginate/TPP nanoparticles across the Caco-2 monolayer by transcytosis.

TMC was modified with the specific ligand CSKSSDYQC peptide (CSK) to prepare ionotropically crosslinked TMC-CSK/TPP nanoparticles, loaded with fluorescein isothiocyanate (FITC)-labelled insulin, targeted to the mucus-producing goblet cells [45]. In transport studies across Caco-2/HT29-MTX co-cultured cell monolayer, simulating mucus-producing intestinal epithelium, the CSK modification showed enhanced drug transport ability, even if the target recognition was partially affected by mucus. In pharmacological and pharmacokinetic studies in diabetic rats, the orally administered CSK-modified nanoparticles produced a stronger hypoglycemic effect than the unmodified ones, prompting the authors to state that the former were sufficiently effective as goblet cell-targeting nanocarriers for oral delivery of insulin.

An oral delivery system for paclitaxel, a mitotic inhibitor used in cancer chemotherapy, was devised by encapsulating the drug in N-(2-hydroxy-3-trimethylammonium) propyl chitosan chloride (HTCC) nanoparticles prepared by the O/W/O double emulsion temperature-programmed solidification method [72]. CLSM studies suggested that the HTCC nanoparticles could be transported across Caco-2 monolayers via the opening of tight junctions between cells. Also the in vivo absorption of these nanoparticles by the small intestine of rats was shown. These transport properties of nanoparticles were ascribed to their positive surface charge, which was also considered responsible for an enhanced nanoparticle uptake by carcinoma cells. Biodistribution studies after oral administration in subcutaneous LLC tumor-bearing mice showed accumulation of paclitaxel-loaded HTCC nanoparticles in liver, spleen, lung, and kidney tissues, which was ascribed to the uptake of nanoparticles by the reticuloendothelial system, and in tumour tissue through the enhanced permeability and retention (EPR) effect. These results are particularly intriguing as they open the prospect of a targeted oral treatment of cancer by nanomedicine.

3.2. Thiolated derivatives

The thiol groups immobilized on these polymers are supposed to give exchange reactions with disulfide bonds within the mucus, or oxidation reactions with cysteine-rich subdomains of mucus glycoproteins [73, 74], both resulting in the formation of disulfide bonds between thiolated chitosan derivatives and the mucus, which improve the polymer mucoadhesivity. Nanoparticles prepared from this type of chitosan derivatives were supposed to be themselves mucoadhesive, and hence, apt to make nanocarriers for oral drug delivery. In fact, enhanced mucoadhesive properties of nanoparticles prepared by gelation of chitosan-N-acetyl cysteine conjugate (chitosan-NAC) with TPP, compared with unmodified chitosan nanoparticles, were found by Wang et al. [23]. Enhanced insulin in vivo absorption via nasal mucosa was found by these authors when insulin-loaded chitosan-NAC/TPP nanoparticles were administered intranasally to rats.

Another thiolated chitosan derivative, chitosan-4-thiobutylamidine (chitosan-TBA) was used by Bernkop-Schnürch et al. [22] to develop a mucoadhesive nanoparticulate delivery system.

Polymer	Gelling agent	Drug	Diameter (nm)	Zeta potential (mV)	Reference
TMC-CSK	TPP	insulin	200-350	3-10	[14]
HTCC	o/w/o double emulsion	paclitaxel	130	21	[72]
TMC	cisplatin-hyaluronate	cisplatin	450	45	[27]
TMC	TPP	OVA	300	20	[15]
TMC	MCC	tetanus toxoid, FITC-BSA	not reported	not reported	[24]
HTCC	poly(aspartic acid)	BSA	200-300	55	[26]
TMC	poly(γ-glutamic acid)	insulin	100	30	[25]
TEC, DMEC	insulin	insulin	200	25	[30]
TMC, DEMC	TPP, insulin	insulin	250	25	[31]
TMC	TPP	FITC-BSA	300	14	[16]
TMC	TPP	OVA	254-300	20-61	[19]
TMC	TPP	FD4	200	-	[17]

Table 1. Main characteristics of nanoparticles based on quaternized chitosans

The polymer was first crosslinked ionotropically by TPP, followed by stabilization of the resulting nanoparticles via formation of inter- and intrachain disulfide bonds by thiol oxidation with H_2O_2. Subsequently, TPP was removed by dialysis. The covalently crosslinked particles would not disintegrate in the acidic medium of the stomach. The adhesion to porcine intestinal mucosa was studied after incorporation of fluorescein diacetate into nanoparticles. The more thiol groups were oxidized, the lower was the nanoparticle mucoadhesivity, nevertheless, even when as much as 90% of all thiols were oxidized the mucoadhesivity of chitosan-TBA nano-particles was twice as high as that of unmodified chitosan nanoparticles.

Polymer	Gelling agent	Drug	Diameter (nm)	Zeta potential (mV)	Reference
chitosan-NAC	TPP	insulin	140-210	19-31	[23]
chitosan-TGA	DNA	DNA	75-120	2-20	[34]
chitosan-TBA	TPP	none	268	4-19	[22]
chitosan-TBA	TPP	none	240	5-11	[21]
thiolated TMC	thiolated HA	OVA	250-350	10-20	[28]
chitosan-TGA	none	pSEAP	212-113	4-8	[33]
glycol chitosan-TGA	TPP	calcitonin	230-330	21-27	[20]

Table 2. Main characteristics of nanoparticles based on thiolated chitosan derivatives

Glycol chitosan coupled with thioglycolic acid (TGA) was ionotropically gelled with TPP to yield nanoparticles, which showed a twofold increase in mucoadhesion to lung tissue after intra-tracheal administration to rats as compared to non-thiolated nanoparticles. Biocompatibility of nanoparticle formulations with lung tissue was demonstrated. Calcitonin-loaded glycol chitosan and glycol chitosan-TGA nanoparticles resulted in a pronounced hypocalcemic effect for at least 12 and 24 h and a bioavailability of 27 and 40%, respectively [20].

Verheul et al. [28] used the thiol groups of thiolated TMC to spontaneously form interchain disulfide crosslinks with the thiols of thiolated hyaluronic acid (HA), after ionic gelation. OVA-loaded stabilized TMC-S-S-HA nanoparticles demonstrated higher immunogenicity than not stabilized particles, indicated by higher IgG titers, in nasal and intradermal vaccination.

Besides showing enhanced mucoadhesivity and cell penetration properties, nanoparticles made of thiolated chitosans have appeared highly effective as gene delivery systems. Thiolated derivatives, prepared from 33-kDa chitosan by coupling with TGA, formed nanocomplexes with plasmid DNA encoding green fluorescent protein (GFP), that were able to bind and protect plasmid DNA from Dnase I digestion. Thiolated chitosan/DNA nanocomplexes induced higher GFP expression in HEK293, MDCK and Hep-2 cell lines than unmodified chitosan. Nanocomplexes of disulfide-crosslinked thiolated chitosan/DNA showed a sustained DNA release and continuous expression in cultured cells lasting up to 60 h post transfection. Intranasal administration of crosslinked thiolated chitosan/DNA nanocomplexes to mice yielded gene expression that lasted at least 14 days [34].

Nanoparticles containing the gene reporter pSEAP (recombinant Secreted Alkaline Phosphatase) were generated, based on a thiolated chitosan conjugate, chitosan-TGA, crosslinked by thiol oxidation with H_2O_2 to form disulfide crosslinks. Transfection of nanoparticles in Caco-2 cells led to increased protein expression compared to unmodified chitosan nanoparticles. Red blood cells lysis tests provided evidence for no cytotoxicity of nanoparticles. On the basis of their experimental results the authors stated that their crosslinked thiolated chitosan nanoparticles showed the potential for being used as a non-viral vector system for gene therapy [33].

3.3. Amphiphilic derivatives

Amphiphilic derivatives resulted when hydrophobic structures were attached to the hydrophilic chitosan backbone. In aqueous milieu these derivatives would self-assemble into nanoparticles to attain thermodynamic stability. Nanoparticles derived from the self-assembly of amphiphilic derivatives were often intended for cancer therapy. Glycol chitosan (hydrophilic)-cholanic acid (hydrophobic) conjugates self-assembled to form nanoparticles, the in vivo tissue distribution, time-dependent excretion and tumor accumulation of which were monitored in tumor-bearing mice by Park et al. [37]. The particles exhibited prolonged blood circulation time, decreased time-dependent excretion from the body, and increased tumor accumulation with increasing polymer molecular weight. The enhanced tumor targeting by nanoparticles made of high molecular weight glycol chitosan-cholanic acid was ascribed to a better in vivo stability, related to an improvement in blood circulation time [37].

Similar nanoparticles as the above, formed from glycol chitosan-cholanic acid conjugate, loaded with the anticancer drug camptothecin, exhibited significant antitumor effects and high tumor targeting ability towards MDA-MB231 human breast cancer xenografts subcutaneously implanted in nude mice. The significant antitumor efficacy of nanoparticles was ascribed to both their prolonged blood circulation and high accumulation in tumors through the EPR effect [39].

The cellular uptake mechanism and the intracellular fate of nanoparticles formed from glycol chitosan hydrophobically modified with cholanic acid have been reported [40]. These particles showed an enhanced distribution in the whole cells, compared to the parent hydrophilic glycol chitosan polymer. In vitro experiments with endocytic inhibitors suggested that the cellular uptake of these nanoparticles involved several distinct pathways, e.g., clathrin-mediated endocytosis, caveolae-mediated endocytosis, and macropinocytosis. Such a property, along with low toxicity and biocompatibility suggested these hydrophobically modified glycol chitosan nanoparticles as a versatile carrier for the intracellular delivery of therapeutic agents [40].

A further hydrophobically modified chitosan derivative from which self-assembled nanoparticles were obtained was oleoyl chitosan. The toxicity profile of the relevant nanoparticles, evaluated in vitro via hemolysis test and MTT assay, was within acceptable limits. When loaded with the antitumor drug doxorubicin, oleoyl chitosan nanoparticles exhibited inhibitory rates on different human cancer cells (A549, Bel-7402, HeLa, and SGC-7901) significantly higher than the drug solution [43].

Folic acid was conjugated with O-carboxymethyl chitosan via the bifunctional 2,2'-(ethylenedioxy)-bis-(ethylamine) to obtain an amphiphilic chitosan derivative that would self-assemble into nanoparticles. Folate-mediated endocytosis significantly enhanced the cellular targeting of nanoparticles, thus facilitating apoptosis of cancer cells (HeLa, B16F1). Doxorubicin could be loaded into the nanoparticles. It was observed that survival in cancer cells treated with doxorubicin-loaded nanoparticles was lower than that of normal cells in similar concentrations [75].

The ability of nanoparticles prepared by self-assembly of chitosan amphiphiles to promote oral absorption of hydrophobic and hydrophilic drugs in rats was recently investigated by Siew et al. [42], using quaternary ammonium palmitoyl glycol chitosan as the basic material. The nanoparticles were found to enhance the oral absorption (Cmax) of griseofulvin and cyclosporine A (hydrophobic) and, to a lesser extent, of ranitidine (hydrophilic). Hydrophobic drug absorption was facilitated by the nanomedicine by: (a) increasing the drug dissolution rate, (b) adhering to and penetrating the mucus layer, thus allowing intimate contact between the drug and the GI epithelium absorptive cells, and (c) enhancing transcellular drug transport. As for the absorption of the hydrophilic ranitidine, despite an 80% increase of Cmax there was no appreciable opening of tight junctions by the nanoparticles. No uptake of this type of nanoparticles by epithelial cells is reported [42].

Polymer	Drug	Diameter (nm)	Zeta potential (mV)	Reference
quaternary ammonium palmitoyl glycol chitosan	griseofulvin cyclosporin A ranitidine .	100-500	not report-ed	[42]
glycol chitosan-5β-cholanic acid	none	300-400	10	[40]
O-carboxymethyl chitosan-2,2¹,(ethylene dioxy)-bis-(ethylamine)-folic acid	doxorubicin	150-200	10-20	[75]
glycol chitosan-5β-cholanic acid	none	230-310	10-11	[37]
glycol chitosan-5β-cholanic acid	camptothe-cin	250-350	not report-ed	[39]

Polymer	Drug	Diameter (nm)	Zeta potential (mV)	Reference
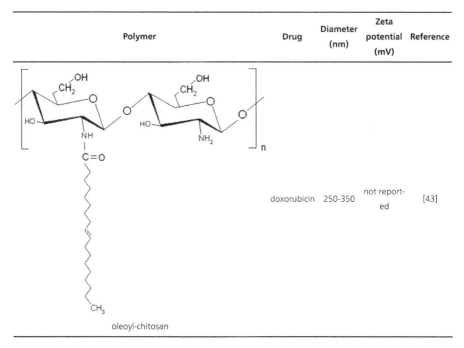 oleoyl-chitosan	doxorubicin	250-350	not report-ed	[43]

Table 3. Main characteristics of nanoparticles based on anphiphilic chitosans

4. Concluding remarks

Three families of chitosan derivatives have been synthesized and used to prepare nanoparticles for pharmaceutical application, namely, polycations obtained by introducing quaternary ammonium groups on the polymer backbone; thiolated derivatives, and amphiphilic deriva-tives obtained by attaching hydrophobic structures to the chitosan or glycol chitosan backbone. The nanoparticles prepared from the quaternary ammonium-chitosan derivatives, especially via the PEC formation method, have shown improved stability and physical properties (smaller size, higher zeta potential) compared to nanoparticles from unmodified chitosan. The thiolated derivatives offered the opportunity to stabilize the nanoparticles by covalent crosslinks formed from interchain thiol oxidation to disulfide, which made the particles stable in the GI environment. The critical aggregation concentration of the amphiphilic hydrophob-ically modified chitosan derivatives is usually very low, which implies stability of the self aggregates in dilute conditions, such as those encountered by the nanoparticles in the organ-ism. The nanoparticulate systems prepared from chitosan derivatives have generally shown acceptable cytotoxicity. In accord with the known behavior of particles of a size smaller than 500 nm, they have shown endocytic uptake by cells. Smaller particles with higher zeta potential have shown more aptitude to endocytosis. Ionotropically crosslinked TMC nanoparticles are a potential vehicle for transport of proteins across mucosal epithelia, as they have been found to open the tight junctions between epithelial cells. Indeed, nanoparticles based on quaternized chitosan are a promising vehicle for the oral administration of insulin, especially if the chitosan derivative is conjugated with the specific ligand CSKSSDYQC peptide. Also interesting is the nanosystem based on the quaternary ammonium-chitosan conjugate HTCC, which was orally absorbed by the rat small intestine and subsequently accumulated in carcinoma tissue by the EPR effect. These results are particularly intriguing as they open the prospect of a targeted oral treatment of cancer by nanomedicine. Nanoparticles prepared from thiolated chitosan derivatives have shown a particular mucoadhesivity implying a suitability for making nanocarriers for transmucosal protein delivery. Also this type of nanoparticles have appeared highly effective as gene delivery systems and have shown the potential for being used as a non-viral vector system for gene therapy. Nanoparticles derived from the self-assembly of amphiphilic chitosan derivatives were often intended for cancer therapy. Glycol chitosan hydrophobically modified with cholanic acid yielded nanoparticles with comparatively high in vivo stability, responsible for a prolonged blood circulation time, which led to high accumulation in tumors through the EPR effect. This type of nanoparticles can be taken up by cells through distinct pathways, which points to this system as a versatile carrier for the intracellular delivery of therapeutic agents. Folic acid, conjugated with *O*-carboxymethyl chitosan to obtain doxorubicin-loaded self-assembled nanoparticles, could mediate particle endocytosis by cancer cells with consequent cell apoptosis. In conclusion the present survey has endorsed the concept that chitosan derivatization can lead to new basic materials for nanosystems with unique pharmaceutical performances.

Abbreviations

BSA Bovine serum albumin

CAC Critical aggregation concentration

CLSM Confocal laser scanning microscopy

CSK CSKSSDYQC peptide

DEMC *N,N*-diethyl *N*-methyl chitosan

DMEC *N,N*-dimethyl *N*-ethyl chitosan

EPR Enhanced permeability and retention effect

FD4 Fluorescein isothiocyanate dextran, molecular weight 4400 Da

FITC Fluorescein isothiocyanate

GFP Green fluorescent protein

GI Gastrointestinal

HA Hyaluronic acid

HTCC *N*-(2-hydroxy-3-trimethylammonium) propyl chitosan chloride

LLC Lewis lung carcinoma

MCC Mono-*N*-carboxymethyl chitosan

NAC *N*-acetyl cysteine

NALT Nasal associated lymphoid tissue

OVA Ovalbumin

PEC Polyelectrolyte complex

pSEAP Recombinant secreted alkaline phosphatase

TBA Thiobutyl amidine

TEC *N*-triethyl chitosan

TGA Thioglycolic acid

TMC N-trimethyl chitosan

TPP Sodium tripolyphosphate

Author details

Ylenia Zambito[*]

Address all correspondence to: zambito@farm.unipi.it

Dipartimento di Farmacia, Università di Pisa, Italy

References

[1] Lee, K. Y, Ha, W. S, & Park, W. H. Blood compatibility and biodegradability of parti‐ ally N-acylated chitosan derivatives. Biomaterials (1995). , 16-1211.

[2] Muzzarelli RAAHuman enzymatic activities related to the therapeutic administra‐ tion of chitin derivative. Cellular and Molecular Life Scince (1997). , 53-131.

[3] Onishi, H, & Machida, Y. Biodegradation and distribution of water-soluble chitosan in mice. Biomaterials (1999). , 20-175.

[4] Chandy, T, & Sharma, C. P. Chitosan as a biomaterial. Artificial Cells and Artificial Organs (1990). , 18-1.

[5] Aspeden, T. J, Mason, J. D, Jones, N. S, Lowe, J, Skaugrud, O, & Illum, L. Chitosan solutions on in vitro and in vivo mucociliary transport rates inhuman turbinates and volunteers. Journal of Pharmaceutical Sciences (1997). , 86-509.

[6] Illum, L, Farraj, N. F, & Davis, S. S. Chitosan as a novel nasal delivery system for peptide drugs. Pharmaceutical Research (1994). , 11-1186.

[7] Illum, L, Jabbal-gill, I, Hinchcliffe, M, Fisher, A. N, & Davis, S. S. Chitosan as a novel nasal delivery system for vaccines. Advanced Drug Delivery Reviews (2001). , 51-81.

[8] Junginger, H. E, & Verhoef, J. C. Macromolecules as safe penetration enhancers for hydrophilic drugs-a fiction? Pharmaceutical Sciences Technology Today (1998). , 1-370.

[9] Borchard, G. Lueßen HL, de Boer AG, Verhoef JC, Lehr CM, Junginger HE. The potential of mucoadhesive polymers in enhancing intestinal peptide drug absorption: III. Effects of chitosan glutamate and carbomer on epithelial tight junctions in vitro. Journal of Controlled Release (1996). , 39-131.

[10] Di Colo GZambito Y, Burgalassi S, Nardini I, Saettone MF. Effect of chitosan and of N-carboximethylchitosan on intraocular penetration of topically applied ofloxacin. International Journal of Pharmaceutics (2004). , 273-37.

[11] Peniche, H, & Peniche, C. Chitosan nanoparticles: a contribution to nanomedicine. Polymer Intenational (2001). , 60-883.

[12] Wang, J. J, Zeng, Z. W, Xiao, R. Z, Xie, T, Zhou, G. L, Zhan, X. R, & Wang, S. L. Recent advances of chitosan nanoparticles as drug carriers. International Journal of Nanomedicine (2011). , 6-765.

[13] Calvo, P, Remunan-lopez, C, Vila-jato, J. L, & Alonso, M. J. Novel hydrophilic chitosan-polyethylene oxide nanoparticles as protein carriers Journal of Polymer Scince (1997). , 63-125.

[14] Jin, Y, Song, Y, Zhu, X, Zhou, D, Chen, C, Zhang, Z, & Huang, Y. Goblet cell-targeting nanoparticles for oral insulin delivery and the influence of mucus on insulin transport. Biomaterials (2012). , 33-1573.

[15] Slütter, B, & Jiskoot, W. Dual role of CpG as immune modulator and physical cross-linker in ovalbumin loaded N-trimethyl chitosan (TMC) nanoparticles for nasal vaccination. Journal of Controlled Release (2010). , 148-117.

[16] Chen, F, Zhang, Z. R, Yuan, F, Qin, X, Wang, M, & Huang, Y. In vitro and in vivo study of N-trimethyl chitosan nanoparticles for oral protein delivery. Intenational Journal of Pharmaceutics (2008). , 349-226.

[17] Sandri, G, Bonferoni, M. C, Rossi, S, Ferrari, F, Gibin, S, & Zambito, Y. Di Colo G, Caramella C. Nanoparticles based on N-trimethylchitosan: Evaluation of absorption

properties using in vitro (Caco-2 cells) and ex vivo (excised rat jejunum) models. European Journal of Pharmaceutics and Biopharmaceutics (2007). , 65-68.

[18] Dehousse, V, Garbacki, N, Jaspart, S, Castagne, D, Piel, G, Colige, A, & Evrard, B. Comparison of chitosan/siRNA and trimethylchitosan/siRNA complexes behaviour in vitro. International Journal of Biological Macromolecules (2010). , 46-342.

[19] Amidi, M, Romeijn, S. G, Borchard, G, Junginger, H. E, Hennink, W. E, & Jiskoot, W. Preparation and characterization of protein-loaded N-trimethyl chitosan nanoparticles as nasal delivery system. Journal of Controlled Release (2006). , 111-107.

[20] Makhlof, A, Werle, M, Tozuka, Y, & Takeuchi, H. Nanoparticles of glycol chitosan and its thiolated derivative significantly improved the pulmonary delivery of calcitonin. International Journal of Pharmaceutics (2010). , 397-92.

[21] Bernkop-schnurch, A, Heinrich, A, & Greimel, A. Development of a novel method for the preparation of submicron particles based on thiolated chitosan. European Journal of Pharmaceutics and Biopharmaceutics (2006). , 63-166.

[22] Bernkop-schnürch, A, Weithaler, A, Albrecht, K, & Greimel, A. Thiomers: Preparation and in vitro evaluation of a mucoadhesive nanoparticulate drug delivery system. Intenational Journal of Pharmaceutics (2006). , 317-76.

[23] Wang, X, Zheng, C, Wu, Z, Teng, D, Zhang, X, Wang, Z, & Li, C. Chitosan-NAC nanoparticles as a vehicle for nasal absorption enhancement of insulin. Journal of Biomedical Materials Research Part B: Applied Biomaterials (2009). , 88-150.

[24] Sayin, B, Somavarapu, S, Li, X. W, Sesardic, D, Senel, S, & Alpar, O. H. TMC-MCC (N-trimethyl chitosan-mono-N-carboxymethyl chitosan) nanocomplexes for mucosal delivery of vaccines. European Journal of Pharmaceutical Sciences (2009). , 38-362.

[25] Mi, F. L, Wu, Y. Y, Lin, Y. H, Sonaje, K, Ho, Y. C, Chen, C. T, Juang, J. H, & Sung, H. W. Oral delivery of peptide drugs using nanoparticles self-assembled by poly(γ-glutamic acid) and a chitosan derivative functionalized by trimethylation. Bioconjugate Chemistry (2008). , 19-1248.

[26] Wang, T. W, Xu, Q, Wu, Y, Zeng, A. J, Li, M, & Gao, X. Quaternized chitosan (QCS/ poly (aspartic acid) nanoparticles as a protein drug-delivery system. Carbohydrate Research (2009). , 344-908.

[27] Cafaggi, S, Russo, E, Stefani, R, Parodi, B, Caviglioli, G, Sillo, G, Bisio, A, Aiello, C, & Viale, M. Preparation, characterisation and preliminary antitumour activity evaluation of a novel nanoparticulate system basedon a cisplatin-hyaluronate complex and N-trimethyl chitosan. Invest New Drugs (2011). , 29-443.

[28] Verheul, R. J, Slütter, B, Bal, S. M, Bouwstra, J. A, Jiskoot, W, & Hennink, W. E. Covalently stabilized trimethyl chitosan-hyaluronic acid nanoparticles for nasal and intradermal vaccination. Journal of Controlled Release (2011). , 156-46.

[29] Bayat, A, Larijani, B, Ahmadian, S, Junginger, H. E, & Rafiee-tehrani, M. Preparation and characterization of insulin nanoparticles using chitosan and its quaternized derivatives. Nanomedicine (2008). , 4-115.

[30] Bayat, A, Dorkoosh, F. A, Dehpour, A. R, Moezi, L, Larijani, B, Junginger, H. E, & Rafiee-tehrani, M. Nanoparticles of quaternized chitosan derivatives as a carrier for colon delivery of insulin: Ex vivo and in vivo studies. Intenational Journal of Pharmaceutics (2008). , 356-259.

[31] Sadeghi AMMDorkoosh FA, Avadi MR, Saadat P, Rafiee-Tehrani M, Junginger HE. Preparation, characterization and antibacterial activities of chitosan, N-trimethyl chitosan (TMC) and N-diethylmethyl chitosan (DEMC) nanoparticles loaded with insulin using both the ionotropic gelation and polyelectrolyte complexation methods. International Journal of Parmaceutics (2008). , 355-299.

[32] Jintapattanakit, A, Junyaprasert, V. B, Mao, S, Sitterberg, J, Bakowsky, U, & Kissel, T. Peroral delivery of insulin using chitosan derivatives: A comparative study of polyelectrolyte nanocomplexes and nanoparticles. International Journal of Pharmaceutics (2009). , 342-240.

[33] Martien, R, Loretz, B, Sandbichler, A. M, & Bernkop-schnürch, A. Thiolated chitosan nanoparticles: transfection study in the Caco-2 differentiated cell culture. Nanotechnology (2008).

[34] Lee, D, Zhang, W, Shirley, S. A, Kong, X, Hellermann, G. R, Lockey, R. F, & Mohapatra, S. S. Thiolated chitosan/DNA nanocomplexes exhibit enhanced and sustained gene delivery. Pharmaceutical Research (2007). , 24-157.

[35] Yoo, H. S, Lee, J. E, Chung, H, Kwon, I. C, & Jeong, S. Y. Self-assembled nanoparticles nanoparticles containing hydrophobically modified glycol chitosan for gene delivery. Journal of Controlled Release (2005). , 103-235.

[36] Kim, J. H, Kim, Y. S, Kim, S, Park, J. H, Kim, K, Choi, K, Chung, H, Jeong, S. Y, Park, R. W, Kim, I. S, & Kown, I. C. Hydrophobically modified glycol chitosan nanoparticles as carriers for paclitaxel. Journal of Controlled Release (2006). , 111-228.

[37] Park, K, Kim, J. H, Nam, Y. S, Lee, S, Nam, H. Y, Kim, K, Park, J. H, Kim, I. S, Choi, K, Kim, S. Y, & Kwon, I. C. Effect of polymer molecular weight on the tumor targeting characteristics of self-assembled glycol chitosan nanoparticles. Journal of Controlled Release (2007). , 122-305.

[38] Kim, J. H, Kim, Y. S, Park, K, Kang, E, Lee, S, Nam, H. Y, Kim, K, Park, J. H, Chi, D. Y, Park, R. W, Kim, I. S, Choi, K, & Kwon, I. C. Self-assembled glycol chitosan nanoparticles for the sustained and prolonged delivery of antiangiogenic small peptide drugs in cancer terapy. Biomaterials (2008). , 29-1920.

[39] Min, K. H, Park, K, Kim, Y. S, Bae, S. M, Lee, S, Jo, H. G, Park, R. W, Kim, I. S, Jeong, S. Y, Kim, K, & Kwon, I. C. Hydrophobically modified glycol chitosan nanoparticles-

encapsulated camptothecin enhance the drug stability and tumor targeting in cancer therapy. Journal of Controled Release (2008). , 127-208.

[40] Nam, H. Y, Kwon, S. M, Chung, H, Lee, S. Y, Kwon, S. H, Jeon, H, Kim, Y, Park, J. H, Kim, J, Her, S, Oh, Y. K, Kwon, I. C, Kim, K, & Jeong, S. Y. Cellular uptake mechanism and intracellular fate of hydrophobically modified glycol chitosan nanoparticles. Journal of Controlled Release (2009). , 135-259.

[41] Chen, K. J, Chiu, Y. L, Chen, Y. M, Ho, Y. C, & Sung, H. W. Intracellularly monitoring/imaging the release of doxorubicin from pH-responsive nanoparticles using Förster resonance energy transfer. Biomaterial (2011). , 32-2586.

[42] Siew, A, Le, H, Thiovolet, M, Gellert, P, Schatzlein, A, & Uchegbu, I. Enhanced oral absorption of hydrophobic and hydrophilic drugs using quaternary ammonium palmitoyl glycol chitosan nanoparticles. Molecular Pharmaceutics (2012). , 9-14.

[43] Zhang, J, Chen, X. G, Li, Y. Y, & Liu, C. S. Self-assembled nanoparticles based on hydrophobically modified chitosan as carriers for doxorubicin. Nanomedicine: Nanotechnology, Biology, and Medicine (2007). , 3-258.

[44] Tan, Y. L, & Liu, C. G. Self-aggregated nanoparticles from linoleic acid modified carboxymethyl chitosan: Synthesis, characterization and application in vitro. Colloids and Surfaces B: Biointerface (2009). , 69-178.

[45] Jin, Y, Song, Y, Zhu, X, Zhou, D, Chen, C, Zhang, Z, & Huang, Y. Goblet cell-targeting nanoparticles for oral insulin delivery and the influence of mucus on insulin transport. Biomaterials (2012). , 33-1573.

[46] Schipper, N. G, Varum, K. M, & Artusson, P. Chitosans as absorption enhancers for poorly absorbable drugs. 1. Influence of molecular weight and degree of acetylation on drug transport across human intestinal epithelial (Caco-2) cells. Pharmaceutical Research (1996). , 13-1686.

[47] Kotzé, A. F, & De Leeuw, B. J. Lueßen HL, de Boer AG, Verhoef JC, Junginger HE. Chitosans for enhanced delivery of therapeutic peptides across intestinal epithelia: in vitro evaluation in Caco-2 cell monolayers. Internationa Journal of Pharmaceutics (1997). , 159-243.

[48] Lueßen HLRentel CO, Kotzé AF, Lehr CM, de Boer AG, Verhoef JC, Junginger HE. Mucoadhesive polymers in peroral peptide drug delivery. IV. Polycarbophil and chitosan are potent enhancers of peptide transport across intestinal mucosae in vitro. Journal of Controlled Release (1997). , 45-15.

[49] Lueßen HLde Leew BJ, Langmeÿer MWE, de Boer AG, Verhoef JC, Junginger HE. Mucoadhesive polymers in peroral peptide drug delivery. VI. Carbomer and chitosan improve the intestinal absorption of the peptide drug buserelin in vivo. Pharmaceutical Research (1996). , 13-1668.

[50] Illum, L, Farraj, N. F, & Davis, J. J. Chitosan as novel nasal delivery system for peptide drugs. Pharmaceutical Research (1994). , 11-1186.

[51] Tengamnuay, P, Sahamethapat, A, Sailasuta, A, & Mitra, A. K. Chitosans as nasal absorption enhancers of peptides: comparison between free amine chitosans and soluble salts. International Journal of Pharmaceutics (2000). , 197-53.

[52] Sinswat, P, & Tengamnuay, P. Enhancing effect of chitosan on nasal absorption of salmon calcitonin in rats: comparison with hydroxypropyl- and dimethyl-β-cyclodextrins. Intenational Journal of Pharm (2003). , 257-15.

[53] Hinchcliffe, M, Jabbal-gill, I, & Smith, A. Effect of chitosan on the intranasal absorption of salmon calcitonin in sheep. Journal of Pharmacy and Pharmacology (2005). , 57-681.

[54] Zhang, Y. J, Ma, C. H, Lu, W. L, Zhang, X, Wang, X. L, Sun, J. N, & Zhang, Q. Permeation-enhancing effects of chitosan formulations on recombinant hirudin-2 by nasal delivery in vitro and in vivo. Acta Pharmacologica Sinica (2005). , 26-1402.

[55] Di Colo GBurgalassi S, Chetoni P, Fiaschi MP, Zambito Y, Saettone MF. Gel-forming erodible inserts for ocular controlled delivery of ofloxacin. International Journal of Pharmaceutics (2001). , 215-101.

[56] Schipper NGMVarum KM, Stemberg P, Ocklind G, Lennernäs H. Chitosans as absorption enhancers of poorly absorbable drugs. 3: Influence of mucus on absorption enhancement. European Journal of Pharmaceutical Sciences (1999). , 8-335.

[57] Florea, B. I, Thanou, M, Junginger, H. E, & Borchard, G. Enhancement of bronchial octreotide absorption by chitosan and N-trimethyl chitosan shows linear in vitro/in vivo correlation. Journal of Controlled Release (2006). , 110-353.

[58] Sandri, G, Rossi, S, Bonferoni, M. C, Ferrari, F, & Zambito, Y. Di Colo G, Caramella C. Buccal penetration enhancement properties of N-trimethyl chitosan: Influence of quaternization degree on absorption of a high molecular weight molecule. International Journal of Pharmaceutics (2005). , 297-146.

[59] Kotzé, A. F, Luessen, H. L, De Leew, B. J, De Boer, B. G, & Verhoef, J. C. Junginger HE. N-trimethyl chitosan chloride as a potential absorption enhancer across mucosal surfaces: in vitro evaluation in intestinal epithelial cells (Caco-2). Pharmaceutical Research (1997). , 14-1197.

[60] Kotzé, A. F, Thanou, M, Luessen, H. L, De Boer, B. G, Verhoef, J. C, & Junginger, H. E. Enhancement of paracellular drug transport with highly quaternized N-trimethyl chitosan chloride in neutral environments: in vitro evaluation in intestinal epithelial cells (Caco-2). Journal of Pharmaceutical Sciences (1999). , 88-253.

[61] Thanou, M, Verhoef, J. C, Marbach, P, & Junginger, H. E. Intestinal absorption of octreotide: N-trimethyl chitosan chloride (TMC) ameliorates the permeability and ab-

sorption properties of the somatostatin analogue in vitro and in vivo. Journal of Pharmaceutical Sciences (2000). , 89-951.

[62] Thanou, M, Florea, B. I, Langemeyer, M. W, & Verhoef, J. C. Junginger HE. N-trimethyl chitosan chloride (TMC) improves the intestinal permeation of the peptide drug buserelin in vitro (Caco-2 cells) and in vivo (rats), Pharmaceutical Research (2000). , 17-27.

[63] Hamman, J. H, Stander, M, & Kotzé, A. F. Effect of the degree of quaternization of N-trimethyl chitosan chloride on absorption enhancement: in vivo evaluation in rat nasal epithelia. Internationa Journal of Pharmaceutics (2002). , 232-235.

[64] Florea, B. I, Thanou, M, Junginger, H. E, & Borchard, G. Enhancement of bronchial octreotide absorption by chitosan and N-trimethyl chitosan shows linear in vitro/in vivo correlation. Journal of Controlled Release (2006). , 110-353.

[65] Di Colo G,Burgalassi S,. Zambito Y, Monti D, Chetoni P. Effects of different N-trimethyl chitosans on in vitro/in vivo ofloxacin transcorneal permeation. Journal of Pharmaceutical Sciences (2004). , 93-2851.

[66] Zambito, Y, & Zaino, C. Di Colo G. Effects of N-trimethylchitosan on transcellular and paracellular transcorneal drug transport. European Journal of Pharmaceutics and Biopharmaceutics (2006). , 64-16.

[67] Hamman, J. H, & Schultz, C. M. Kotzé AF. N-trimethyl chitosan chloride: optimum degree of quaternization for drug absorption enhancement across epithelial cells. Drug Development and Industrial Pharmacy (2003). , 29-161.

[68] Avadi, M. R, Zohuriaan-mehr, M. J, Younessi, P, Amini, M, Rafiee-tehrani, M, & Shafiee, A. Optimized synthesis and characterization of N-triethylchitosan. Journal of Bioactive Compatible Polymers (2003). , 18-469.

[69] Bayat, A. Sadeghi AMM, Avadi MR, Amini M, Rafiee-Tehrani M, Shafiee A, Majlesi R, Junginger HE. Synthesis of N,N-dimethyl N-ethylchitosan as a carrier for oral delivery of peptide drugs. Journal of Bioactive Compatible Polymers (2006). , 21-433.

[70] Avadi, M. R. Sadeghi AMM, Tahzibi A, Bayati KH, Pouladzadeh M, Zohuriaan-mehr MJ, Rafiee-Tehrani M. Diethylmethyl chitosan as antimicrobial agent: synthesis, characterization and antibacterial effects. European Journal of Polymers (2004). , 40-1355.

[71] Ludwig, A. The use of mucoadhesive polymers in ocular drug delivery. Advanced Drug Delivery Review (2005). , 57-1595.

[72] Lv, P. P, Wei, W, Yue, H, Yang, T. Y, Wang, L. Y, & Ma, G. H. Porous quaternized chitosan nanoparticles containing paclitaxel nanocrystals improved therapeutic efficacy in non-small-cell lung cancer after oral administration. Biomacromolecules (2011). , 12-4230.

[73]　Kast, C. E, & Bernkop-schnurch, A. Thiolated polymers- thiomers: development and in vitro evaluation of chitosan-thioglycolic acid conjugates. Biomaterials (2001). , 22-2345.

[74]　Leitner, V. M, Walker, G. F, & Bernkop- Schnürch, A. Thiolated polymers: evidence for the formation of disulfide bonds with mucus glycoproteins. European Journal of Pharmaceutics and Biopharmaceutics (2003). , 56-207.

[75]　Sahu, S, Mallick, S. K, Santra, S, Maiti, T. K, Ghosh, S. K, & Pramanik, P. In vitro evaluation of folic acid modified carboxymethyl chitosan nanoparticles loaded with doxorubicin for targeted delivery. Journal of Materials Science: Materials in Medicine (2010). , 21-1587.

pH-Sensitive Nanocrystals of Carbonate Apatite- a Powerful and Versatile Tool for Efficient Delivery of Genetic Materials to Mammalian Cells

Ezharul Hoque Chowdhury

Additional information is available at the end of the chapter

1. Introduction

Delivery of a functional DNA to mammalian cells is an attractive approach for genetic manipulation of the cells in biomedical research as well as in gene therapy for treating critical human diseases. Following delivery to the cytoplasm, a foreign gene enters the nucleus and is transcribed to the corresponding mRNA, which is subsequently transported to the cytoplasm for translation into a specific protein. However, a gene-silencing element, such as an antisense onligonucleotide or a small interfering RNA blocks the transcription of a target mRNA. Thus, nucleic acid delivery has been an essential tool either to turn on or off the expression of a particular gene in basic research laboratories.

Intensive research in the last three decades led to the development of a number of viral and non-viral vectors. However, an ideal vector in terms of safety and efficacy is still lacking. Synthetic non-viral vectors, such as cationic polymers, lipids and peptides, are relatively safe, but extremely inefficient. On the other hand, viral systems are by far the most effective means of DNA delivery to mammalian cells, but some major limitations including toxicity, immunogenicity, restricted targeting of specific cell types, restricted DNA carrying capacity, production and packaging problems, recombination and high cost, limit their successful applications in basic research and clinical medicine. The effectiveness of a viral particle is the result of its highly evolved and specialized structure basically composed of a protein coat surrounding a nucleic acid core. Such a highly organized structure can prevent viral particles from unwanted interactions with serum components, while promoting subsequent internalization by cells, escape from endosomes, and release of genetic material from the particle either before or after entering the nucleus. Development of a non-viral approach having the beneficial virus-like properties and lacking the disadvantageous aspects would emerge as the most attractive one for implementation in research laboratories and gene therapy.

A major barrier to the non-viral delivery is low uptake of DNA across the plasma membrane of a cell owing to the inappropriate and ineffective interactions of the DNA delivery vehicle with the cell membrane. Negatively charged DNA molecules are usually condensed with cationic reagents to allow formation of the complexes carrying net positive charges. The resulting complexes can interact electrostatically with anionic heparan sulfate proteoglycans (syndecans) on cell surface and reach the cytoplasmic side in the form of endosomes through endocytosis [1]. The extremely low pH and enzymes within the late endosomes usually bring about degradation of entrapped DNA and associated complexes. Finally, DNA that survives both endocytic processing and cytoplasmic nucleases must dissociate from the condensed complexes either before or after nuclear translocation through nuclear pore or during cell division.

Many therapeutic applications demand a vehicle with capability of delivering transgene(s) to a selective cell type in order to increase the expression efficacy and alleviate any side effect. A common strategy in non-viral case involves attachment of a targeting moiety onto a polycation (lipid or polymer) backbone which finally condenses the DNA through ionic interactions. Targeting moiety can enable the resulting DNA carrier to bind to a receptor, lectin, antigen or cell-adhesion molecule on plasma membrane prior to internalization via endocytosis or phagocytosis. Polylysine, the first backbone used for gene delivery has been conjugated to a diverse set of cell-specific ligands, such as asialoorosomucoid [2], transferrin [3], epidermal growth factor (EGF) [4], mannose [5], fibroblast growth factor (FGF) [6] and antibodies [7] for targeting, respectively, hepatocytes via asialoglycoprotein receptors, transferrin receptor-positive cells, EGF receptor-carrying cells, macrophages through membrane lectins, FGF receptor-bearing cells and lymphocytes via surface-bound antigens. In the similar fashions, polymers like polyethylenimine and liposomes have been coupled to other cell surface receptor-specific ligands in addition to those described above, such as integrin-binding peptide conjugated onto PEI to target integrins on cell surfaces [8] and vitamin folate conjugated onto liposomes through a polyethylene spacer to target folate receptor-bearing cells [9].

Cell adhesion molecules (integrin, syndecan, cadherin, selectin) which are a diverse group of cell surface proteins mediating interactions between cells, and between cells and the extracellular matrix, are valuable targets for precise gene delivery to haematopoietic cells, airway epithelial cells, tumor cells and vascular endothelial cells using synthetically designed non-viral vectors [10].

Recently, we have reported on the development of a safe, efficient nano-carrier system of carbonate apatite which can assist both intracellular delivery and release of DNA leading to very high level of trans-gene expression in cancer and primary cells [11-13]. We have also revealed a new approach of organic-inorganic hybrid carrier devised by complexing fibronectin and E-cadherin-Fc chimera electrostatically with nano-particles of carbonate apatite [14, 15]. Specific recognition to cell surface integrin and E-cadherin molecules through double ligand-coated nano-particles, resulted in synergistic acceleration of transgene delivery and consequential expression into embryonic stem cells. Instead of simultaneous mixing of DNA and cell-adhesive molecules in particle-preparation medium and subsequent incubation, stepwise addition and incubation of DNA and the protein molecules, results in improved DNA loading and decreased particle diameter with ability of recognizing stem cell surface for more efficient transgene delivery. Activation of PKC which might up-regulate both integrin and E-cadherin, enhances transgene expression in mouse embryonic carcinoma cells.

2. Materials and Methods

2.1. Reagents

Plasmids, pGL3 (Promega) containing a luciferase gene under SV40 promoter and pEGFP-N2 (CLONTECH Laboratories, Inc.) having a green fluorescence protein gene under CMV promoter were propagated in the bacterial strain XL-1 Blue and purified by QIAGEN plasmid kits. Lipofectamine 2000 and DMEM were purchased from Invitrogen and Gibco BRL, respectively. Fibronectin was bought from Sigma and expression as well as purification of E-cad-Fc fusion proteins was done according to the previously described report [16].

2.2. Cell Culture

HeLa cells were cultured in 75-cm^2 flasks in Dulbecco's modified Eagle's medium (DMEM, Gibco BRL) supplemented with 10% fetal bovine serum (FBS), 50 μg penicillin ml^{-1}, 50μg streptomycin ml^{-1} and 100μg neomycin ml^{-1} at 37°C in a humidified 5% CO_2-containing atmosphere. F9, a mouse teratocarcinoma stem cell line and EB3, a mouse embryonic stem cell line were cultured in gelatin-coated 25-cm^2 flasks. F9 cells were maintained in Dulbecco's modified Eagle's medium (DMEM, Gibco BRL) supplemented with 10% fetal bovine serum (FBS) at 37°C in a humidified 5% CO_2-containing atmosphere. Feeder-free murine ES cells were maintained in KNOCKOUT-DMEM (Invitrogen), supplemented with 1 mM L-glutamine, 1% nonessential amino acids (Invitrogen), 0.1 mM β-mercaptoethanol (Sigma Chemical), 10% FBS and 1,000 units/ml leukemia inhibitory factor (LIF) (Chemicon). All media contained 50 μg/ml penicillin, 50 μg/ml streptomycin, and 100 μg/ml neomycin.

2.3. Transfection of cells

Cells from the exponentially growth phase were seeded at 50,000 cells per well into 24-well plates the day before transfection. 3 to 6 μl of 1 M CaCl$_2$ was mixed with 2 μg of plasmid DNA in 1 ml of fresh serum-free HCO3$^-$ - buffered (pH 7.5) medium (DMEM) and incubated for 30 min at 37°c for complete generation of DNA/carbonate apatite particles. For generation of ECM protein-embedded carbonate apatite particles, fibronectin and E-cad-Fc proteins were added either alone or together to a final concentration of 5 μg/ml, to Ca^{2+} and DNA-containing DMEM followed by incubation at 37°c for 30 min. Medium with generated ECM protein-associated or non-associated, DNA-containing particles was added with 10% FBS to the rinsed cells. After 4 hr incubation, the medium was replaced with serum supplemented medium and the cells were cultured for 1 day. Luciferase gene expression was monitored by using a commercial kit (Promega) and photon counting (TD-20/20 Luminometer, USA). Each transfection experiment was done in triplicate and transfection efficiency was expressed as mean light units per mg of cell protein. For lipofectamine-mediated transfection, protocol provided by Invitrogen was followed in a 24-well plate. Cells were incubated with DNA/lipofactamine complexes in serum-free media for 4 hr and like above, grown for 1 day after replacement with fresh serum media.

For transfection with calcium phosphate-DNA co-precipitation, briefly, 12 µg of plasmid DNA was added to 300 µl of a solution containing 250 mM $CaCl_2$. This solution was added to 300µl of a 2×HBS (50 mM Hepes, 140 mM NaCl, 1.5 mM $Na_2HPO_4.2H_2O$, pH 7.05) and mixed rapidly by gentle pipetting twice. The DNA/CaPi mixture was incubated at room temperature for the period of time indicated. After addition of 100 µl of the incubated mixture drop-wise to 1 ml serum supplemented media of each well, cells were incubated for 4 hr and like above, after replacement with fresh serum media, grown for 1 day.

2.4. MTT assay

HeLa cells were transfected and cultured for 1 day as described above. 30 µl of MTT solution (5mg/ml) was added to each well and incubated for 4 hrs. 0.5 ml of DMSO was added after removal of media. After dissolving crystals and incubating for 5 min at 37^0C, absorbance was measured in a microplate reader at 570 nm with a reference wavelength of 630 nm.

2.5. Chemical analysis

Following generation of carbonate apatite as described above, using 6 mM Ca^{2+} and no DNA, precipitated particles were lyophilized after centrifugation and washing with distilled deionized water. Other apatite particles generated as described above, were also similarly lyphilized. Calcium and phosphorus contents were determined using SPS 1500 VR Atomic Absorption Spectrophotometer. Carbon and fluorine were estimated by CHNS-932 (Leco, USA) and SX-elements micro analyser, YS-10 (Yanaco, Japan), respectively.

2.6. Infrared spectroscopy

Fourier transform-infrared spectroscopy of apatite particles prepared as described above, was performed using FT/IR-230, JASCO. The samples were ground in a mortar and approximately 1 mg was thoroughly mixed with 300 mg of ground spectroscopic grade KBr. Transparent pellets were prepared in a KBr die with an applied load of 8000 kg, under a vacuum of 0.5 torr.

2.7. X-ray diffraction

The x-ray diffraction powder reflections of the particles prepared as described above, were recorded using M18XHF-SRA diffractometer system.

2.8. Particle size measurements

For visualization by a scanning electron microscope (SEM), a drop of DNA-carbonate apatite suspension prepared according to the instructions in transfection protocol, was added to a carbon-coated SEM stage and dried, followed by observation by a high resolution SEM (S-800, Hitachi, Japan). Dynamic light scattering (DLS) measurement for particle suspension was carried out with a Super-dynamic Light Scattering Spectrophotometer, 'Photal' (Otsuka Electronics) at 75 mW Ar laser.

2.9. Confocal laser scanning microscopy

pGL3 vector was labeled with PI at a PI/DNA ratio of 1:1 and particles generated with this labeled plasmid (described in transfection protocol), were incubated with HeLa cells for 6 hours. Acidic compartments were labeled with 5μM LysoSensor, according to the instructions provided by Molecular Probes, and membrane-bound precipitates were removed by 5 mM EDTA in PBS before observation by LEICA TCS-NT.

2.10. SDS-PAGE and Western blotting

Following generation of carbonate apatite as described above using 3 mM Ca^{2+} and required amount of fibronectin or E-cad-Fc chimera and no DNA and centrifugation at 15000 rpm for 5 min at 4^0C, precipitated particles were washed with water with several centrifugation steps to remove unbound proteins and dissolved with 50 mM EDTA in PBS for subsequent analysis by 7.5% SDS-PAGE in reducing condition. In order to see particle-bound fibronectin, after SDS-PAGE, the gel was stained with Coumassie blue, washed and dried. For detection of particle-associated E-cad-Fc, proteins after being run by SDS-PAGE were transferred to PVDF membrane (Immobilon, Millipore) and 80 mA current was applied for 90 min to complete transfer of the proteins. The PVDF membrane was washed with PBS (-)-containing 0.1% Tween 20 and then blocked for 1 hr at room temperature by "Blocking One" (Nacalai Tesque, Japan). The membrane was incubated with horseradish peroxidase (HRP)-conjugated anti-mouse IgG for 1 hr and washed with PBS-T three to four times to completely remove non-specific interactions. Enhanced chemiluminescence system (Amersham Bioscience) was used for visualization.

2.11. DNA labelling, fluorescence microscopy and flow cytometry

Plasmid DNA was labelled non-covalently with propidium iodide (PI) using 1:1 weight ratio of DNA to PI in the particle preparation medium. Labelled DNA inside the cells was observed by a fluorescence microscope (Olympus-IX71), following 4 hr incubation of differentially formulated particle suspensions with F9 cells and removing extracellularly bound particles by 5 mM EDTA in PBS. For flow cytometric analysis using FACS Calibur (Becton, Dickinson and Company), 1 day after transfection with pEGFP plasmid DNA, F9 cells were collected in a sorter buffer following treatment with trypsin-EDTA and repeated centrifugation and washing of the resulting cell pellet with PBS (-) (2 times).

3. Results and Discussion

3.1. Generation of carbonate apatite particles

Addition of only 3 mM Ca^{2+} to the HCO_3^- - buffered cell culture medium (DMEM or William E, pH 7.5) and incubation at 37^0C for 30 min, resulted in microscopically visible particles. Generation of these particles only in HCO_3^--, but not in Hepes-buffered media or solution (pH 7.5) containing the same amount of exogenous Ca^{2+} and phosphate (0.9 mM), indicates the possible involvement of carbonate along with phosphate and Ca^{2+} in particle formation. Elemental analysis proved the existence of C (3%), P (17%) and Ca^{2+} (32%) and FT-IR spectra (Fig. 1a) identified carbonate, as evident from the peaks between 1410 and 1540 cm^{-1} and at approximately 880 cm^{-1}, along with phosphate in the particles, as shown by the peaks at 1000-1100 cm^{-1} and 550-650 cm^{-1}. X-ray diffraction patterns (Fig. 1b) indicated less crystalline nature, represented by broad diffraction peaks of the particles, compared to that of hydrox-yaptite (Fig. 1c) – an intrinsic property of carbonate apatite [12].

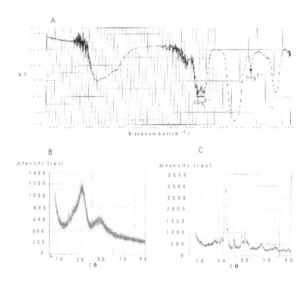

Figure 1. Infrared spectra of generated carbonate apatite (A) and X-ray diffraction patterns of carbonate apatite (B) and hydroxyapatite (C).

3.2. Influences of pH and temperature on generation of effective particles of carbonate apatite

We have investigated a long range of pH (7.0 to 7.9) of the HCO_3^- –buffered medium as well as incubation temperatures (25 °C to 65 °C) in order to make particles by exogenously added Ca^{2+} and subsequently transfect HeLa cells using the generated particles. Interestingly, the optimal Ca^{2+} concentrations required for generation of effective number of DNA/carbonate apatite particles leading to the high transfection efficiency, were inversely related to the pHs of the media (Fig. 2-a) and the incubation temperatures (Fig. 2-b). Thus, while 4 mM Ca^{2+} was sufficient to induce particle formation at pH 7.4 by incubating the Ca^{2+}-supplemented buffered medium for 30 min at 37 °C, only 1 mM^{2+} was enough to stimulate particle genera-tion to the similar level at pH 7.9. Like pH, incubation temperatures have also profound and sensitive effects on particle formulation and subsequent trans-gene delivery. Thus, at the incubation temperature of 37 °C, 3 mM Ca^{2+} was able to induce the proper "supersaturation" whereas at 65 °C, only 1 mM Ca^{2+} could stimulate "supersaturation" development to a similar extent – a prior need for generation of the particles. The decline below the high efficiency level of transfection was due to the formation of too few particles (microscopically observed) since increase in pH or temperature contributed to the development of "supersaturation" by increasing the ionization of phosphate and carbonate in the solution. The new system of particle synthesis is, therefore, very flexible since it allows us to make particles at a wide range of pH and temperatures. The analysis also indicates that induction of "supersaturation" as required for particle formation, can be delicately controlled by manipulating the parameters.

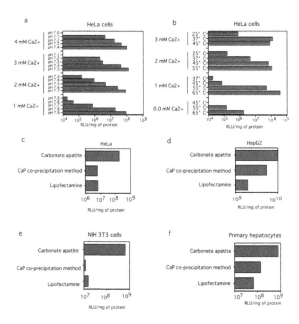

Figure 2. Regulation of trans-gene delivery and expression facilitated by carbonate apatite particles. Regulation of trans-gene expression by the nanoparticles of carbonate apatite generated at a wide range of pH and temperature. DNA/carbonate apatite particles were generated by addition of 1 to 4 mM Ca^{2+} and 2 µg plasmid DNA to 1 ml HCO_3^- (40 mM)-buffered DMEM medium with a pH range from 7.0 to 7.9, followed by incubation for 30 min either at 37 °C (a) or at 25 °C to 65 °C (b). Transfection of HeLa cells, HepG2, NIH3T3 and primary hepatocytes was performed in the same manner as mentioned in 'Materials and methods' section.

3.3. Tranfection efficiency and cell viability assessment

To evaluate the role of carbonate apatite as a powerful carrier of genetic material, we compared transfection efficiency of different techniques including two frequently used ones-CaP co-precipitation method and lipofection. In HeLa cell, for example, luciferase expression level for carbonate apatite-mediated transfection was over 25-fold higher than for lipofection and CaP co-precipitation method (Fig. 2c). Nano gram level of DNA was even sufficient for efficient transgene expression (Fig. 2c). Transfection efficiency was also significantly high in HepG2 (Fig. 2d), NIH 3T3 cells (Fig. 2e) and mouse primary hepato-cytes (Fig. 2f). We performed MTT assay in HeLa cells (not shown here) to clarify that high transfection efficiency was accompanied by high viability of the cells [12].

3.4. Estimation of particle sizes and cellular uptake of particle-associated plasmid DNA

To explore why carbonate apatite is so efficient as a vector for gene delivery, we investigat-ed two basic properties of carbonate apatite [12]. Carbonate, when present in the apatite structure, limits the size of the growing apatite crystals and increases the dissolution rate [12]. We carried out scanning electron microscopic observation of generated carbonate apa-tite (Fig. 3A) which revealed reduced growth of the crystals, most of which had diameters of 50 to 300 nm. We verified this size limiting effect of carbonate by observing cellular uptake of the PI (propidium iodide)-labeled plasmid DNA adsorbed to the apatites, since large par-ticles are phagocytosed less efficiently than small ones [12]. DNA was carried into the cells by carbonate apatite (Fig. 3B-c) at least 10 times more efficiently than hydroxyapatite, gener-ated by 1 min incubation (Fig. 3B-d). Longer period (30 min) incubation resulted in large hy-droxyapatite particles [12], showing significantly reduced transfection efficiency [12] (Fig. 2A) due to extremely low cellular uptake of DNA [12]. Our findings, therefore, clearly sug-gest that carbonate apatite is superior over hydroxyapatite for its intrinsic property of pre-venting crystal growth, leading to high efficiency cellular uptake of DNA.

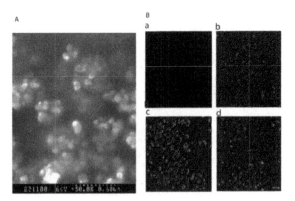

Figure 3. A, scanning electron microscopy, showing limited growth of generated carbonate apatite cryatals. Scale bar, 600 nm. B, cellular uptake of PI-labeled plasmid DNA associated with carbonate apatite and hydroxyapatite. a, no up-take of DNA (control), since endocytosis was blocked by energy depletion (50 mM 2-deoxy glucose and 1 mM Na-azide). DNA/carbonate apatite particles were prepared in 1 ml serum-free media (described in legend to Fig. 3) using 6 mM Ca^{2+} and 2 µg DNA. 40 ng (b) and 200 ng (c) of DNA in 20 µl and 100 µl of 1ml suspension respectively, were allowed for cellular uptake for 4 hr. d, 2 µg of DNA adsorbed to hydroxyapatite (described in experimental protocol) was allowed for uptake for the same period of time. Bar indicates 50 µM.

3.5. Endosomal escape of plasmid DNA carried by nanoparticles

To evaluate the role of endosomal escape of DNA in transgene expression, following endocytosis of PI-labeled plasmid DNA, we labeled endosomes with LysoSensor (a fluorescence probe for endosomes). Following 6 hr of DNA uptake by cells, a significant portion of DNA (red colour) appeared to be released from endosomes (green colour) after colocalization of plasmid DNA with endosomes (Fig. 4).

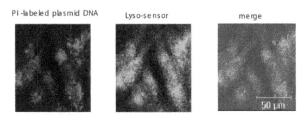

Figure 4. Endosomal escape of endocytosed PI–labeled DNA, as evident after colocalization with a fluorescence probe (Lyso-Sensor) for endosomes.

3.6. Relationship of endosomal pH and crystalline properties of particles affecting transfection

Treatment with bafilomycin A1, a specific inhibitor of v-ATPase (a proton pump for acidification of endocytic vesicles) resulted in drastic reduction of transfection efficiency in HeLa cells (Fig. 5A), which indicated that acidic environment might be necessary for solubilization of carbonate apatite to release DNA from the apatite. To establish this notion, we generated fluoridated carbonate apatite to see the effect of solubility of the particles on transfection efficiency, since incorporation of fluoride reduces the solubility of the apatite [12]. Surprisingly, transfection efficiency was reduced gradually to a significant extent (100 fold) with increasing fluoride level in carbonate apatite (Fig. 5B).

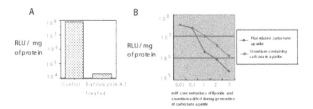

Figure 5. A, Effect of bafilomycin A1 (an inhibitor of v-ATPase) on transfection. HeLa cells were incubated with DNA/ carbonate apatite particles and 200 nM bafilomycin A1 for 6 hr. After washing with 5 mM EDTA in PBS, cells were grown for 1 day and luciferase expression was detected. B, Changes in luciferase expression for increasing concentrations of F- (0.01 to 3 mM) and strontium (0.01 to 3 mM) added during generation of DNA/carbonate apatite particles.

To establish a relationship between transfection efficiency and dissolution rates of the apatites, turbidity (320 nm) measurement was done as an indicator of their solubilization, following an acid load in solution of generated apatites. Carbonate apatite generated in presence of increasing concentrations of NaF, showed gradual decrease in dissolution rates, as evident from changes in turbidity, following adjustment of pH from 7.5 to 7.0 with 1 N HCl (Fig. 6 A, B), which is consistent with gradually reduced transfection efficiency of fluoridated carbonate apatites (Fig. 5 B). With decreasing pH from 7.0 to 6.8, carbonate apatite was completely solubilized within 1 min, whereas fluoridated carbonate apatite was partially dissolved (Fig. 6 B).

To examine whether dissolution rates of apatites are correlated with their degree of crystallization, we studied x-ray diffraction of the apatites (Fig. 7), which clearly indicates that apatite with higher degree of crystallization, had lower solubility (Fig. 6A). In other words, apatites with higher crystallinity (Fig. 7) showed lower transfection efficiency (Fig. 5 B). The gradual increase in crystallinity owing to increased level of incorporated fluoride in carbonate apatite (Fig. 7) resulted in gradual decrease in transfection efficiency (Fig. 5B).

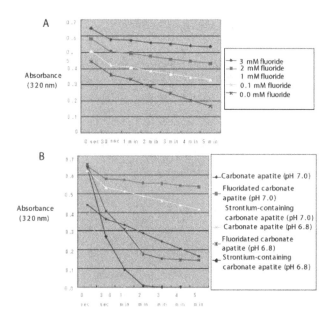

Figure 6. A, Dissolution rates (at pH 7.0) of fluoridated carbonate apatites prepared by addition of 0-3 mM F during generation of carbonate apatite at pH 7.5 (described in experimental protocol), were studied by turbidity measurement at 320 nm of apatite suspensions just after being adjusted to the pH 7.0 with 1 N HCl. B, Dissolution rates of carbonate apatite, fluoridated carbonate apatite and strontium-containing carbonate apatite at pHs of 7.0 and 6.8.

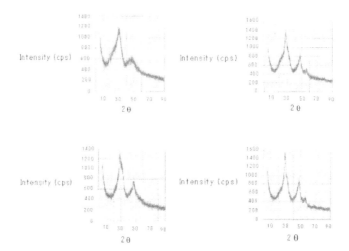

Figure 7. X-ray diffraction patterns of carbonate apatite (A) and fluoridated carbonate apatites, containing 0.65% (B), 1.43% (C) and 2.5% (D). Carbonate apatite was generated by addition of 6 mM Ca^{2+} and fluoridated carbonate apatites by addition of 1 mM (B), 2 mM (C) and 3 mM (D) NaF along with 6 mM Ca^{2+} to HCO_3^- -buffered medium (pH7.5), followed by incubation at 37°C

To establish that decreased transfection efficiency was only due to decreased solubility of fluoridated carbonate apatite, but not by any other fluoride-mediated effects, we examined the effects of strontium which, when incorporated into carbonate apatite, is known to improve the crystallinity and reduce the solubility of the apatite, but to a lesser extent than fluoride [12]. As expected, addition of strontium chloride during preparation of carbonate apatite reduced its dissolution rate but to a level less than that observed for fluoride (Fig 6B). Moreover, transfection efficiency was gradually decreased with increasing concentrations of strontium chloride during generation of DNA/carbonate apatite particles (Fig. 5B). Taken together, our findings suggest that intracellular release of DNA through dissolution of apatite should play a major role in carbonate apatite-mediated transfection.

3.7. Immobilization of cell-adhesive molecules on nano-particle surface

Since embryonic stem cells produce substantial amount of fibronectin-specific integrins as well as E-cadherin as transmembrane proteins [17], we hypothesized that if the nano-particles of carbonate apatite could be complexed with fibronectin and E-cadherin, either individually or together, they might recognize in the immobilized state the corresponding receptors on cell surface in order to facilitate quick internalization of the composite particles across the plasma membrane through endocytosis. These nano-apatite particles possess anion- and cation-binding domains which enable them to bind to both acidic and basic amino acids of protein molecules [18, 19]. On the other hand, fibronectin as well as E-cadherin are rich in acidic amino acid residues [19, 20] which make them excellent candidates for possible binding with the apatite particles. We have examined whether these "cell adhesive molecules" could, in deed, bind to the particles, by SDS-PAGE and Western blot analysis, following generation of apatite-protein composites and decomplexation through EDTA-mediated particle dissolution. Whereas binding affinity of the particles for fibronectin was relatively lower requiring higher amount of initially added fibronectin as observed by SDS-PAGE, almost all E-cad-Fc was found to be associated with the particles as verified by Western blot analysis (Fig 8). Very high affinity for E-cadherin could be interpreted by the previous report that E-cadhein has many exposed acidic residues in several loop structures responsible for binding divalent cation Ca^{2+} [20].

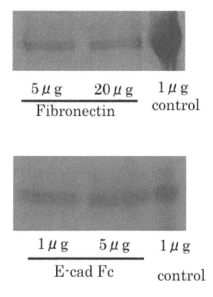

Figure 8. Analysis of the binding of cell-adhesive proteins to nano-particles. Particles were prepared by addition of 3 µl of 1 M $CaCl_2$ and 5 to 20 µg of fibronectin or 1 to 5 µg of E-cad-Fc to 1 ml bicarbonate-buffered DMEM and incubation for 30 min at 37°C. Generated particles were centrifuged at 15000 rpm for 5 min and washed 2 times with H_2O to remove the unbound proteins, followed by EDTA treatment to dissolve the particles. SDS-PAGE and Western blot analysis were performed in order to see, respectively, particle-associated fibronectin (A) or E-cad-Fc (B).

3.8. Enhanced cellular uptake of DNA by immobilized cell-adhesive molecules

In order to explore whether apatite particles functionalized with fibronectin and E-cad-Fc can facilitate enhanced delivery of apatite-associated plasmid DNA across the plasma membrane, we examined cellular uptake of the DNA labeled with propidium iodide (PI) [19], following 4 hr incubation of F9 cells with various particle formulations. As shown in Fig. 9, while with only apatite particles, delivery of PI-labeled DNA into the cells was extremely low, complexation of the particles with either fibronectin or E-cad-Fc resulted in significantly improved DNA delivery, suggesting that immobilized fibonectin or E-cad-Fc retained their functionalities in order to recognize specific cell surface integrin or E-cadherin, respectively for enabling subsequent internalization of the whole particle composite through endocytosis [19, 21]. Moreover, the apatite particles when complexed with both fibronectin and E-cad-Fc, demonstrated more pronounced DNA delivering activity compared to the particles embedded with either fibronectin or E-cad-Fc, indicating a synergistic effect of the multifunctional particles on endocytosis through simultaneous recognition of extracellular domains of specific integrin as well as E-cadherin molecules.

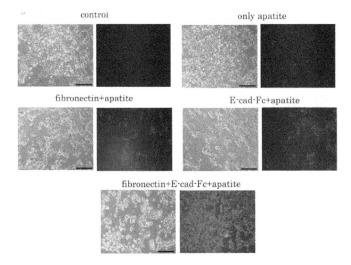

Figure 9. Effects of particle-immobilized proteins on cellular internalization of plasmid DNA. Particles were prepared by addition of 3 μl of 1 M CaCl₂, 2 μg of PI-labelled plasmid DNA and 5 μg of fibronectin and/or 5 μg of E-cad-Fc to 1 ml bicarbonate-buffered DMEM and incubation for 30 min at 37°C. F9 cells were incubated with the generated particles for 4 hr, washed with 5 mM EDTA in PBS and visualized by a fluorescence microscope (scale bar, 50 μm).

3.9. Quantitation and validation of trans-gene expression facilitated by cell-adhesive molecules

Since expression of a trans-gene is the result of overcoming a number of barriers including entry into the cells, release from the particle and endosomes and finally nuclear translocation [17, 18], we have investigated whether improved DNA delivery as a result of integrin- and E-cadherin-mediated endocytosis of composite particles (Fig. 9) contributed to the similar extent to final protein expression. Quantitative luciferase expression analysis indicated that particles complexed with fibronectin or E-cad-Fc promoted trans-gene expression with a value which was almost 20 times higher than that achieved for the particles only (Fig 10). A prior optimization study demonstrated that 1 to 5 µg/ml of fibronectin as well as E-cad-Fc conferred the best transfection efficiency and was, therefore, maintained for all subsequent experiments. Finally, synergistic activity of fibronectin and E-cad-Fc which caused huge cellular uptake of DNA (Fig. 9), further accelerated gene expression efficiency with a value almost 3 times higher than that observed for commercially available lipofectamine (Fig. 10). With increasing the total amount of initially added DNA up to 4 µg, a further increase in trasfection efficiency was observed (data not shown here) possibly due to the higher loading of DNA into the crystals with the consequence of more DNA getting inside the cells. The high level of expression could directly be observed by fluorescence microscopy which demonstrated many GFP-expressing F9 cells (Fig. 11). Fluorescence Activated Cell Sorting (FACS) analysis demonstrated that almost 60% cells were GFP-positive following transfection with the particles carrying, in addition to pEGFP plasmid DNA, both fibronectin and E-cad-Fc (Fig 11). MTT assay was performed in F9 cells to clarify that high transfection efficiency was not accompanied by significant toxicity of the cells (data not shown here). In order to establish that such organic-inorganic hybrid particles promote trans-gene delivery and expression through specific interactions with cell-surface molecules (integrin or E-cadherin), we added increasingly high amounts of free fibronectin to the preformed particle suspension carrying both fibronectin and E-cadherin and incubated with the cells for the same period of time (4 hr) as followed in usual transfection procedure. Transfection efficiency decreased as the concentration of free fibronectin increased from 5 to 100µg/ml, indicating the involvement of specific interactions between immobilized fibronectin and the corresponding specific integrin receptors (Fig 12). At a sufficiently high concentration (300 µg/ml), free fibronectin drastically reduced luciferase expression suggesting that high amount of fibronectin molecules not only saturate their specific integrins and block binding of immobilized fibronectin needed for particle internalization, but also shield cell-surface E-cadherin and prevent specific binding of particle surface-embedded E-cad-Fc chimera leading to very low cellular uptake of particle-associated DNA and diminished luciferase expression. Since embryonic stem cells are the final target for genetic modification in regenerative medicine, we applied the new transfection approach to mouse embryonic stem cells. As shown in Fig. 13, only apatite particles were extremely inefficient in transfecting the cells, whereas fibronectin-bound particles to some extent promoted GFP expression and fibronectin and E-cad-Fc-bound particles to a significant extent accelerated trans-gene expression, thus proposing that the synergistic effect is a universal way of accelerating trans-gene delivery and expression using inorganic nano-particle-associated cell recognizable proteins. Quantitative luciferase expression in embryonic stem cells indicated that particles complexed with fibronectin and E-cad-Fc individually, promoted trans-gene expression with efficiency approximately 9 and 7 times higher, respectively, than that achieved with the particles only (Fig. 14). However, when the particles were associated with both fibronectin and E-cadherin-Fc, a synergistic effect resulted in remarkable level of transgene expression leading to almost 40 and 28 times higher efficiency than that obtained by apatite particles and widely used lipofectamine 2000 system [14].

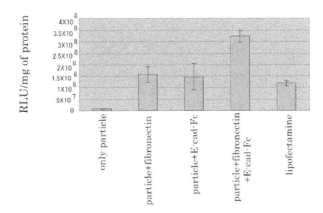

Figure 10. Comparison of luciferase expression for differentially formulated particles. Particles were prepared by addition of 3 µl of 1 M CaCl$_2$, 2 µg of luciferase plasmid DNA and 5 µg of either fibronectin, E-cad-Fc or both to 1 ml bicarbonate-buffered DMEM and incubation for 30 min at 37°C. F9 cells were incubated with the generated particles for 4 hr and after replacement of particle-containing media with fresh media, further incubated for 1 day in order to quantitate luciferase expression. Transfection efficiency was normalized after estimation of total proteins in cell lysate.

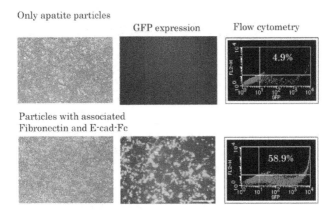

Figure 11. Comparison of GFP expression between only particles and fibronectin/E-cad-Fc-embedded-particles. Particles were prepared by addition of 3 µl of 1 M CaCl$_2$, 2 µg of pEGFP plasmid DNA and 5 µg of fibronectin and 5 µg of E-cad-Fc to 1 ml bicarbonate-buffered DMEM and incubation for 30 min at 37°C. F9 cells were incubated with the generated particles for 4 hr and after replacement of particle-containing media with fresh media, further incubated for 1 day in order to both observe and quantitate GFP expression by fluorescence microscopy and flow cytometry, respectively (scale bar, 50 µm).

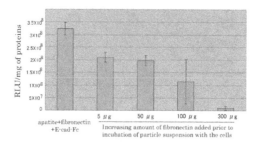

Figure 12. Blocking of integrin-mediated trans-gene delivery by excess free fibronectin. Particles were prepared by addition of 3 μl of 1 M CaCl₂, 2 μg of luciferase plasmid DNA and 5 μg of fibronectin and 5 μg of E-cad-Fc to 1 ml bicarbonate-buffered DMEM and incubation for 30 min at 37°C. F9 cells were incubated with the generated particles in presence or absence of increasingly high concentrations of free fibronectin for 4 hr and after replacement of particle-containing media with fresh media, further incubated for 1 day in order to quantitate luciferase expression. Transfection efficiency was normalized after estimation of total proteins in cell lysate.

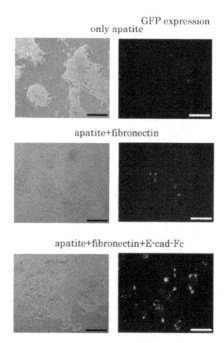

Figure 13. Enhancement of GFP expression in mouse embryonic stem cells with fibronectin/E-cad-Fc-embedded-particles. Particles were prepared by addition of 3 μl of 1 M CaCl₂, 2 μg of pEGFP plasmid DNA and 5 μg of fibronectin and 5 μg of E-cad-Fc to 1 ml bicarbonate-buffered DMEM and incubation for 30 min at 37°C. Embryonic stem cells were incubated with the generated particles for 4 hr and after replacement of particle-containing media with fresh media, further incubated for 1 day in order to see GFP expression by a fluorescence microscope (scale bar, 50 μm).

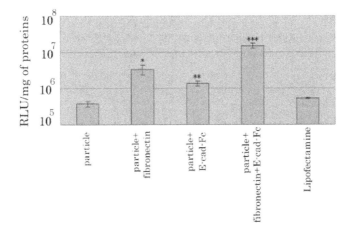

Figure 14. Comparison of luciferase expression for differentially formulated apatite particles and liposomes. Particles were prepared by addition of 3 μl of 1 M $CaCl_2$, 2 μg of luciferase plasmid DNA and 2 μg of either fibronectin, E-cad-Fc or both to 1 ml bicarbonate-buffered DMEM and incubation for 30 min at 37°C. Embryonic stem cells were incubated with the generated particles for 4 hr and after replacement of particle-containing media with fresh media, further incubated for 1 day in order to quantitate luciferase expression. Transfection efficiency was normalized after estimation of total proteins in cell lysate. Transfection by lipofectamine was performed according to the instructions provided by Invitrogen.

3.10. DNA binding with differentially formulated cell adhesive protein-embedded particles

Since direct mixing of DNA and cell-adhesive proteins in Ca^{2+} and PO_4^{3-}-containing medium prior to induction of particle formation by incubation at 37°C for 30 min, could interfere with maximum DNA loading due to the competitive binding of the proteins to the growing crystals, we investigated DNA binding efficiency by first adding DNA to the particle-preparation medium prior to time-dependent addition of the proteins [22]. As shown in Fig. 15, in the direct mixing process (control), DNA binding is much higher for E-cadherin-Fc compared to fibronectin, indicating that E-cadherin-Fc facilitates DNA loading probably by accelerating particle growth because turbidity of particle suspension was higher for E-cadherin-Fc than for fibronectin (not shown). It is worth mentioning that only particles have also higher affinity towards DNA (almost 40%) that the particles associated with fibronectin which showed lower turbidity than the particles (mentioned before), suggesting again that particle growth has a significant role in the observed DNA binding efficiency. When cell adhesive proteins were added after 5, 10 and 20 min from the start of incubation of DNA-containing particle-preparation medium, followed by incubation for an additional 25, 20 and 10 min respectively, DNA binding to the particles was enhanced to a significant extent for fibronectin, E-cadherin and fibronectin/E-cadherin-Fc compared to the control, suggesting than a competitive inhibition of DNA binding happens in the direct mixing procedure while delaying addition of the proteins to the growing crystals and DNA favors optimal DNA binding to the particles. Decreased DNA binding to the particles with which E-cadherin and fibronectin/E-cadherin-Fc were incubated for only 1 min, could be due to the reduced growth of the particles for too long time absence of E-cadherin-Fc in particle-preparation medium.

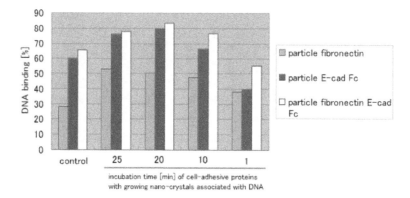

Figure 15. Binding affinities of DNA to differentially formulated cell adhesive protein-embedded particles. Particles in the control samples were prepared by addition of 3 μl of 1 M CaCl₂, 2 μg of luciferase plasmid DNA and 2 μg of either fibronectin, E-cad-Fc or both to 1 ml bicarbonate-buffered DMEM and incubation at 37°C for 30 min. Formation of the particles in experimental samples was done by addition of fibronectin, E-cadherin-Fc or both after 5, 10, 20 and 29 min from the start of incubation of DNA-containing particle preparation medium, followed by incubation for an additional 25, 20, 10 and 1 min respectively. F9 cells were incubated with the generated particles for 4 hr and after replacement of particle-containing media with fresh media, further incubated up to 1 day for quantitation of luciferase expression. Transfection efficiency was normalized after estimation of total proteins in cell lysate.

3.11. Size determination for differentially formulated cell adhesive protein-embedded particles

Particle growth kinetics is correlated to the size of the finally formed particles and excessive growth lead to big size particles being inefficient for intracellular DNA delivery [11]. Since E-cadherin-Fc favors particle growth by making bridges among the neighboring E-cadherin-anchored crystals [14], prolonged incubation together with DNA for generation of functional particles might lead to large complex particles. As shown in Fig. 16, fibronectin association maintained the average particle diameter close to 300 nm whereas E-cadherin-Fc or fibronectin/E-cadherin-Fc induced the particle growth with an average diameter of approximately 900 nm. However, addition of E-cadherin-Fc or fibronectin/E-cadherin-F after 5, 10, 20 and 29 min from the start of incubation of DNA-containing particle-preparation medium, followed by incubation for an additional 25, 20, 10 and 1 min respectively, resulted in the particles of decreasing sizes with a minimum average value of approximately 300 nm. On the other hand, time-dependent association of fibronectin having no role in particle growth induction, demonstrated no significant change in overall particle diame-ter, suggesting that particle growth is the size-determining factor for cell-adhesive protein-embedded particles.

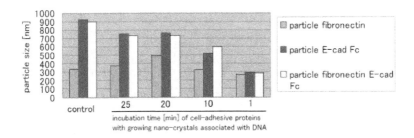

Figure 16. Estimation of sizes for differentially formulated cell adhesive protein-embedded particles. Following prepa-ration of different particles as mentioned in the legend to Figure 4, dynamic light scattering (DLS) measurement was performed with a Super-dynamic Light Scattering Spectrophotometer.

3.12. Cellular delivery of DNA in association with cell adhesive protein-embedded particles

Both DNA binding to the particles and particle size contribute to the overall uptake of DNA by cells. As shown in Fig. 17, only particles were very inefficient in delivering pro-pidium (PI)-labeled plasmid DNA into F9 cells whereas particles being associated with fibronectin or E-cadherin-Fc significantly increased cellular delivery of labeled DNA in a 4 hr uptake study. Moreover, particles when complexed with both fibronectin and E-cad-herin-Fc in direct mixing with DNA, synergistically accelerated delivery of PI-labeled DNA into the cells. Particles prepared by addition of fibronectin or fibronectin/E-cadherin-Fc after 5, 10 and 20 min from the start of incubation of labeled DNA-containing particle preparation medium and incubation for an additional 25, 20 and 10 min respectively, medi-ated increased cellular delivery of labeled DNA, indicating that transgene delivery is well-controlled by the sizes as well as the DNA-loading efficiency of cell adhesive protein-embedded particles. Reduced DNA uptake level for the small size particles with which cell-adhesive proteins were incubated for a very short time (1 min) could be accounted for their inefficient binding with the cell-recognition molecules. The reason for low DNA up-take for the particles to which only E-cadherin-Fc was adsorbed in a time-dependent man-ner, is still not clear and might be related to the serum instability of the complex particles at the time of transgene delivery.

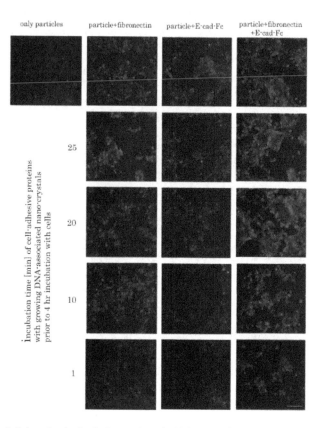

Figure 17. Differentially formulated cell adhesive protein-embedded particles for cellular delivery of DNA. Particles in the control samples were prepared by addition of 3 μl of 1 M CaCl$_2$, 2 μg of PI-labelled plasmid DNA and 2 μg of either fibronectin, E-cad-Fc or both to 1 ml bicarbonate-buffered DMEM and incubation at 37°C for 30 min. Formation of the particles in experimental samples was done by addition of fibronectin, E-cadherin-Fc or both after 5, 10, 20 and 29 min from the start of incubation of DNA-containing particle preparation medium, followed by incubation for an additional 25, 20, 10 and 1 min respectively. F9 cells were incubated with the generated particles for 4 hr, washed with 5 mM EDTA in PBS and visualized by a fluorescence microscope (scale bar, 100 μm).

3.13. Transfection efficiency achieved with cell adhesive protein-embedded particles

Since transgene expression is the result of overcoming a number of barriers including entry into the cells, release from the particles and endosomes, and finally nuclear translocation [11], we checked whether accelerated DNA delivery owing to the improved DNA loading capacity and smaller sizes of fibronectin and E-cadherin-Fc-anchored carbonate apatite particles, contributed to the similar extent to final protein expression (Fig. 18). Quantitative luciferase expression demonstrated that particles generated by addition of fibronectin and fibronectin/E-cadherin-Fc after 5 min from the start of incubation of DNA-containing medium and incubation for an additional 25 min, enhanced 2 and 3-fold higher transgene expression than the control samples prepared by direct mixing with DNA. This is a significant achievement considering the high expression level already achieved with control samples [15]. The decline in luciferase expression for other samples is consistent with the low efficiency of DNA delivery as described before.

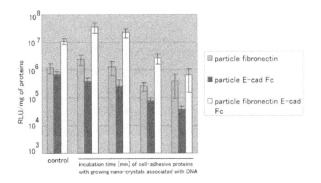

Figure 18. Intracellular expression of luciferase gene delivered by differentially formulated cell adhesive protein-embedded particles. Particles in the control samples were prepared by addition of 3 μl of 1 M $CaCl_2$, 2 μg of PI-labelled plasmid DNA and 2 μg of either fibronectin, E-cad-Fc or both to 1 ml bicarbonate-buffered DMEM and incubation at 37^0C for 30 min. Formation of the particles in experimental samples was done by addition of fibronectin, E-cadherin-Fc or both after 5, 10, 20 and 29 min from the start of incubation of DNA-containing particle preparation medium, followed by incubation for an additional 25, 20, 10 and 1 min respectively. F9 cells were incubated with the generated particles for 4 hr and after replacement of particle-containing media with fresh media, further incubated up to 1 day in order to quantitate luciferase expression. Transfection efficiency was normalized after estimation of total proteins in cell lysate.

3.14. Role of protein kinase C on immobilized fibronectin and E-cad-Fc-mediated gene delivery

Since protein kinase C (PKC) in "inside-out" signaling cascade enhances integrin affinity towards ECM proteins promoting cell adhesion and spreading [23, 24] and up regulates endocytosis and recycling of E-cadherin [21], we have investigated the effect of Phorbol 12-myristate 13-acetate (PMA), a specific activator of PKC on trans-gene delivery mediated by particle-immobilized fibronectin and E-cadherin-Fc. As shown in Fig. 19, while only carbonate apatite particles are very inefficient in transfecting F9 cells even in presence of increasing doses of PMA (0 to 100 nM), fibronectin- or E-cad-Fc-embedded particles showed significant increment in luciferase gene expression (2 to 10 times) depending on PMA concentrations. Surprisingly, particles when associated with both of the "cell adhesive molecules" remarkably enhanced trans-gene expression resulting in almost 8, 14, 20 and 92-fold higher efficiency due to the presence of PMA at 1, 10, 50 and 100 nM concentrations, respectively. Immobilization of either fibronectin or E-cad-Fc on the particles also showed a dramatic increment in transgene expression, indicating clearly that both of the transmembrane proteins integrin and E-cadherin are up-regulated in response to PKC activation to promote efficient internalization of the bio-functional particles across the plasma membrane (data not shown here) and subsequent expression of the particle-associated DNA in cytoplasm [27] (Fig 19).

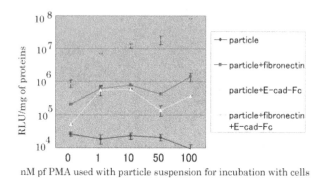

Figure 19. Effects of PMA on trans-gene expression mediated by fibronectin/E-cad-Fc-embedded-particles. Particles were prepared by addition of 3 µl of 1 M CaCl₂ 2 µg of luciferase plasmid DNA and 2 µg of either fibronectin, E-cad-Fc or both to 1 ml bicarbonate-buffered DMEM and incubation for 30 min at 37°C. F9 cells were incubated with the generated particles in presence of increasingly high concentrations of PMA (o to 100 nM) for 1 hr and after replacement of particle- and PMA-containing media with fresh media, further incubated for 1 day in order to quantitate luciferase expression.

3.15. Transfection efficiency achieved in leukemia cells with cell adhesive protein-embedded particles

T cell expresses on its membrane $\alpha 4\beta 1$ and $\alpha 5\beta 1$ integrins which can bind fibronectin during lymphocyte adhesion and migration from vascular compartment to the injured tissues [22]. Moreover, $\alpha_E\beta 7$ integrin on some T cells can interact with epithelial E-cadherin for tissue-specific retention of lymphocytes [22]. We, therefore, aimed to functionalize the surface of DNA-associated nanocrystals with fibronectin and E-cadherin-Fc for transgene delivery through integrin-mediated endocytosis [22].

As shown in Fig. 20, luciferase expression in Jurkat cells was significantly low after delivery of luciferase gene-containing plasmid DNA with the help of carbonate apatite particles. A 3-fold enhancement in transgene expression was observed following delivery with fibronectin-embedded particles. Transgene expression could be further increased to the level (up to 6 times) equivalent to that of lipofection with the particles complexed with both fibronectin and E-cadherin-Fc. Since lymphocytes posses 2 different types of integrins ($\alpha 4\beta 1$ and $\alpha 5\beta 1$)

being able to bind fibronectin [22], particles with electrostatically associated fibronectin could recognize any of the two receptors for efficient endocytosis in Jurkat cells leading to high transgene expression. However, particles with adsorbed E-cadherin-Fc reduced transfection efficiency below the level obtained with particles only, indicating that binding of E-cadherin-Fc probably neutralizes the positive charges of the particles as required for their subsequent interaction with anionic cell surface and additionally, E-cadherin-Fc on the particle surface might have low affinity interaction with the cell membrane integrin ($\alpha_E\beta7$). On the other hand, the highest gene expression obtained with the particles complexed with both fibronectin and E-cadherin-Fc could be interpreted by the strong affinity of the composite particles towards the cell membrane due to the specific and synchronized recognition of the two different ligands on particle surface to their corresponding integrin receptors on plasma membrane, resulting in fast endocytosis of the particles along with DNA.

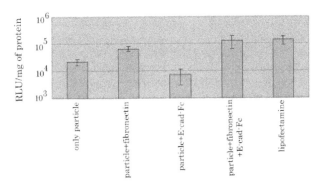

Figure 20. Comparison of luciferase expression among differentially formulated apatite particles. Particles were prepared by addition of 3 μl of 1 M $CaCl_2$, 2 μg of luciferase plasmid DNA and 2 μg of either fibronectin, E-cad-Fc or both to 1 ml bicarbonate-buffered DMEM and incubation for 30 min at 37°C. Jurkat cells were incubated with the generated particles for 1 day followed by quantitation of luciferase expression. Transfection efficiency was normalized after estimation of total proteins in cell lysate. Transfection by lipofectamine was performed according to the instructions provided by Invitrogen. Reproducibility of the result was established by performing same the experiment in another day.

4. Conclusions

Stem cells possessing the inherent capability of transforming into many cell types, have been shown tremendous potential for cell-based therapies in regenerative medicine for neurological disease or injury [28], diabetes [29] and myocardial infarct [30]. The *in vitro* differentiated derivatives of stem cells are thought to be able to repair or replace damaged cells, tissues or organs. However, compared to embryonic stem cells, adult stem cells are likely more difficult to be implemented into useful therapies considering their limited pluripotency. Transgene delivery could be a powerful strategy for specific differentiation of embryonic stem cells since several transcription factors have been demonstrated to regulate stem cell differentiation to specific cell types of heart, pancreas, liver and neurons [31-36]. On the other hand, tumor cells such as leukemia and lymphoma cells are obvious and attractive targets for gene therapy. Gene transfer and expression for cytokine and immunomodulatory molecules in various kinds of tumor cells have been shown to mediate tumor regression and anti-metastatic effects [37-40]. Moreover, genetically modified leukemia cells expressing co-stimulatory molecules or cytokines are likely to have significant therapeutic roles for patients with leukemia [41, 42].

Among the existing approaches for transgene delivery, viral systems suffer from their potential life-threatening effects of immunogenicity and carcinogenicity whereas non-viral ones, although safe, possess significant limitation in terms of efficacy [43]. Development of a safe as well as an efficient carrier is, therefore, an urgent requirement for effective implementation of the stem cells in regenerative medicine and the leukemia (or lymphocytes) in cancer treatment.

We have established a novel type of non-viral gene delivery systems based on pH-sensitive inorganic nanoparticles and revealed an innovative strategy for surface-functionalization of these biodegradable nanoparticles through their ionic interactions with "cell-adhesive molecules". Moreover, the new approach has directly been applied for highly efficient delivery and expression of a trans-gene into "hard-to-transfect" embryonic stem cells- a success with tremendous future for stem-cell based therapeutic development. The involvement of E-cadherin and fibronectin in intercellular and extracellular interactions of cultured undifferentiated embryonic stem cells may exclude the possibility of stem cell differentiation following transfection with the new nano-apatite carriers associated with E-cad-Fc and fibronectin. More the same approach has successfully used to transfect the leukemia cells having potential application in cancer therapy.

Acknowledgements

This work has financially been supported by a research grant (Project ID 02-02-09-SF0013) of the Ministry of Science, Technology and Innovation (MOSTI), Malaysia.

Author details

Ezharul Hoque Chowdhury*

Address all correspondence to: md.ezharul.hoque@med.monash.edu.my

Jeffrey Cheah School of Medicine and Health Sciences, Faculty of Medicine, Nursing and Health Sciences, Monash University (Sunway Campus), Australia

References

[1] Kopatz, I., Remy, J. S., & Behr, J. P. (2004). A model for non-viral gene delivery: through syndecan adhesion molecules and powered by actin. *Journal Gene Medicine*, 6, 769-776.

[2] Wu, G. Y., & Wu, C. H. (1997). Receptor-mediated in vitro gene transformation by a soluble DNA carrier system. *Journal Biological Chemistry*, 262, 4432-4439.

[3] Cotton, M., Längle-Rouault, F., Kirlappos, H., Wagner, E., Mechtler, K., Zenke, M., Beug, H., & Birnstiel, M. L. (1990). Transferrin-polycation-mediated introduction of DNA into human leukemic cells: stimulation by agents that affect the survival of transfected DNA or modulate transferrin receptor levels. *Proceedings of the National Academy of Sciences*, 87, 4033-4037.

[4] Schaffer, D. V., & Lauffenburger, D. A. (1998). Optimization of cell surface binding enhances efficiency and specificity of molecular conjugate gene delivery. *Journal Biological Chemistry*, 273, 28004-28009.

[5] Erbacher, P., Bousser, M. T., Raimond, J., Monsigny, M., Midoux, P., & Roche, A. C. (1996). Gene transfer by DNA/glycosylated polylysine complexes into human blood monocyte-derived macrophages. *Human Gene Therapy*, 7, 721-729.

[6] Hoganson, D. K., Chandler, L. A., Fleurbaaij, G. A., Ying, W., Black, ME, Doukas, J., Pierce, G. F., Baird, A., & Sosnowski, BA. (1998). Targeted delivery of DNA encoding cytotoxic proteins through high-affinity fibroblast growth factor receptors. *Human Gene Therapy*, 9, 2565-2575.

[7] Buschle, M., Cotton, M., Kirlappos, H., Mechtler, K., Schaffner, G., Zauner, W., & Birnstiel, M. L. (1995). Receptor-mediated gene transfer into human T lymphocytes via binding of DNA/CD3 antibody particles to the CD3 T cell receptor complex. *Human Gene Therapy*, 6, 753-761.

[8] Erbacher, P., Remy, J. S., & Behr, J. P. (1999). Gene transfer with synthetic virus-like particles via the integrin-mediated endocytosis pathway. *Gene Therapy*, 6, 138-145.

[9] Wang, S., Lee, R. J., Cauchon, G., Gorenstein, D. G., & Low, P. S. (1995). Delivery of antisense oligodeoxyribonucleotides against the human epidermal growth factor receptor into cultured KB cells with liposomes conjugated to folate via polyethylene glycol. *Proceedings of the National Academy of Sciences*, 92, 3318-3322.

[10] Parkes, R. J., & Hart, S. L. (2000). Adhesion molecules and gene transfer. *Advanced Drug Delivery Reviews*, 44, 135-152.

[11] Chowdhury, E. H. (2007). pH-sensitive nano-crystals of carbonate apatite for smart and cell-specific transgene delivery. *Expert Opinion Drug Delivery*, 4, 193-196.

[12] Chowdhury, E. H., Maruyama, A., Kano, A., Nagaoka, M., Kotaka, M., Hirose, S., Kunou, M., & Akaike, A. (2006). pH-sensing nano-crystals of carbonate apatite: ef-

fects on intracellular delivery and release of DNA for efficient expression into mammalian cells. *Gene*, 376, 87-94.

[13] Chowdhury, E. H., Kutsuzawa, K., & Akaike, T. Designing Smart Nano-apatite Composites: The Emerging era of non-viral gene delivery. *Gene Therapy and Molecular Biology*, 9, 301-316.

[14] Kutsuzawa, K., Maruyama, K., Akiyama, Y., Akaike, T., & Chowdhury, E. H. (2008). Efficient transfection of mouse embryonic stem cells with cell-adhesive protein-embedded inorganic nanocarrier. *Analytical Biochemistry*, 372, 122-124.

[15] Kutsuzawa, K., Chowdhury, E. H., Nagaoka, M., Maruyama, K., Akiyama, Y., & Akaike, T. (2006). Surface functionalization of inorganic nano-crystals with fibronectin and E-cadherin chimera synergistically accelerates trans-gene delivery into embryonic stem cells. *Biochemical and Biophysical Research Communications*, 350, 514-520.

[16] Shirayoshi, Y., Okada, T. S., & Takeichi, M. (1983). The calcium-dependent cell-cell adhesion system regulates inner cell mass formation and cell surface polarization in early mouse development. *Cell*, 35, 631-638.

[17] Oka, M., Tagoku, K., Russell, T. L., Nakano, Y., Hamazaki, T., Meyer, E. M., Yokota, T., & Terada, N. (2002). CD9 is associated with leukemia inhibitory factor-mediated maintenance of embryonic stem cells. *Molecular Biology of the Cell*, 13, 1274-1281.

[18] Chowdhury, E. H., Zohra, F. T., Tada, S., Kitamura, C., & Akaike, T. (2004). Fibronectin in collaboration with Mg^{2+} enhances transgene expression by calcium phosphate coprecipitates. *Analytical Biochemistry*, 335, 162-164.

[19] Chowdhury, E. H., Nagaoka, M., Ogiwara, K., Zohra, F. T., Kutsuzawa, K., Tada, S., Kitamura, C., & Akaike, T. (2005). Integrin-supported fast rate intracellular delivery of plasmid DNA by extracellular matrix protein embedded calcium phosphate complexes. *Biochemistry*, 44, 12273-12278.

[20] Overduin, M., Harvey, T. S., Bagby, S., Tong, K. I., Yau, P., Takeichi, M., & Ikura, M. (1995). Solution structure of the epithelial cadherin domain responsible for selective cell adhesion. *Science*, 267, 386-389.

[21] Le Joseph, T. L., Yap, S. R., , A. S., & Stow, J. L. (2002). Protein kinase C regulates endocytosis and recycling of E-cadherin. *American Journal of Physiology- Cell Physiology*, 283, C489-C499.

[22] Kutsuzawa, K., Maruyama, K., Akiyama, Y., Akaike, T., & Chowdhury, E. H. (2008). The influence of the cell-adhesive proteins E-cadherin and fibronectin embedded in carbonate-apatite DNA carrier on transgene delivery and expression in a mouse embryonic stem cell line. *Biomaterials*, 29, 370-376.

[23] Kolanus, W., & Seed, B. (1997). Integrins and inside-out signal transduction: converging signals from PKC and PIP3. *Current Opinion in Cell Biology*, 9, 725-731.

[24] Besson, A., Wilson, T. L., & Yong, V. W. (2002). The anchoring protein RACK1 links protein kinase Cepsilon to integrin beta chains. Requirements for adhesion and motility. *Journal Biological Chemistry*, 277, 22073-22084.

[25] Stephens, L. E., Sonne, J. E., Fitzgerald, M. L., & Damsky, C. H. (1993). Targeted deletion of beta 1 integrins in F9 embryonal carcinoma cells affects morphological differentiation but not tissue-specific gene expression. *Journal of Cell Biology*, 123, 1607-1620.

[26] Maeno, Y., Moroi, S., Nagashima, H., Noda, T., Shiozaki, H., Monden, M., Tsukita, S., & Nagafuchi, A. (1999). alpha-catenin-deficient F9 cells differentiate into signet ring cells. *American Journal of Pathology*, 154, 1323-1328.

[27] Kutsuzawa, K., Maruyama, K., Akiyama, Y., Akaike, T., & Chowdhury, E. H. (2007). Protein kinase C activation enhances transfection efficacy of cell-adhesive protein-anchored carbonate apatite nanocrystals. *Analytical Biochemistry*, 37, 116-117.

[28] Webber, D. J., & Minger, S. L. (2004). Therapeutic potential of stem cells in central nervous system regeneration. *Current Opinion in Investigational Drugs*, 5, 714-719.

[29] Hussain, M. A., & Theise, N. D. (2004). Stem-cell therapy for diabetes mellitus. *Lancet*, 364, 203-205.

[30] Mathur, A., & Martin, J. F. (2004). Stem cells and repair of the heart. *Lancet*, 364, 183-192.

[31] Duncan, S. A., Navas, MA, Dufort, D., Rossant, J., & Stoffel, M. (1998). Regulation of a transcription factor network required for differentiation and metabolism. *Science*, 281, 692-695.

[32] Li, J., Ning, G., & Duncan, S. A. (2000). Mammalian hepatocyte differentiation requires the transcription factor HNF-4alpha. *Genes and Development*, 14, 464-474.

[33] Ishizaka, S., Shiroi, A., Kanda, S., Yoshikawa, M., Tsujinoue, H., Kuriyama, S., Hasuma, T., Nakatani, K., & Takahashi, K. (2002). Development of hepatocytes from ES cells after transfection with the HNF-3beta gene. *FASEB Journal*, 16, 1444-1446.

[34] Dohrmann, C., Gruss, P., & Lemaire, L. (2000). Pax genes and the differentiation of hormone-producing endocrine cells in the pancreas. *Mechanisms of Development*, 92, 47-54.

[35] Kim, S. K., & Hebrok, M. (2001). Intercellular signals regulating pancreas development and function. *Genes and Development*, 15, 111-127.

[36] Xian, H. Q., & Gottlieb, D. I. (2001). Peering into early neurogenesis with embryonic stem cells. *Trends in Neurosciences*, 24, 685-686.

[37] Adams, S. W., & Emerson, S. G. (1998). Gene therapy for leukemia and lymphoma. *Hematology/Oncology Clinics of North America*, 12(3), 631-48.

[38] Schakowski, F., Buttgereit, P., Mazur, M., Märten, A., Schöttker, B., Gorschlüter, M., & Schmidt-Wolf, I. G. (2004). Novel non-viral method for transfection of primary leukemia cells and cell lines. *Genetic Vaccines and Therapy*, 2(1), 1.

[39] Szeps, M., Erickson, S., Gruber, A., Castro, J., Einhorn, S., & Grandér, D. (2003). Effects of interferon-alpha on cell cycle regulatory proteins in leukemic cells. *Leukemia and Lymphoma*, 44(6), 1019-25.

[40] Finke, S., Trojaneck, B., Lefterova, P., Csipai, M., Wagner, E., Kircheis, R., Neubauer, A., Huhn, D., Wittig, B., & Schmidt-Wolf, I. G. (1998). Increase of proliferation rate and enhancement of antitumor cytotoxicity of expanded human CD3+ CD56+ immunologic effector cells by receptor-mediated transfection with the interleukin-7 gene. *Gene Therapy*, 5(1), 31-9.

[41] Notter, M., Willinger, T., Erben, U., & Thiel, E. (2001). Targeting of a B7-1 (CD80) immunoglobulin G fusion protein to acute myeloid leukemia blasts increases their costimulatory activity for autologous remission T cells. *Blood*, 97(10), 3138-45.

[42] Kato, K., Cantwell, MJ, Sharma, S., & Kipps, T. J. (1998). Gene transfer of CD40-ligand induces autologous immune recognition of chronic lymphocytic leukemia B cells. *Journal of Clinical Investigation*, 101(5), 1133-1141.

[43] Chowdhury, E. H., & Akaike, T. (2005). Bio-functional inorganic materials: an attractive branch of gene-based nano-medicine delivery for 21st century. *Current Gene Therapy*, 5, 669-676.

Permissions

The contributors of this book come from diverse backgrounds, making this book a truly international effort. This book will bring forth new frontiers with its revolutionizing research information and detailed analysis of the nascent developments around the world.

We would like to thank Rosario Pignatello, for lending his expertise to make the book truly unique. He has played a crucial role in the development of this book. Without his invaluable contribution this book wouldn't have been possible. He has made vital efforts to compile up to date information on the varied aspects of this subject to make this book a valuable addition to the collection of many professionals and students.

This book was conceptualized with the vision of imparting up-to-date information and advanced data in this field. To ensure the same, a matchless editorial board was set up. Every individual on the board went through rigorous rounds of assessment to prove their worth. After which they invested a large part of their time researching and compiling the most relevant data for our readers. Conferences and sessions were held from time to time between the editorial board and the contributing authors to present the data in the most comprehensible form. The editorial team has worked tirelessly to provide valuable and valid information to help people across the globe.

Every chapter published in this book has been scrutinized by our experts. Their significance has been extensively debated. The topics covered herein carry significant findings which will fuel the growth of the discipline. They may even be implemented as practical applications or may be referred to as a beginning point for another development. Chapters in this book were first published by InTech; hereby published with permission under the Creative Commons Attribution License or equivalent.

The editorial board has been involved in producing this book since its inception. They have spent rigorous hours researching and exploring the diverse topics which have resulted in the successful publishing of this book. They have passed on their knowledge of decades through this book. To expedite this challenging task, the publisher supported the team at every step. A small team of assistant editors was also appointed to further simplify the editing procedure and attain best results for the readers.

Our editorial team has been hand-picked from every corner of the world. Their multi-ethnicity adds dynamic inputs to the discussions which result in innovative outcomes. These outcomes are then further discussed with the researchers and contributors who give their valuable feedback and opinion regarding the same. The feedback is then collaborated with the researches and they are edited in a comprehensive manner to aid the understanding of the subject.

Apart from the editorial board, the designing team has also invested a significant amount of their time in understanding the subject and creating the most relevant covers. They scrutinized every image to scout for the most suitable representation of the subject and create an appropriate cover for the book.

The publishing team has been involved in this book since its early stages. They were actively engaged in every process, be it collecting the data, connecting with the contributors or procuring relevant information. The team has been an ardent support to the editorial, designing and production team. Their endless efforts to recruit the best for this project, has resulted in the accomplishment of this book. They are a veteran in the field of academics and their pool of knowledge is as vast as their experience in printing. Their expertise and guidance has proved useful at every step. Their uncompromising quality standards have made this book an exceptional effort. Their encouragement from time to time has been an inspiration for everyone.

The publisher and the editorial board hope that this book will prove to be a valuable piece of knowledge for researchers, students, practitioners and scholars across the globe.

List of Contributors

V. Tereshko
School of Computing, University of the West of Scotland, Paisley, UK

A. Gorchakov
MISTEM, Mogilev, Belarus

I. Tereshko and V. Abidzina
Department of Physics, Belarusian-Russian University, Mogilev, Belarus

V. Red'ko
Department of Physical Methods of Control, Belarusian-Russian University, Mogilev, Belarus

Juan V. Cauich-Rodríguez, Lerma H. Chan-Chan, Fernando Hernandez-Sánchez and José M. Cervantes-Uc
Centro de Investigación Científica de Yucatán A.C., Grupo de Biomateriales e Ingeniería de Tejidos, Mexico

Siwar Sakka, Jamel Bouaziz and Foued Ben Ayed
Laboratory of Industrial Chemistry, National School of Engineering, Sfax University, Sfax, Tunisia

Frank Xue Jiang
Unilever Research & Development, Shanghai, P.R. China

Xiaohong Wang
Key Laboratory for Advanced Materials Processing Technology, Ministry of Education & Center of Organ Manufacturing, Department of Mechanical Engineering, Tsinghua University, Beijing, P.R. China
Business Innovation Technology (BIT) Research Centre, School of Science and Technology, Aalto University, Aalto, Finland
State Key Laboratory of Materials Processing and Die & Mould Technology, Huazhong, University of Science and Technology, Wuhan, P.R. China

Shaojun Yuan
Multi-phases Mass Transfer & Reaction Engineering Lab, College of Chemical Engineering, Sichuan University, Chengdu, China
School of Materials Science and Engineering, Nanyang Technological University, Singapore

Gordon Xiong and Cleo Choong
School of Materials Science and Engineering, Nanyang Technological University, Singapore

Ariel Roguin
Department of Cardiology, Rambam Medical Center, B. Rappaport Faculty of Medicine, Technion – Israel Institute of Technology, Israel

Swee Hin Teoh
School of Chemical and Biomedical Engineering, Nanyang Technological University, Singapore

Antonello A. Romani
Department of Surgery, O.U. of General Surgery, University Hospital of Parma, Italy

Luigi Ippolito
Department of Pathology and Medicine of Laboratory University Hospital Parma, Italy

Federica Riccardi
Department of Medicine poly-specialist 2, University Hospital Parma, Italy

Silvia Pipitone and Angelo F. Borghetti
Department of Experimental Medicine, University of Parma, Italy

Marina Morganti and Maria Cristina Baroni
Department of Internal Medicine and Biomedical Sciences, University of Parma, Italy

Ruggero Bettini
Department of Pharmacy, University of Parma, Italy

M. Lotfi
Faculty of Medicine of Monastir, Tunisia, Laboratory of biophysics, Avicenne Avenue, Tunisia

M. Nejib
Higher Institute of Agronomy of Chott Meriem, Laboratory of animal sciences, Sousse, Tunisia

M. Naceur
Ecole Polytechnique of Montreal, Canada

Ylenia Zambito
Dipartimento di Farmacia, Università di Pisa, Italy

Ezharul Hoque Chowdhury
Jeffrey Cheah School of Medicine and Health Sciences, Faculty of Medicine, Nursing and Health Sciences, Monash University (Sunway Campus), Australia

Printed in the USA
CPSIA information can be obtained
at www.ICGtesting.com
JSHW011500221024
72173JS00005B/1149

9 781632 380289